RADIOGRAPHY
in Veterinary Technology

RADIOGRAPHY
in Veterinary Technology

FOURTH EDITION

Lisa M. Lavin, MBA, CVT

Vice President and Chief Operating Officer
Spinal Designs International, Incorporated
Minneapolis, Minnesota

With 506 illustrations

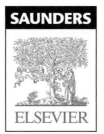

SAUNDERS

ELSEVIER

SAUNDERS
ELSEVIER

11830 Westline Industrial Drive
St. Louis, Missouri 63146

RADIOGRAPHY IN VETERINARY TECHNOLOGY ISBN-13: 978-1-4160-3189-5
Copyright © 2007, 2003, 1999, 1994 by Saunders, an imprint of Elsevier Inc. ISBN-10: 1-4160-3189-8

Notice

Knowledge and best practice in Radiography are constantly changing. As new research and experience broaden our knowledge, changes in practice, treatment and drug therapy may become necessary or appropriate. Readers are advised to check the most current information provided (i) on procedures featured or (ii) by the manufacturer of each product to be administered, to verify the recommended dose or formula, the method and duration of administration, and contraindications. It is the responsibility of the practitioner, relying on their own experience and knowledge of the patient, to make diagnoses, to determine dosages and the best treatment for each individual patient, and to take all appropriate safety precautions. To the fullest extent of the law, neither the Publisher nor the Author assumes any liability for any injury and/or damage to persons or property arising out or related to any use of the material contained in this book.

Previous editions copyrighted 2003, 1999, 1994

ISBN-13: 978-1-4160-3189-5
ISBN-10: 1-4160-3189-8

Editorial Director: Linda Duncan
Managing Editor: Teri Merchant
Publishing Services Manager: Pat Joiner
Project Manager: Jennifer Clark
Design Direction: Julia Dummitt
Text Designer: Julia Dummitt

Printed in the United States of America

Last digit is the print number: 9 8 7 6 5 4 3 2 1

For
Janet M. Lavin

John S. Mattoon, DVM, Dipl ACVR
Associate Professor of Radiology
Veterinary Clinical Sciences
College of Veterinary Medicine
Washington State University, Pullman, Washington

Susan L. McClanahan, RT(R)
Radiation Supervisor, Department of Radiation Control Section
State Department of Health, Minneapolis, Minnesota

Patricia A. Walter, DVM, MS, Dipl ACVR
Associate Professor of Radiology
College of Veterinary Medicine
University of Minnesota, St. Paul, Minnesota

Preface to the Fourth Edition

Technology continues to move forward and advance our efforts to provide the best care for our patients. Radiography has made its way into the digital age. With the advent of veterinary-specific digital imaging equipment at lower costs, veterinary medicine is able to use the benefits of digital radiography. With this evolution, we have added an additional chapter to this text (Chapter 22) entitled *Digital Radiography*. While conventional radiography is still considered the mainstay in veterinary imaging, it is wise to understand the principles of advanced technology and its implications for our future.

My gratitude is extended to many who have assisted in the production of the fourth edition of this text. This edition is a compilation of three previous editions and includes input from many individuals over many years. Many thanks to Greg Knoblauch of the University of Minnesota Veterinary College for his support in updating photographs for this edition. I also want to thank Dr. John Mattoon for his contribution of Chapter 22. Despite his incredibly busy schedule, Dr. Mattoon was gracious with his time and energy to round out this text with an excellent summary of the world of digital radiography. Last, but certainly not least, my deepest appreciation goes to my family. With their steadfast support, I am convinced that anything is possible.

Lisa M. Lavin, MBA, CVT

Preface to the Third Edition

Radiography is a unique art form. Knowing the technical principles is only the beginning to becoming an accomplished radiographic artist. This text provides an excellent technical foundation for radiography, but it is the individual's responsibility to take the technical facts and turn them into the tools necessary to produce artwork. My advice to new and experienced technicians concerning radiography: Don't be discouraged! Becoming an artist in the field of radiography does not happen overnight. Developing the necessary skill and finesse can take years. It takes practice to develop the ability to manipulate all the variables in radiography. These variables include the wide range of species and body types, various makes and models of x-ray equipment, and the hundreds of potential errors that can occur in the darkroom. For those who have mastered the ability to juggle all those variables and produce beautiful, diagnostic radiographs—I salute you. To those who aspire to such skill—I salute you as well.

Many thanks are extended to those who assisted in the production of the third edition of this text. This edition is a compilation of two previous editions and the input from many individuals over several years. I especially thank Michelle Mero-Reidel of the University of Minnesota Veterinary Medical Graphics Department for her continued support in producing excellent photographs for publication. I also acknowledge and thank the entire staff of the 3M Animal Care Department. The 3M staff has been an invaluable source of support and friendship. Last, but certainly not least, my deepest appreciation goes to my family (this means you too, Mom!). It is their patience and support that bring flight to my wings.

Lisa M. Lavin, MBA, CVT

Preface to the Second Edition

The generous acceptance and continued support of the first edition of this text have prompted the preparation of this new edition. With the advent of advanced technology and its extension to private veterinary clinics, I have added Chapter 21, discussing Alternative Imaging Technology. A number of minor changes have been made to simplify Part I, specifically in Chapters 8 and 9 on Radiographic Technique Evaluation and Developing a Technique Chart.

I firmly believe that teachers learn the most from their students. Having been a teacher for more than 12 years, I can honestly say that my students can take most of the credit for this text. It was the student who did not understand a concept who forced me to find a way to explain it. The inception and continuation of this book are the result of the students' search for knowledge, and my ongoing goal it to bring clarity to the subject of radiography.

Many people were involved with the second edition. The University of Minnesota Veterinary Teaching Hospital has been an invaluable resource, adding to the depth and presentation of this edition. I am grateful to Dr. Patricia Walter for her spectacular addition of Chapter 21. Dr. Walter has been a valuable visionary, colleague, and friend. Thanks are also extended to Dr. Dan Feeney for his continued editorial support. In addition, special thanks are extended to the staff of the Medical Imaging Unit: Cindy Henrikson, Connie Callfas, Marcia Kocourek, Debra White, Annie Smith, Greg Knoblauch, John Nielsen, Katie Bend-Rubenstien, and Barb Talbot.

My deepest appreciation is extended to my family. If it were not for the support at home, my career journey would not be possible.

Lisa M. Lavin, MBA, CVT

$\mathcal{P}$reface to the $\mathcal{F}$irst $\mathcal{E}$dition

A radiograph is an image recorded on a special film consisting of shadows formed by structures and objects in the path of the x-ray beam. A radiograph is in essence a "shadowgraph."

One does not need to be a student of physics to grasp the concepts of radiography. Radiography requires the comprehension of key, integral concepts that form a cerebral foundation. This foundation can then be a building block for further understanding and the subsequent production of high-quality radiographs.

Radiography is like no other realm in veterinary technology. Unlike a urinalysis or a blood analysis, the product of radiography can be considered a piece of art work. Technical staff members can take pride in the results of their efforts.

Much confusion exists about a number of key areas of radiography. These areas include the physics of radiography, patient positioning, and technique evaluation. These areas are presented extensively in this text. To generate better understanding of the material, theoretical concepts are explained in a practical manner. One of the outstanding features of this text is its simplicity, with the intention to minimize confusion concerning the subject of radiography.

This text serves not only as a learning aid but also as a reference source. Licensed technicians may find this material to be a bridge between what is learned in school and what is applied in practice.

The primary goal in veterinary radiography is to produce radiographs of diagnostic quality on the first attempt. This goal serves three purposes: (1) to decrease radiation exposure to the patient and veterinary personnel; (2) to decrease the cost of the study for the client; and (3) to produce diagnostic data for rapid interpretation and treatment of the patient. The purpose of this text, therefore, is to provide information on veterinary radiographic technique to achieve this goal.

It is not by trial and error that we achieve quality … but a conscious understanding of the variables that transform an ordinary image into a work of art.

Lisa M. Lavin, MBA, CVT

Contents

PART 1   RADIOGRAPHIC THEORY AND EQUIPMENT, 1

1   X-Ray Production, 3

2   Anatomy of the X-Ray Machine, 9

3   Radiation Safety, 23

4   Exposure Factors, 35

5   Radiographic Quality, 43

6   Image Receptors, 59

7   Film Processing, 73

8   Radiographic Technique Evaluation, 89

9   Developing a Technique Chart, 97

10   Quality Assurance/Quality Control, 105

11   Technical Artifacts and Errors: Case Studies, 125

PART 2   RADIOGRAPHIC IMAGING, 143

12   General Principles of Positioning, 145

13   Small Animal Forelimb, 153

14   Small Animal Pelvis and Hind Limb, 173

15   Small Animal Skull, 191

16   Small Animal Spine, 207

17   Small Animal Soft Tissue, 223

18   Special Procedures, 233

19   Large Animal Radiography, 251

20   Avian and Exotic Radiography, 291

21   Alternative Imaging Technologies, 311

22   Digital Radiography, 329

Answers to Review Questions, 349

Index, 353

RADIOGRAPHY

in Veterinary Technology

part 1

Radiographic Theory and Equipment

chapter 1

X-ray Production

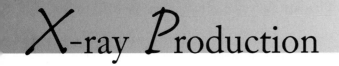

CHAPTER OUTLINE

Definition of X-rays
Physical Properties of X-ray Electromagnetic Radiation

Generation of X-rays
Discovery of X-rays

OBJECTIVES

Upon completion of this chapter, the reader should be able to do the following:

- Define x-rays
- Define electromagnetic radiation
- List and describe the two characteristics of electromagnetic radiation
- Describe the anatomy of an atom

- State the significance of the wavelength of x-rays
- List the seven physical properties of x-rays
- Describe how x-rays are generated
- Name the man who discovered x-rays

GLOSSARY

Anode: A positively charged electrode.

Atom: A basic part of matter that consists of a nucleus and a surrounding cloud of electrons.

Atomic number: The number of protons in an atom's nucleus.

Cathode: A negatively charged electrode.

Electromagnetic radiation: A method of transporting energy through space, distinguished by wavelength, frequency, and energy.

Electromagnetic spectrum: Electromagnetic radiation grouped according to wavelength and frequency.

Electron: A negatively charged particle that travels around the nucleus.

Excitation: A process in which an electron is moved to a higher energy level within the atom.

Fluorescence: The ability of a substance to emit visible light.

Frequency: The number of cycles of the wave that pass a stationary point in a second.

Gamma rays: Electromagnetic radiation emitted from the nucleus of radioactive substances.

Infrared rays: Electromagnetic radiation, beyond the red end of the visible spectrum, characterized by long wavelengths.

Ionization: A process in which an outer electron is removed from the atom so that the atom is left positively charged.

Neutron: A neutral particle located in the nucleus of an atom.

Photons: A bundle of radiant energy (synonymous with quanta).

Proton: A positively charged particle located in the nucleus of an atom.

Quanta: A bundle of radiant energy (synonymous with photons).

Radiant energy: Energy contained in light rays or any other form of radiation.

Radiograph: A visible photographic record on film produced by x-rays passing through an object.

Shell: An electron's orbital path and energy level.

Ultraviolet rays: Electromagnetic radiation, beyond the violet end of the visible spectrum, that is characterized by short wavelengths.

Vacuum: An area from which all air has been removed.

Wavelength: The distance between two consecutive corresponding points on a wave.

X-rays: A form of electromagnetic radiation similar to visible light but of a shorter wavelength.

X-ray beam: A number of x-rays traveling together through space at a rapid speed.

DEFINITION OF X-RAYS

Knowledge of the nature and behavior of x-rays is the first step in understanding the production of a **radiograph.** The veterinary radiographer does not need detailed knowledge of the underlying radiologic physics, but a basic understanding of certain principles is necessary to produce quality radiographs.

X-rays are defined as a form of electromagnetic radiation similar to visible light but of much shorter wavelength. **Electromagnetic radiation** is a method of transporting energy through space and is distinguished by its wavelength, frequency, and energy. Essentially, there are two characteristics of electromagnetic radiation: particles and waves.

We will first consider the wave. All **radiant energy** travels in a waveform along a straight path and is measured by its wavelength. In a series of waves the distance between two consecutive, corresponding points on a wave is called the **wavelength** (Fig. 1-1). Electromagnetic radiation that has a short wavelength has a high frequency. Electromagnetic radiation that has a long wavelength has a low frequency. **Frequency** is measured by the number of cycles of the wave that pass a stationary point per second

(cycles per second). The higher the frequency, the more penetrating power the energy has through space and matter.

All forms of electromagnetic radiation are grouped according to their wavelength and frequency in what is called the **electromagnetic spectrum.** Examples of electromagnetic radiation are radio waves, television waves, radar, **infrared rays,** the visible spectrum of light, **ultraviolet rays,** x-rays, and **gamma rays** (Fig. 1-2).

Electromagnetic radiation behaves as a particle, as well as a wave. **Atoms** consist of small particles called **protons, neutrons,** and **electrons.** An atom has a nucleus with a surrounding cloud of electrons (Fig. 1-3). The nucleus of an atom contains protons, which are positively charged,

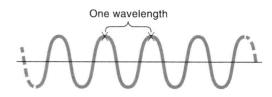

Figure 1-1 *Wavelength motion showing two corresponding points on consecutive waves.*

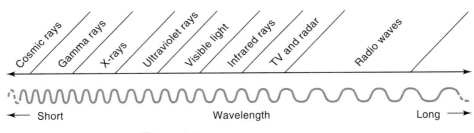

Figure 1-2 *The electromagnetic spectrum.*

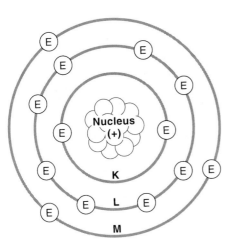

Figure 1-3 *Model of an atom.*

and neutrons, which are neutral. Electrons, which are negatively charged, travel around the nucleus in specific orbits, which are called **shells.** X-rays are produced when charged particles (electrons) are slowed down or stopped by the atoms of a target area. This process occurs inside the x-ray tube to create an **x-ray beam.**

An x-ray beam is composed of bundles of energy that travel in a wave. These bundles of energy, or **quanta,** are referred to as **photons.** The photons have no mass or electrical charge. Photons consist of pure energy and are transported, or "carried," by the wave.

Electromagnetic radiation can carry a wide range of energies. The energy of the radiation is proportional to the wavelength. The shorter the wavelength, the greater the energy. Therefore in radiography, x-rays that have a shorter wavelength penetrate farther than rays that have longer wavelengths.

PHYSICAL PROPERTIES OF X-RAY ELECTROMAGNETIC RADIATION

The physical properties of x-ray electromagnetic radiation, listed as follows, have diagnostic, medical, and research applications:

1. Wavelength is variable and is related to the energy of the radiation.

2. Travel is in a straight line. Direction can be altered, but the new path is also in a straight line.
3. Because of the extremely short wavelength, x-rays can penetrate materials that absorb or reflect visible light. They are gradually absorbed the farther they pass through an object. The amount of absorption depends on the **atomic number,** the physical density of the object, and the energy of the x-rays.
4. Certain substances have the property of **fluorescence** (i.e., they can emit visible light). Crystalline substances such as calcium tungstate or rare-earth phosphors fluoresce (emit light) within the visible spectrum after absorbing electromagnetic radiation of a shorter wavelength (i.e., x-rays).
5. X-rays produce an invisible image on photographic film that can be made visible by processing the film.
6. X-rays have the ability to excite or ionize the atoms and molecules of the substances including gases through which they pass. **Excitation** is a process in which an electron is moved to a higher energy level within the atom. Energy is required to initiate this change. **Ionization** is a process in which an outer electron is completely removed from the atom so that the atom is left positively charged. This process requires more energy than excitation.
7. X-rays can cause biologic changes in living tissue. A biologic change occurs either by direct action of excitation and ionization on important molecules in cells or indirectly as a result of chemical changes occurring near the cells. Affected cells may be damaged or killed.

GENERATION OF X-RAYS

X-rays are generated when fast-moving electrons (small particles bearing a negative charge) collide with any matter. This is best achieved in an x-ray tube. The x-ray tube consists of two electrodes, a **cathode** and an **anode,** that have opposite electrical charges. Because electrons have a negative charge at the cathode, they are attracted to the positive pole (anode) in the tube, and they collide with the positively charged target. This collision results in the production of x-radiation and a great amount of heat. Heat is the result of the interaction of the electrons and the atoms in the target. In fact, in diagnostic x-ray tubes,

99% of the energy from fast-moving electrons is converted into heat and 1% into x-ray energy.

DISCOVERY OF X-RAYS

On November 8, 1895, Wilhelm Conrad Roentgen discovered x-rays, an invaluable contribution to science. A professor of physics, Roentgen was the director of the new Physical Institute of the University of Würzburg, Germany. "Gas" tubes were being used at the time to conduct experiments with cathode rays. A **vacuum** was created in the tube by pumping out the air, and a current of electrons was passed through the tube. The tube consisted basically of a cathode (negative electrical charge) and an anode (positive electrical charge). The difference in electrical charge potential between the two electrodes caused the electrons to accelerate toward the tube end, where they interacted with the glass, producing x-rays.

Roentgen then wrapped the glass tube with dark paper, and during activation he saw a greenish illumination from a piece of cardboard across the room. The cardboard was painted with a fluorescent material called barium platinocyanide. This fluorescent material had been used previously to detect cathode rays. After further investigation, Roentgen presented a written report to the Society of Physics and Medical Sciences at the University of Würzburg on November 28, 1895. With his findings, he also submitted a radiograph of the hand of his wife, which he had produced with his own x-ray tube (Fig. 1-4).

By 1896, thousands of manuscripts and many books on x-rays had been published. X-rays were used immediately for medical and surgical diagnosis. And by as early as April 1896, changes in skin color caused by exposure to x-rays, similar to a sunburn, were reported. This discovery of skin color changes resulted in the use of x-rays for radiation therapy.

In recognition of Roentgen's discovery, he was awarded the Nobel Prize in 1901. This was the first Nobel Prize awarded in the field of physics.

Interestingly, a professor Goodspeed in Philadelphia had also made the discovery of x-rays in 1890, but he did not recognize their medical significance.

KEY POINTS

1. Energy travels in waves, the length of which is measurable.
2. X-rays with a shorter wavelength have a higher frequency and penetrate farther than rays having longer wavelengths.
3. X-radiation is a form of electromagnetic radiation produced when electrons moving with great speed collide with matter.
4. The ability of x-rays to excite and ionize molecules within cells can cause severe damage or death to those cells.
5. The first written report concerning x-rays and their use for medical and surgical diagnosis was made in 1895. The author and discoverer was Wilhelm Roentgen.

REVIEW QUESTIONS

1. The negatively charged particle of an atom is the:
   a. proton.
   b. neutron.
   c. electron.
   d. nucleus.

2. As x-rays pass through materials, they have the ability to:
   a. cause some substances to fluoresce (emit visible light).
   b. completely remove an electron from an atom, leaving the atom positively charged.
   c. cause chemical changes that can kill cells.
   d. All of the above.

3. Which of the following statements is true?
   a. X-rays with longer wavelengths penetrate farther than rays with shorter wavelengths.
   b. X-rays with shorter wavelengths penetrate farther than rays with longer wavelengths.
   c. Electromagnetic radiation with lower *higher* frequency has more penetrating power through space and matter.
   d. Gamma rays are required for the production of a radiograph.

4. Electrons travel:
   a. toward the cathode in an x-ray tube.
   b. away from the anode in an x-ray tube.
   c. toward the anode in an x-ray tube.
   d. within the nucleus of an atom.

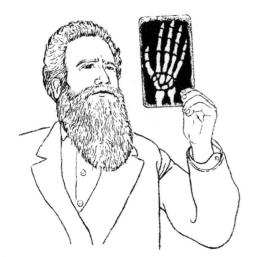

Figure 1-4 *Roentgen viewing a radiograph of his wife's hand.*

5. In x-ray tubes, the majority of energy produced by the movement of electrons is in the form of:
   a. light.
   b. heat.
   c. sound.
   d. x-ray energy.

6. On the electromagnetic spectrum, in relation to visible light, x-rays:
   a. have a longer wavelength.
   b. have a lower frequency.
   c. have a shorter wavelength.
   d. are closer in wavelength to infrared rays than light waves.

7. Bundles of energy that travel in a wave are called:
   a. protons.
   b. photons.
   c. quanta.
   d. Both b and c are correct.

8. True or false (circle one).
   X-ray electromagnetic radiation travels in a straight line, the direction of which can be altered.

9. True or false (circle one).
   A radiograph is synonymous with an x-ray.

Suggested Readings

Ball JL, Moore AD: *Essential physics for radiographers,* Boston, 1980, Blackwell Scientific.

Durez Y, Sieband MP, Jacobsen AF: *Production of x-rays—applications to medical radiography,* Madison, Wis, 1978, University of Wisconsin.

Eastman Kodak Company: Kodak: *The fundamentals of radiography,* ed 12, Rochester, NY, 1980, Kodak.

Johns HE, Cunningham JR: *The physics of radiology,* ed 4, Springfield, Ill, 1983, Charles C. Thomas.

Sprawls P: *The physical principles of diagnostic radiology,* Baltimore, 1977, University Park Press.

chapter 2

Anatomy of the X-ray Machine

CHAPTER OUTLINE

The X-ray Tube
Possible Areas of Tube Failure
Technical Components of the X-ray Machine

OBJECTIVES

Upon completion of this chapter, the reader should be able to do the following:

- State the purpose of the x-ray tube
- List the five elements necessary for x-ray production
- Describe the anatomy of the x-ray tube
- State the purpose and construction of the cathode
- Describe the basic construction of the anode
- Give reasons for the use of tungsten, molybdenum, and copper in the construction of the x-ray tube
- List methods of heat dissipation within the x-ray tube housing
- List and describe the two types of anodes
- Define heel effect

- Define and describe the focal spot
- Define the line-focus principle
- List the possible areas of x-ray tube failure
- List the electrical components of an x-ray machine
- State the purpose of the autotransformer, step-up transformer, line-voltage compensator, step-down transformer, and timer switch
- State and define the methods of rectification
- Describe x-ray tube rating and the three-phase generator
- List the components of the x-ray machine and console

Acceleration: The increase in speed over time.

Actual focal spot: The area of the focal spot consisting of a coiled wire that is perpendicular to the surface of the target.

Alloy: A mixture of metals.

Anode: A positively charged electrode that acts as a target for the electrons from the cathode. Electrons interacting with the anode produce heat and x-rays.

Arcing: A phenomenon in which metal deposits on the inner wall of the envelope act as a secondary anode, thereby attracting electrons from the cathode.

Autotransformer: Provides a variable yet predetermined voltage to the high-voltage step-up transformer. It acts as the kilovoltage selector.

Cathode: A negatively charged electrode that provides a source of electrons.

Collimator: A restricting device used to control the size of the primary x-ray beam.

Console: The control panel of the x-ray machine.

Effective focal spot: The area of the focal spot that is visible through the x-ray tube window and directed toward the x-ray film.

Filament: Part of a low-energy circuit in the cathode that, when heated, releases electrons from their orbits.

Focal spot: The small area of the target with which electrons collide on the anode.

Focusing cup: A recessed area where the filament lies, directing the electrons toward the anode.

Full-wave rectification: Creates an almost constant electrical potential across the x-ray tube, converting the positive electrical current pulses to 120 times per second compared with the normal rate of 60 times per second.

Glass envelope: A glass vacuum tube that contains the anode and cathode of the x-ray tube.

Half-wave rectification: A method of converting alternating to direct current in which half of the current is lost.

Heel effect: A decrease of x-ray intensity on the anode side of the x-ray beam caused by the anode target angle.

Kilovoltage: The amount of electrical energy being applied to the anode and cathode to accelerate the electrons from the cathode to the anode (1 kilovolt [kV] = 1000 volts [V]).

Kilovoltage peak (kVp): The peak energy of the x-rays, which determines the quality (penetrating power) of the x-ray beam.

Line-focus principle: The effect of making the actual focal spot size appear smaller when viewed from the position of the film because of the angle of the target to the electron stream.

Line-voltage compensator: Adjusts the incoming line voltage to the autotransformer so that the voltage remains constant.

Milliamperage (mA): The amount of electrical energy being applied to the filament. Milliamperage describes the number of x-rays produced during the exposure.

Molybdenum: A metal commonly used in focusing cups because of its high melting point and poor conduction of heat.

Penumbra: Partial outer shadow of an object being imaged by illumination.

Rectification: Process of changing alternating current to direct current.

Rotating anode: An anode that turns on an axis to increase x-ray production while dissipating heat.

Stationary anode: A nonmoving anode, usually found in dental and small portable radiography units.

Step-down transformer: Reduces the x-ray machine input voltage from 110 or 220 V to 10 V to prevent burnout of the cathode filament.

Step-up transformer: Increases the incoming voltage of 110 or 220 V to thousands of volts (i.e., kilovolts).

Target: Anode.

Timer switch: Controls the length of exposure.

Tungsten: A common metal used in the filament of a cathode.

Valve tubes: Allow the flow of electrons in one direction only. Commonly called self-rectifiers.

X-ray tube: A mechanism consisting of an anode and a cathode in a vacuum that produces a controlled x-ray beam.

THE X-RAY TUBE

X-rays are generated in an **x-ray tube.** The purpose of the x-ray tube is to produce a controlled x-ray beam. The tube must be responsive to manual control so that both the amount and the penetrating power of the radiation produced are accurately controlled. To better understand the x-ray tube, we need to consider the necessary elements for the production of x-rays.

X-ray Production

The following elements are necessary for x-ray production:

1. A source of electrons
2. A method of accelerating the electrons
3. An obstacle-free path for the passage of high-speed electrons

4. A target in which the electrons can interact, releasing energy in the form of x-rays
5. An envelope (tube) to provide a vacuum environment, eliminating the air molecule obstacles from the electron stream and preventing rapid oxidation of the elements.

The x-ray tube consists of a **cathode** side (with a negative electrical charge) and an **anode** side (with a positive electrical charge) encased in a **glass envelope,** which is evacuated to form a vacuum (Fig. 2-1).

In the tube, a stream of fast-moving electrons is produced at the cathode and directed to the anode. As the electrons collide and interact with the atoms of the **target** on the anode, a great amount of energy is produced; 1% of this energy is in the form of roentgen radiation (x-rays), and 99% is released as heat. A thin window area, located on the dependent portion of the tube, acts as a doorway for the exit of the x-rays. The entire tube is encased in a metal housing to prevent the escape of stray radiation and to protect the glass envelope from physical damage.

Cathode

The purpose of the cathode is to provide a source of electrons and direct these electrons toward the anode (Fig. 2-2). The cathode consists of a coiled wire **filament** that emits electrons when heated. The filament in most x-ray tubes measures approximately 0.2 cm in diameter and 1 cm in length. It is mounted on rigid wires that support it and carry the electrical current that is used to heat the filament. The filament of the cathode is similar to the filament of a light bulb (Fig. 2-3). When a filament is heated, electrons are held less tightly by the nucleus of the atoms of the metal. In other words, the electrons become excited. When the energy level exceeds the binding energy, a cloud of electrons is formed and made available to travel to the anode.

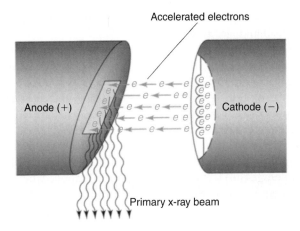

Accelerated electrons

Anode (+)

Cathode (−)

Primary x-ray beam

Figure 2-2 *Flow of electrons from the cathode to the anode.*

The filament is constructed of **tungsten** because of its high melting point (3370° C) and high atomic number. The atomic number is the number of protons in the nucleus of an atom. This number is matched by an equal number of electrons traveling around the nucleus. A high atomic number is proportionate to the potential electron availability. A metal of this type is also necessary because of the great amount of heat produced at the filament. Some x-ray tubes, usually those used in small portable and mobile units, have a single filament. Most modern tubes have two filaments mounted side by side. One is

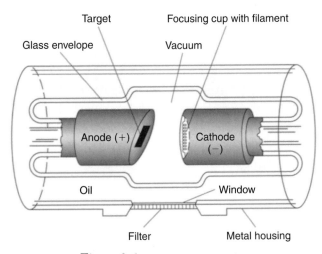

Target

Focusing cup with filament

Glass envelope

Vacuum

Anode (+)

Cathode (−)

Oil

Window

Filter

Metal housing

Figure 2-1 *X-ray tube construction.*

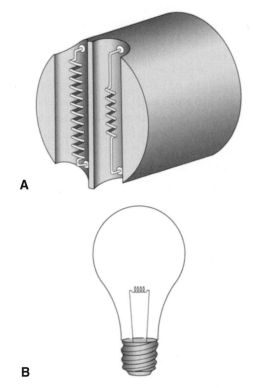

A

B

Figure 2-3 **A,** *Cathode filament construction showing a small (fine) and large (coarse) filament within the focusing cup.* **B,** *Light bulb containing a filament similar to the filament within the focusing cup of an x-ray tube.*

smaller than the other, and each has a different capacity for heat and electron emission.

The filament is located in a concave cup called the **focusing cup.** The focusing cup is made of **molybdenum** because it has a high melting point and is a poor conductor of heat. As a result of the shape and electrical charge of the focusing cup, the electrons are confined and directed toward the anode side of the tube.

The filament is heated by a low-energy circuit. The amount of energy in the circuit is referred to as **milliamperage (mA).** As the milliamperage is applied and the filament is heated, electrons are released from their atomic orbits. The quantity of electrons produced depends on the heat of the filament. Because of its negative electrical charge, the electron cloud is attracted to the anode side of the tube. The electron stream must be accelerated to create an impact great enough to produce x-rays. **Acceleration** of the electrons is controlled by the **kilovoltage** applied between the anode and the cathode. Milliamperage and kilovoltage are discussed in more detail in Chapter 4.

Anode

The basic construction of the anode consists of a beveled target placed on a cylindric base. The target is composed of tungsten, which can withstand and dissipate high temperatures. The base of the target usually is made of copper. Copper acts as a conductor of heat and draws the heat away from the tungsten target. Temperatures in excess of 1000° C occur during x-ray production. If the heat were not removed efficiently, the metal on the target would melt, and the tube would be useless. Approximately 99% of the energy released at the impact of the electrons, in diagnostic radiography is in the form of heat. Only 1% is in the form of x-rays.

Other methods of cooling the x-ray tube include surrounding the glass tube with oil within the metal housing. The oil transfers the heat away from the anode. For tubes designed for heavy-duty radiography, the oil in the tube housing often is circulated through a heat exchanger.

In specialized radiography, targets other than tungsten are used. One such material, molybdenum, is used for mammography in a human application of radiography.

Types of Anodes. The construction of the anode varies greatly. This variance is the main factor that differentiates one x-ray tube from another. The difference in anode type is associated with the maximum level of heat dissipation possible. The two main types are the **stationary anode** and the **rotating anode.**

STATIONARY ANODE. Stationary, or "fixed," anodes are found in dental and small portable radiography units. These units have a relatively small capacity for x-ray production (Fig. 2-4). As shown in Figure 2-5, the tungsten target area of the stationary anode is embedded on a cylinder of copper, with the face of the target angled

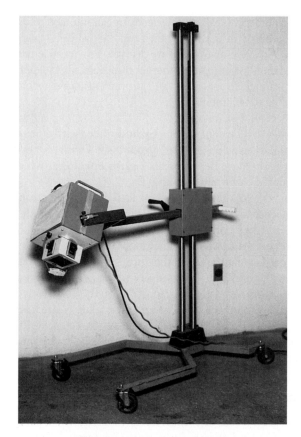

Figure 2-4 *Portable x-ray unit.*

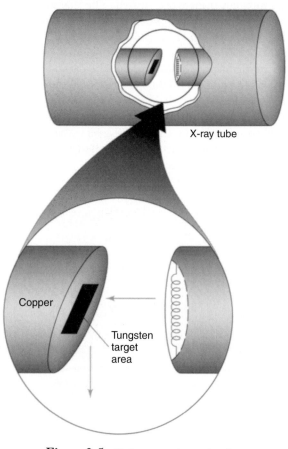

X-ray tube

Copper

Tungsten target area

Figure 2-5 *Stationary anode construction.*

down toward the window. The angle may range from 15 to 23 degrees, altering the "focal spot" size. The focal spot is the small area of the target with which the electrons collide. The focal spot is discussed in detail later.

The primary limitation of the stationary anode is its inability to withstand large amounts of heat. Repeated bombardment by electrons and subsequent heat production can damage the target. Damage commonly seen from this repeated bombardment is a pitting of the target surface. Once a target has been damaged in such a way, the x-rays produced from that area scatter in undesirable directions (Fig. 2-6). Radiographs produced by an x-ray tube with a pitted target area appear lighter than expected.

With the rapid development of increasingly powerful generators, temperature requirements far exceeded the capabilities of the stationary anode. This limitation prompted a search for a more efficient target area and resulted in the development of the rotating anode.

ROTATING ANODE.   The rotating anode is disk shaped and rotates on an axis through the center of the tube (Fig. 2-7). The disk is approximately 3 inches in diameter with a beveled edge. It is composed of tungsten or some similar **alloy** that can withstand high temperatures. The spindle on which the anode is mounted usually is made of molybdenum. Molybdenum dissipates the heat produced on electron impact. This heat reduction is necessary to reduce the heat flow to the rotor and bearing mechanism that spins the anode.

The filament is positioned to direct the electron stream at the beveled target area of the rotating disk. The target area with which the x-rays collide remains constant, while the anode disk rapidly rotates. The anode rotates approximately 3350 times per minute during the exposure. The rotation continually provides a cooler surface for the electron stream. A rotating disk distributes heat over a larger area yet still provides a small focal spot.

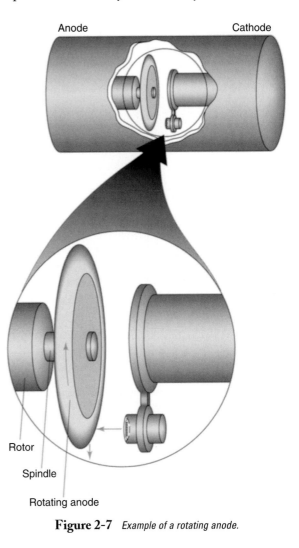

Figure 2-7 *Example of a rotating anode.*

Spreading the electron stream over a larger area also can be accomplished by decreasing the angle of the target. However, the smallness of the anode angle is limited. In a diagnostic x-ray tube, the target usually is angled at about 20 degrees from vertical. A small anode target angle results in an excessive falling off of intensity on the anode side of the x-ray beam. In other words, the x-ray beam is stronger toward the cathode side than the anode side. This variation of intensity of the primary x-ray beam is called the **heel effect** (Fig. 2-8). A small anode angle accentuates the heel effect. Decreasing the angle of the target also decreases the field size of the x-ray beam, thereby altering the focal spot.

Focal Spot.   The small area of the target with which the electrons collide is called the **focal spot** (Fig. 2-9). The size of the focal spot has an important effect on the formation of the x-ray image.

X-ray photons collide and leave the entire focal spot area. If the focal spot were the size of a pinpoint, the radiographic image produced would have great image clarity. As the focal spot becomes larger, the "shadow unsharpness" is increased. Any focal spot larger than a

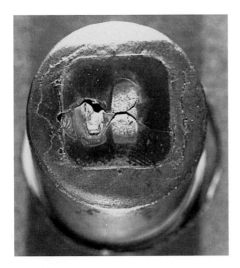

Figure 2-6 *Pitted anode target area showing scatter radiation resulting from the uneven target surface.*

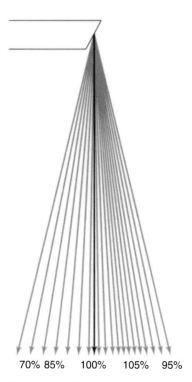

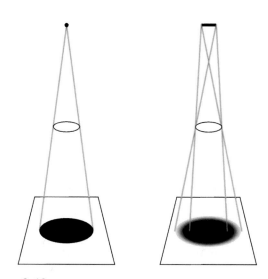

Figure 2-10 *Diagram showing the effect of the size of the focal spot on image sharpness—the penumbra effect. A small focal spot produces a sharp image, whereas a larger focal spot causes the penumbra effect, which blurs the projected image.*

70% 85% 100% 105% 95%

Figure 2-8 *Demonstration of the heel effect. The intensity of the primary x-ray beam is not uniform throughout all areas of the beam; the intensity is greater toward the cathode side of the x-ray beam because of the angle of the anode target area.*

pinpoint forms a **penumbra,** or halo effect, on a radiographic image (Fig. 2-10). Unfortunately, the focal spot size must be larger than a pinpoint to withstand the heat generated when the anode is bombarded with electrons. Each focal spot has definite dimensions; in most veterinary units, focal spots cover an area of 1 to 2 mm^2.

A stationary anode is limited to a larger focal spot to accommodate higher temperatures. The rotating anode can have a small focal spot and yet withstand a greater amount of heat.

EFFECTIVE FOCAL SPOT. If a person were to lie on an x-ray table and look into the window of the x-ray tube, the area of the focal spot called the **effective focal spot** would be visible. The **actual focal spot** is the area that is perpendicular to the surface of the target area (Fig. 2-11). This difference between the actual and effective focal spot is the result of the **line-focus principle.** The actual focal spot is useless to a radiographer because the effective x-ray beam should be directed in a downward angle (toward the x-ray film). However, the actual focal spot size is important in determining anode heat capacity.

The actual focal spot also influences the heel effect. As stated previously, the target with a small angle accentuates the heel effect. More x-rays leave the x-ray tube on the cathode side than on the anode side. This causes a variation in exposure to x-ray film.

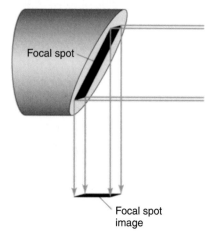

Figure 2-9 *The focal spot is the area in which the electrons collide with the target.*

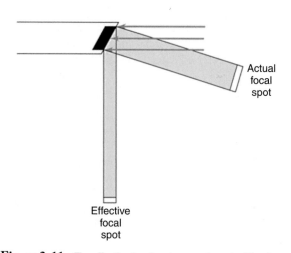

Figure 2-11 *The effective focal spot versus the actual focal spot.*

The heel effect can be used to advantage in some circumstances. When radiographing an anatomic area that varies in thickness (e.g., a ventrodorsal abdominal view of a dog with a deep thorax), the larger area can be positioned under the cathode side of the tube. The greater intensity toward the cathode side allows better radiographic exposure of the larger area. The cathode and anode ends of an x-ray tube housing usually are labeled near the area where the main electrical cables are attached.

POSSIBLE AREAS OF TUBE FAILURE

According to current price listings, the x-ray tube can range in cost from $2500 to $35,000. Because of this high replacement cost, the x-ray tube should be cared for properly. The life of a radiographic tube largely depends on the manner in which it is used. The majority of damaged tubes returned to manufacturers have been damaged as the result of technical error.

Cathode Failure

The most common cause of x-ray tube failure is filament evaporation. Filament failure can occur in any x-ray tube.

As the tube is fired with normal use, the filament is heated with each exposure. The filament of the cathode is similar to the filament in a light bulb. When a light bulb is "turned on," the filament is heated and emits light. When the filament of the cathode is heated, it emits electrons. With each use, the life of the filament is decreased. The higher the temperature and the longer the length of time that the filament is heated, the greater the chance that the filament will evaporate. When the filament of the cathode is destroyed, no electron cloud can be produced, and therefore no flow of electrons is transferred from the cathode to the anode. The film remains unexposed and appears transparent to light after development.

Current x-ray units have a mechanism that can prolong the life of a tube. This mechanism is known as a "standby current." The standby current preheats the filament to a low temperature when placed in the "on" position. The filament is "on standby" before the exposure is necessary. The filament is not heated to a sufficient temperature to produce an electron cloud until the preexposure button is depressed.

The preexposure switch protects the filament in some respects, but the machine should be turned off when not in use. Even the relatively low heat to which the filament is subjected on standby can damage the filament over a long period.

The switch should not be left in the "ready" position for any extended period. By heating the filament before the exposure for any time longer than necessary, the prolonged high temperature during operation can promote evaporation as well.

A common problem experienced in practice is depressing the preexposure button before actually exposing the film. This problem results from inadequate preparation at the time of exposure. The proper exposure settings should be selected before final positioning of the animal. Animals tend to move out of position at the least opportune time. By presetting the proper technique required for the anatomic area before final patient positioning, excess time for animal movement is reduced.

The best practice to lengthen the filament life is to evaluate all aspects of the radiographic procedure before activating the preexposure button. Thus the preheating time or repeated filament preheating also is reduced. By decreasing the amount of time in the preexposure phase, the life of an x-ray tube can be increased.

If an x-ray tube has an evaporated filament, it will be apparent not only on the film but also on the machine's control panel. Under normal circumstances, the milliamperage or milliamperage-seconds (mAs) meter on the console moves to indicate the exposure technique set. In filament failure, no movement of the mA meter needle is seen.

Anode Bearing Failure

In x-ray tubes with a rotating anode, the preexposure button has two purposes: (1) It heats the filament, and (2) it rotates the anode disk at top speed in preparation for the oncoming electrons.

As with other parts of the x-ray tube, bearings in the rotating anode mechanism can be damaged from heat. Unnecessary use of the preexposure button can result in heat accumulation while the anode is spinning. As the heat builds during rotation, the bearings become worn over time, and their life is shortened.

Bearing failure can be detected by a change in the noise produced as the anode spins. The usual noise increases over time as a result of use and is fostered by thermal overloading of the tube and housing. Eventually the bearings may decrease anode speed or even stop it. In the case of a slower rotation speed, the anode target eventually overheats. If the bearings cease to rotate, no noise is heard when the preexposure button is depressed. When the bearings fail, anode target failure soon follows.

Anode Target Failure

As stated earlier, the target can be damaged by excessive heat exposure, which can occur as the result of inadequate heat dissipation or exceeding the melting point during exposure. Damage to the target area is caused by melting of the surface, resulting in a roughened surface. As electrons hit this rough surface, the intensity of the x-ray beam produced is not uniform (see Fig. 2-6).

A damaged target can cause major frustration for the radiographer. The x-ray tube remains functional, but the exposures and therefore the film density (blackness) vary among uses. The radiation produced with each exposure is not constant. To prevent damage to the anode, high **kilovoltage peak (kVp)** and low mAs techniques should be used as often as possible. Exposures made with low mA settings produce fewer heat units than equivalent exposures made with high mA settings. The number of electrons available to affect the anode determines the amount of heat produced.

Use of a warm-up procedure is another method to prevent anode damage. If heat is introduced to an anode too quickly, the target area does not expand uniformly and may even crack. If the anode is warmed gradually, such damage is less likely to occur. Manufacturers specify warm-up procedures in equipment manuals.

Glass Envelope Damage

The glass envelope can become damaged or ineffective in two main ways. The first involves metal deposits that form on the inner lining of the glass as a result of target overheating. These deposits act as a secondary anode and attract the electrons that are produced at the filament. This phenomenon is called **arcing.** Arcing often is unnoticed until exposure techniques with a higher kVp are used. A tube with such deposits may be effective for quite some time if a lower kVp is used.

The second way a glass envelope can become disabled is through the presence of air within the glass housing. In a "gassy tube" the air molecules interact with the electron stream. This interaction results in a decreased number of x-rays produced at the target area. A gassy tube has little value because of the inability to control the exposure factors necessary for a quality radiograph (Fig. 2-12).

Tube Housing Anomalies

A number of malfunctions can occur in the tube housing, but the problems are rare. Two of the various possibilities may be of concern in the veterinary practice.

The first possible malfunction involves a shift of the glass envelope within the metal housing. Such a shift may displace the anode target area partially out of alignment with the window, located on the dependent side of the housing. If this occurs, a portion of the x-ray beam is absorbed by the metal housing, which results in a partially exposed radiograph.

The second potential problem is an oil leak from the metal housing. As stated previously, the oil acts as insulation and assists in heat dissipation. Once the oil is depleted, overheating and eventual destruction of the tube are imminent.

TECHNICAL COMPONENTS OF THE X-RAY MACHINE

Each x-ray apparatus consists of more than the x-ray tube. The x-ray machine comprises many complex mechanisms

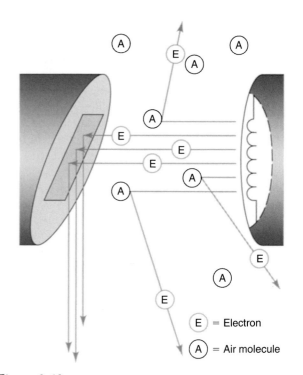

Figure 2-12 *Air molecules colliding with the electron stream in a "gassy" x-ray tube.*

E = Electron

A = Air molecule

that allow the radiographer to produce quality radiographs consistently and accurately.

Electrical Components

As described at the beginning of the chapter, the filament in the cathode must be heated. Once it is heated and an electron cloud is available, a source of power to push the cloud toward the anode target area is necessary. These two events must not only occur but also be controlled. Transformers, timers, and generators are necessary to control the power, time, and amount of release from the x-ray beam.

High-Voltage Circuit. The purpose of the high-voltage circuit is to provide the high electrical potential necessary to transport the electron stream from the cathode to the anode. The high-voltage circuit comprises two transformers: the **autotransformer** and the **step-up transformer.**

The step-up transformer increases the incoming voltage of 110 or 220 V to thousands of volts (kilovoltage). An extremely high potential (kVp) is necessary to transport the electron stream at a speed fast enough to produce x-rays at the anode target impact. The average table-based x-ray machine has a range of 40 to 120 kVp, whereas most portable x-ray machines have a range of 60 to 90 kVp.

The kVp selection switch on the x-ray machine's control panel is connected to the autotransformer to control the amount of kVp potential across the x-ray tube. The autotransformer mechanism is placed between the kVp selector and the high-voltage transformer (Fig. 2-13). The purpose of the autotransformer is to provide a variable yet predetermined voltage to the high-voltage step-up transformer. The high voltage can be preselected at the autotransformer before the exposure is made. Thus the autotransformer is the kVp selector.

The **line-voltage compensator** is associated with the autotransformer. This mechanism adjusts the incoming line voltage to the autotransformer so that the primary coil voltage remains constant. This compensation occurs automatically in newer x-ray units.

Low-Voltage (Filament) Circuit. The purpose of the filament circuit is to provide the electricity (amperage) necessary to heat the filament. The amount of heat at the filament determines how many electrons are available to travel toward the anode. Because the tungsten filament has little resistance to excessive heat, minimal energy is necessary to achieve an adequate temperature for electron emission. A simple **step-down transformer** is placed between the cathode filament and the x-ray machine input voltage. The average incoming line voltage to most x-ray machines is 110 or 220 V. This extreme voltage would cause the filament to vaporize instantly. The step-down transformer reduces the voltage of the incoming line to approximately 10 V.

The step-down mechanism is connected to the mA control of the x-ray machine's control panel. Control over

the amperage in the cathode filament is directly proportional to the number of x-rays produced over a given period.

Timer Switch. A mechanism is necessary to control the amount of time during which high voltage is applied across the x-ray tube. The duration of x-ray generation is controlled by controlling the time of high-voltage transfer. The device used to control the length of exposure is the **timer switch.**

Exposure time is an important variable in veterinary radiography. Shorter exposure times are necessary because of the chance of motion caused by animal movement. Exposure times of 1/30 of a second (0.3 second) or shorter are necessary to decrease the potential for motion on the finished radiograph.

Rectification. When an alternating 60-cycle voltage is applied to the x-ray machine, electrons flow from the cathode to the anode only when the positive deflection of the cycle is applied to the anode. As stated in Chapter 1, all electromagnetic radiation travels in a waveform. During the negative half of every cycle, no electrons are generated within the x-ray tube.

Rectification is the process of changing an alternating current to a direct current. The x-ray tube may perform its own rectification, known as **half-wave rectification.** As a machine performs its own rectification, one half of the current is lost and a marked increase in heat occurs at

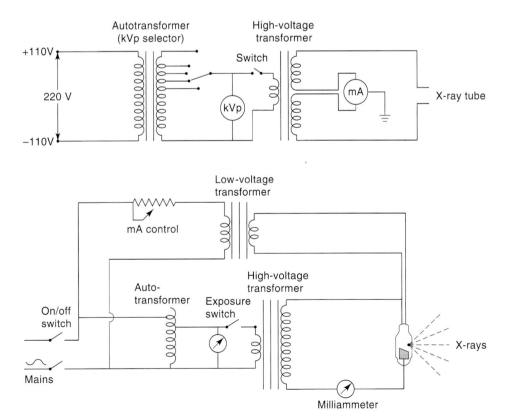

Figure 2-13 *Autotransformer electrical circuit.*

the anode. If the anode becomes too hot, it may form an electron cloud and pass a current from the anode to the cathode. If an electron beam is accelerated toward the filament at the cathode from the anode, severe damage—even filament vaporization—can occur. Because of this possibility, valve tubes or silicon rectifiers are used to play the role of a rectifier.

Rectifiers allow the flow of electrons in one direction only. The use of **valve tubes** or self-rectifiers prolongs the life of the x-ray tube. However, the efficiency of a self-rectified system and that of valve tube or solid-state rectification do not differ appreciably.

Half-wave rectification also is made possible by placing two rectifiers in a series within the tube. The two sequential rectifiers prevent a reverse flow of the current and subsequent overheating of the cathode. This method provides some protection to the x-ray tube but does not allow the use of more of the electrical current (Fig. 2-14, *A*). This type of rectification is used in most small dental and portable units.

The alternating current can be converted into a direct current without losing any amount of electricity. **Full-wave rectification** creates an almost constant electric potential across the x-ray tube (Fig. 2-14, *B*). The addition of four valve tubes or silicon rectifiers to the high-voltage circuit increases the efficiency of the electrical potential by 100%. The electrical current pulses 120 times per second, compared with the 60 times per second obtained with half-wave rectification. Full-wave rectification results in twice the x-ray production and decreased exposure times.

X-ray Tube Rating

X-ray tube rating is based on four factors: (1) focal spot size; (2) target angle; (3) anode speed; and (4) electrical current, either single- or three-phase operation. The effects of focal spot size, target angle, and anode speed on x-ray tube efficiency were discussed earlier. This section discusses the maximum usage of the electrical supply, which increases the x-ray tube rating.

Each type of x-ray tube has an individual tube rating. X-ray tube ratings dictate the maximum combinations of kilovolt peak (kVp), milliamperes (mA), and time that can safely be used without overloading the tube. This rating is expressed in kilowatts. Remember that the watt

(W) is the unit of electric power, with the kilowatt being equal to 1000 W.

Both electrical and thermal limitations exist for a given x-ray tube. The electrical current potential must be increased to increase the x-ray–producing potential of the x-ray tube. In the United States, commercial electrical power ranges from 115-V to 230-V, 60-cycle alternating current. As discussed in the section on rectification, electrons flow from the cathode to the anode only when the positive deflection of the electrical cycle is applied to the anode. A generator is used to increase the potential power of the electrical supply.

Three-Phase Generator

Most modern table-based x-ray machines have a three-phase generator, which produces an almost constant electrical potential difference between the anode and the cathode. This almost constant electrical current is produced by superimposing three single-phase currents so that they are 120 degrees out of phase. In other words, each phase is 120 degrees behind the next with no deep valleys between the electrical pulses (Fig. 2-15).

The advantages of an x-ray tube with a three-phase generator versus a single-phase generator follow:

1. More power is available to the x-ray tube per unit time, and therefore shorter exposure can be used.
2. Intensity of the x-radiation generated is considerably higher.
3. Radiation quality is greater because it contains fewer low-energy x-rays.
4. Tube utilization is more efficient because the target is not subjected to bombardment of low-energy electrons, which creates only heat in the anode target area.

High-Frequency Generators

As previously discussed, single-phase generators are limited by their low power capacity. Three-phase generators were developed to overcome the shortcomings of the single-phase systems, but for many private veterinary practices, three-phase generators are too expensive and their installation costs are high because of the electrical requirements. The development of the high-frequency generator provides the veterinary field an affordable, efficient way to produce twice the amount of radiation per unit of time than that produced by a single-phase unit.

High-frequency technology provides a high electrical-to-radiographic energy conversion. In conventional single-phase (self-rectified) units an electrical wave proceeds to the x-ray tube 60 times per second and is converted to radiographic energy. In the high-frequency unit, many thousands of waves per second flow to the x-ray tube and are converted to radiographic energy. When the high-frequency unit is energized, the electrical frequency of

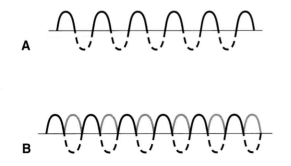

Figure 2-14 *A,* Half-wave rectification. *B,* Full-wave rectification.

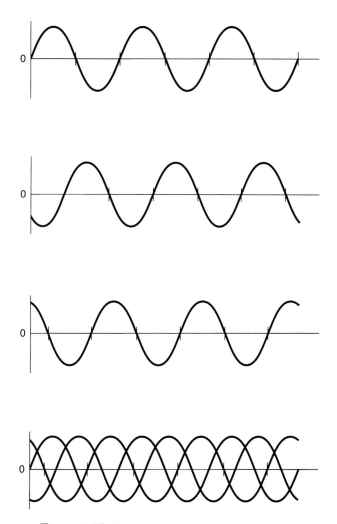

Figure 2-15 *Three-phase alternating current waveforms.*

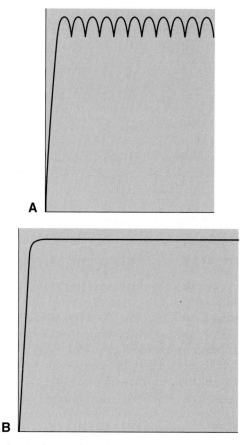

Figure 2-16 *A, Three-phase output. B, 100-kHz high-frequency output.*

the unit reaches a constant potential. In effect, the electrical energy delivered takes the form of a square wave (Fig. 2-16). A full-wave rectified high-frequency unit possesses the highest energy conversion possible for a radiographic system.

The Collimator

A **collimator** is a restricting device used to control the size of the primary x-ray beam. The beam emerges from the x-ray tube in a diverging manner. If uncontrolled, the beam could extend to considerable width. Most x-ray machines incorporate some type of x-ray beam restriction to limit the beam to the essential size. Collimation prevents unnecessary irradiation of the patient or persons involved in restraining the patient and reduces scatter radiation.

Many older or simpler x-ray machines incorporate a lead plate or cone over the aperture of the tube to alter the size of the x-ray beam (Fig. 2-17). Each plate or cone has a different-sized circular hole that alters the size of the window from which the x-rays emerge. Collimation is often described as "coning down" because of the cones.

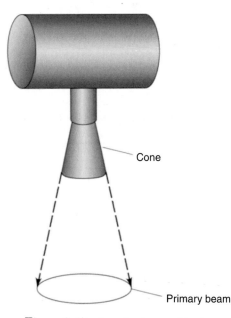

Figure 2-17 *Example of cone collimation.*

A more versatile method of collimation uses adjustable lead shutters, which are permanently attached to the tube housing, correlating with the tube window. A collimator with lead shutters usually incorporates a light source (Fig. 2-18). The light assists visualization of the field

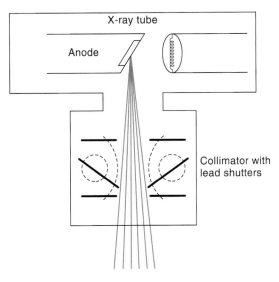

X-ray tube

Anode

Collimator with
lead shutters

Figure 2-18 *Collimator with lead shutters.*

size and accurate positioning of the x-ray beam. The
collimator light often is difficult to visualize in a brightly
lit room and may be most effective in subdued room
light.

Knobs located on the collimator allow for adjustment
of the field size. A good guideline is to always use the
smallest field size possible for any radiograph, as a small
field size decreases the amount of scatter radiation.

The Tube Stand

The tube stand is the apparatus that supports the x-ray
tube during radiographic procedures. The design of the
stand varies immensely, differing in forms of suspension.
Models range from small tabletop stands to larger mobile
or overhead ceiling tract stands (Fig. 2-19).

For veterinary purposes the stand should be durable
and sturdy. Some lighter stands on the market are moved
easily or damaged by boisterous animals. A shaky stand is
a common cause of motion artifact on a radiograph.

The Control Panel

The control panel, or **console,** consists of the many knobs
and switches necessary to operate the x-ray machine. The
radiographer must be familiar with all components on
the face of the panel and understand that not all control
panels are alike (Fig. 2-20). The following is a list of
mechanisms found on most x-ray consoles.

1. *On/off switch.* Provides a closure to the electrical
   circuit to allow the flow of electricity necessary for
   subsequent exposure.
2. *Voltage compensator.* The voltmeter provides manual
   adjustment of the transformer to allow for inconsistent electrical output from the main electrical
   line. The line voltage should be checked whenever
   the machine is turned on.
3. *Kilovoltage selector.* Most modern x-ray machines
   are calibrated so that the desired kilovoltage value
   can be selected. However, in some smaller x-ray
   units, the kilovoltage control is linked automatically
   with a certain milliamperage.
4. *Milliamperage selector.* This component lets the
   radiographer select the desired current to the
   cathode filament. This method of selection varies
   among x-ray machines.

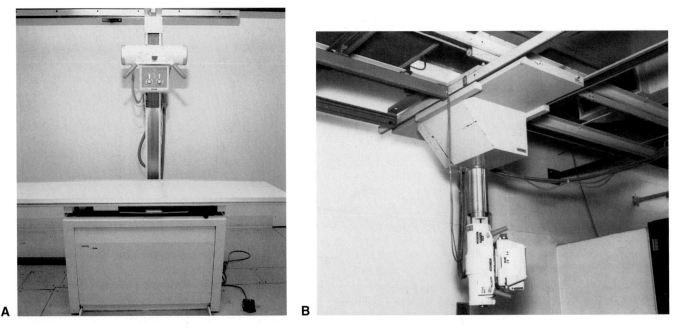

A   B

Figure 2-19 *A, Example of a fixed tube stand construction. B, Example of a ceiling-mounted x-ray unit.*

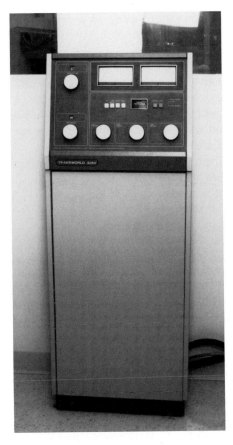

Figure 2-20 *X-ray machine/console.*

5. *Timer.* This mechanism allows the radiographer to preselect the time of each exposure. The timer varies greatly among models of x-ray machines. Examples include a clockwork timer, a synchronous timer, and an electronic timer. The timer enables a short exposure time with accuracy.
6. *Exposure button.* The exposure button is on the face of the control panel or attached to it by a length of cable. In either case the button should be positioned to allow the person making the exposure to be at least 2 m from the tube housing. Many x-ray machines operate on a two-stage button. Two stages are necessary for the cathode filament to be activated and heated to produce the electrons necessary for the exposure. Depression of the first half of the button activates the filament and rotating anode, if present, and after a few seconds, the button is fully depressed to complete the circuit for exposure.
7. *Warning light.* Most control panels have a light that illuminates when an exposure is made and x-rays are being emitted.

Key Points

1. The purpose of the x-ray tube is to produce a controlled x-ray beam.

2. High kilovoltage peak (kVp) and low milliamperage-second (mAs) techniques should be used as often as possible to prevent damage to the anode.
3. X-ray tube failure is usually a result of technical error; x-ray tubes should be cared for properly.
4. The electrical components of the x-ray machine consist of (1) the transformer, (2) the generator, (3) the line-voltage compensator, (4) the timer, and (5) the rectifier.

Review Questions

1. Filaments located in an x-ray tube:
   a. are made of molybdenum.
   b. must have a low melting point and low atomic number.
   c. are found in the anode.
   d. emit electrons when heated.

2. The anode's target:
   a. is composed of tungsten.
   b. reaches temperatures in excess of 1000° C during x-ray production.
   c. usually has a copper base.
   d. All of the above.

3. Which of the following are limitations of the stationary anode?
   a. The target is made of tungsten.
   b. It is unable to withstand large amounts of heat.
   c. If the target becomes pitted, radiographs appear darker.
   d. It is limited to a larger focal spot to accommodate higher temperatures.

4. How can the technician help to prolong the life of the filament in the x-ray tube?
   a. Enter the proper exposure settings in the control panel before the final positioning of the animal.
   b. Leave the x-ray unit on at all times to ensure that the filament is heated when the radiograph is requested.
   c. Always leave the x-ray unit in the standby mode.
   d. The technician can do nothing because filament defects are largely the fault of the manufacturer.

5. Which of the following are possible effects of excessive heat within an x-ray tube?
   a. Bearing failure and decreased anode speed
   b. Roughened target surface
   c. Arcing
   d. All of the above

6. True or false (circle one).
   A small amount of air within the glass envelope is beneficial because it helps to dissipate heat.

7. Veterinary patients have a tendency to move while being positioned for radiographs to be taken. The radiographer should help to safely prevent artifacts of movement by:
   a. using the shortest exposure time possible.
   b. altering the direction in which the x-rays move.
   c. selecting a longer exposure time than is recommended.
   d. sedating all patients before taking radiographs.

8. Which of the following is recommended to reduce unnecessary irradiation of the patient or persons restraining the patient and to decrease scatter radiation?
   a. Opening the collimator as wide as possible
   b. Placement of a lead apron over the area of interest on the patient
   c. Selection of full-wave rectification as opposed to half-wave rectification on the control panel
   d. Adjustment of the collimator so that the smallest field size possible is used

9. X-ray tube ratings are based on target angle, focal spot size, electrical current (single- or three-phase operation), and:
   a. rectification.
   b. its alloy composition.
   c. anode speed.
   d. type of filament.

10. The advantages of using an x-ray machine with a three-phase generator as opposed to a single-phase generator include:
    a. creation of more low-energy electrons bombarding the target, thus producing less heat.
    b. use of shorter exposure times because more power is available to the x-ray tube per unit time.
    c. production of more low-energy x-rays so that radiation quality is increased.
    d. generation of considerably higher intensity of the x-radiation.

Suggested Readings

Ball JL, Moore AD: *Essential physics for the radiographer,* Boston, 1980, Blackwell Scientific.

Curry, ES III, Dowdey JE, Murry RC Jr: *Christensen's physics of diagnostic radiology,* ed 4, Philadelphia, 1990, Lea & Febiger.

Gillette EL, Thrall DE, Lebel JD: *Carlson's veterinary radiology,* ed 3, Philadelphia, 1977, Lea & Febiger.

Gray JE, Winkler NT, Stears J, Frank ED: *Quality control in diagnostic imaging,* Rockville, Md, 1983, Aspen.

Hendee WR, Chaney EL, Rossi RP: *Radiologic physics, equipment and quality control,* St Louis, 1977, Mosby-Year Book.

Kay RS: Modern x-ray tubes, *Vet Tech* 575-577, September 1992.

Terpogossian MM: *The physical aspects of diagnostic radiology,* New York, 1967, Hoeber Medical Division, Harper & Row.

Thompson TT: The abuse of radiographic tubes, *Radiographics* 3: 397-399, 1983.

chapter 3

Radiation Safety

CHAPTER OUTLINE

Hazards of Ionizing Radiation
Maximum Permissible Dose
Patient Exposure

Personnel Monitoring Devices
Practical Application of Radiation Safety

OBJECTIVES

Upon completion of this chapter, the reader should be able to do the following:

- List the tissues most sensitive to radiation-induced damage
- State which personnel are prohibited from assisting in radiographic procedures
- State the two types of tissue damage that can occur from exposure to radiation
- Define maximum permissible dose (MPD) and name the organization that is responsible for setting dose limits
- List and define the units of radiation exposure for absorption

- State the MPD for occupationally exposed personnel
- List and describe the three types of personal exposure dosimeters
- State the three primary methods by which personnel are exposed to radiation during radiography
- List the practical methods that personnel can use to reduce personal exposure during radiography
- State the proper maintenance protocol for protective apparel
- State the risks and safety measures necessary with the use of fluoroscopy

GLOSSARY

Absorbed dose: The quantity of energy imparted by ionizing radiations to matter.

Dose equivalent: The quantity obtained by multiplying the absorbed dose in tissue by the quality factor.

Dosimeter: A device used to measure radiation exposure to personnel.

Dosimetry: Various methods used to measure radiation exposure to personnel.

Film badge: A method of dosimetry consisting of a plastic holder with a radiation-sensitive film in a lightproof package.

Fluoroscopy: A special radiographic diagnostic method in which a "live view" of the internal anatomy is possible.

Genetic damage: Effects of radiation that occur to the genes of reproductive cells.

Gray (Gy): The unit of absorbed dose imparted by ionizing radiations to matter (1 gray equals 100 rad).

Hemopoietic: Anatomic areas where red blood cells are produced.

Leukopoietic: Anatomic areas where white blood cells are produced.

Maximum permissible dose (MPD): The maximum dose of radiation a person may receive in a given time period.

Pocket ionization chamber: A method of dosimetry consisting of a charged ion chamber and electrometer, which can be read immediately to determine the amount of exposure.

Primary beam: The path that the x-rays follow as they leave the tube.

Secondary radiation: Commonly called *scatter radiation*, it is caused by interaction of the primary beam with objects in its path.

Sievert (Sv): The dose of radiation equivalent to the absorbed dose in tissue (1 sievert equals 100 rem).

Somatic damage: Damage to the body induced by radiation that becomes manifest within the lifetime of the recipient.

Thermoluminescent dosimeter (TLD): A method of dosimetry consisting of a chamber containing special compounds that become electrically altered by ionizing radiation.

INTRODUCTION

During each laboratory or diagnostic procedure, safety should be a primary objective. Radiography is no different.

It is a scientific fact that ionizing radiation is hazardous. The exposure to stray radiation is a common occurrence with the use of diagnostic x-rays in veterinary medicine. However, following proper safety precautions can limit the exposure.

The veterinarian must establish and maintain a radiation safety program for the protection of the patient, the client, and the technical staff. Safe operating procedures for each facility should include (1) an adequate technique chart or comparable system, (2) positioning aids, (3) protective clothing and other protective barriers, (4) personnel dosimetry devices, (5) emergency procedures for malfunctioning x-ray equipment, and (6) quality control measurements and tests.

All radiographic equipment including radiation protection devices must meet state regulation requirements, which can vary by state. Regulations can usually be obtained from the state Department of Health.

The radiographer should keep one important concept about ionizing radiation in mind: *Radiation should be respected … not feared.*

HAZARDS OF IONIZING RADIATION

All living cells are susceptible to ionizing radiation damage. Affected cells may be damaged or killed. Cells that are most sensitive to radiation are rapidly dividing cells (e.g., growth cells, gonadal cells, neoplastic cells, and metabolically active cells). Therefore persons younger than 18 years of age and pregnant women should *not* be involved in radiographic procedures. Other tissues that are readily sensitive to radiation include bone, lymphatic, dermis, **leukopoietic** and **hemopoietic** (blood forming), and epithelial tissues.

A vast amount of knowledge has been collected over the years concerning the effects of radiation on the body. Two types of biologic damage can occur from overexposure to radiation: somatic damage and genetic damage.

Somatic damage describes damage to the body that becomes manifest within the lifetime of the recipient. Radiation can produce immediate changes in the cell, although the damage may not be apparent for some time. Because the body has the ability to repair itself, cell damage may never be appreciated or visible. Damage is more extensive when the body is exposed to a single massive dose of radiation than to smaller, cumulatively equivalent repeated exposures. As mentioned earlier, body cells are not equally sensitive to radiation, and the healing process varies among cell types. Examples of somatic damage include cancer, cataracts, aplastic anemia, and sterility.

Genetic damage from radiation occurs as a result of injury to the genes (DNA) of reproductive cells. Ionizing radiation can damage chromosomal material within any cell. The result of the damage is determined by the cell type (i.e., somatic cell or reproductive cell). Damage to reproductive cells can result in the effect known as *gene mutation*. Genetic damage is not detectable until future generations are produced. The offspring of irradiated persons may be abnormally formed because of changes in the hereditary material, resulting in alteration of the individual phenotype (physical appearance). The mutation may be lethal or may be only a visible anomaly. The gene mutation may also stay latent or recessive until the second or third generation.

Mortality from radiation is caused by exposure to extremely high levels of radiation. Exposure to a large, single dose of radiation, as from a hydrogen bomb, is necessary to cause rapid death. A single exposure to a dose of 300 rad (radiation absorbed dose; see later) or more has been shown to be lethal to humans. Further information on death due to radiation exposure can be found in a radiobiology textbook. A technologist working in a practical situation and following proper safety protocol should never receive this level of radiation. Because the body has the ability to repair itself, accumulative smaller doses of radiation are sublethal.

Theoretically, no amount of radiation is nondamaging. Even under the best conditions, some exposure to ionizing radiation will occur. Therefore it is the responsibility of radiographers to limit the exposure of ionizing radiation to patients, clients, and themselves. The exposure received by any individual should never exceed the maximum permissible dose.

MAXIMUM PERMISSIBLE DOSE

The **maximum permissible dose (MPD)** is of great interest to the radiographer. The MPD is the maximum dose of radiation that a person may receive in a given period. The concept of MPD was introduced to denote an amount of irradiation that does not involve a risk to the health of radiation workers so great that it significantly influences future generations or the individuals occupationally exposed. The MPD helps to determine whether procedures and equipment are adequate to provide the degree of protection necessary to stay within the stated limit.

The National Committee on Radiation Protection and Measurements (NCRP) defines the MPD for occupationally and nonoccupationally exposed persons. The NCRP is a nonprofit organization, chartered by Congress and consisting of scientific committees of persons who are experts in a particular area.

The NCRP has issued a practical approach to radiation safety in the workplace through a program known as *ALARA* (as low as reasonably achievable). The process of ensuring that radiation exposures are ALARA may be viewed as an ongoing series of decisions about possible radiation protection actions. A practical approach to the implementation of ALARA in a medical setting must provide a framework for a standard radiation protection program. Thus certain rules and regulations have been designed to achieve ALARA in the veterinary workplace.

The NCRP and most state health codes permit occupationally exposed persons to restrain and position animal patients manually for radiography when absolutely necessary. However, some states prohibit manual restraint of animals during diagnostic radiography by occupationally exposed personnel. In these cases the animal owner or staff personnel who are not routinely involved in radiographic procedures must be used for this purpose.

Another option customary in some states is the use of chemical restraint and positioning devices only (e.g., anesthesia, sandbags, adhesive tape).

Radiation Exposure Units

To quantify the amount of radiation received, radiation exposure units are stated in two categories: absorbed dose and dose equivalent.

1. **Absorbed dose** is the quantity of energy imparted by ionizing radiations to matter per unit mass of the matter. The unit of absorbed dose is the **gray** (Gy). This replaces the previously used unit, which is known as the *rad* (1 Gy = 100 rad).
2. **Dose equivalent** is the quantity obtained by multiplying the absorbed dose in tissue by the quality factor. This equation accounts for the differing biologic effectiveness of equal absorbed doses and other modifying factors. The unit of dose equivalent is the **Sievert** (Sv). The Sievert supersedes the *rem*, which was previously used for this purpose (1 Sv = 100 rem).

State and federal restrictions dictate that occupationally exposed individuals older than 18 years of age and wearing monitoring devices can receive up to 0.05 Sv/year from occupational and background exposure.

Any person younger than age 18 is not allowed to enter the radiographic suite during exposure unless ordered by a medical doctor. These young people are still growing and are more susceptible to radiation damage. Nonoccupationally exposed persons can receive 10% of this figure (0.005 Sv/year). The MPD for the general public is set at a much lower level because they will not be monitored and are not trained to recognize and avoid accidental exposure (Table 3-1).

Booklets that outline the specific requirements and regulations on radiation protection in veterinary medicine

TABLE 3-1

MAXIMUM PERMISSIBLE DOSE (PER CALENDAR YEAR)

	OCCUPATIONALLY EXPOSED (>18 YR)	NONOCCUPATIONALLY EXPOSED (>18 YR)
Whole body	0.05 Sv (5 rem)	0.005 Sv (0.5 rem)
Individual organs and tissues	0.5 Sv (50 rem)	0.05 Sv (5 rem)
Lens of the eye	0.15 Sv (1.5 rem)	0.03 Sv (3 rem)

can be purchased from NCRP for a small fee.* Suggested readings include NCRP #36, *Radiation Protection in Veterinary Medicine* (also see Suggested Readings later).

Patient Exposure

The risk of radiation exposure to the patient has been questioned by animal owners and veterinary personnel for some time. This chapter mainly discusses the radiation risk to people but is not intended to ignore the risk to animals. Animal patients are just as susceptible to irradiation damage as humans, but because veterinary personnel are likely to be involved in many more radiographic procedures than any one patient, the risk to the animal is, in general, less severe. However, the veterinary radiographer should always be conscious of the radiation risk to the fetus and gonads of breeding animals. Shielding the gonads of breeding animals is possible and recommended (Fig. 3-1). Unnecessary and excessive radiography should always be avoided for any patient in general.

PERSONNEL MONITORING DEVICES

The actual amount of radiation received by those engaged in radiography can be monitored **(dosimetry).** Personal exposure monitoring devices **(dosimeters)** should be worn by personnel at all times during radiographic procedures. The monitors are sent regularly to a federally approved laboratory, where they are processed, and the dosage received is reported. The exact routine adopted by each practice may vary and depends on the amount and nature of the radiographic examinations performed. The preferred practice is to wear a dosimeter for 1 month and then submit it for evaluation. A replacement dosimeter is issued immediately so that there is no time when the radiographer is not monitored.

Various types of radiation monitoring devices are used in veterinary medicine. The **film badge** is the most common type used today (Fig. 3-2). A film badge consists of a plastic holder that contains a radiation-sensitive film in a lightproof packaging. The film is sensitive to beta-,

gamma-, and x-radiation of various energies. The films are developed and evaluated by measuring the blackening, caused by exposure, on the film. The film badge is worn on the belt, hand, or collar, depending on the anatomic area considered to be most at risk (e.g., gonads, extremities, thyroid). The same badge is worn for a week, month, or quarter. The length of time depends on the sensitivity of the film and the amount of radiation to which personnel are exposed. Film badges are available in several forms such as ring badges, wrist badges, and clip-on badges. Film badge dosimetry service can be ordered through several federally approved laboratories (Table 3-2).

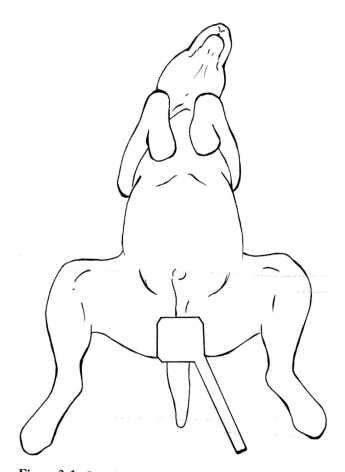

Figure 3-1 *Example of a gonad shield, in this case used to shield the testicles of a dog.*

*NCRP Publications, 7910 Woodmont Avenue, Bethesda, MD 20814.

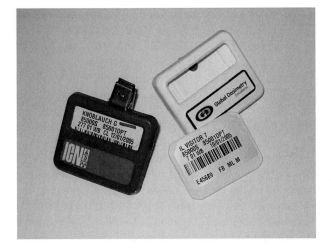

Figure 3-2 *Example of a radiation detection device called a film badge, which consists of a plastic holder containing radiation-sensitive film.*

Other forms of radiation detectors include the **pocket ionization chamber** and the **thermoluminescent dosimeter (TLD).** The pocket ionization chamber is the same size and shape as a pen and fits conveniently in the wearer's pocket. It consists of an ion chamber and an electrometer. The chamber is charged before use, and subsequent exposure to radiation discharges the ions. This discharge is proportional to the amount of radiation received. The exposure can be read immediately from the electrometer, providing an instant determination of the amount of radiation received. The use of this device in medical diagnostic situations is not recommended.

TLDs contain special compounds (e.g., lithium fluoride and calcium fluoride) that are electrically altered by ionizing radiation. The compounds are available in fine crystals, which are placed in small containers (badges) and worn by personnel. After a period of time, the badge is returned to the dosimetry service for heat processing. When the crystal compounds are heated, they emit light directly proportional to the amount of radiation they have absorbed before heating. TLD dosimetry is considered superior to other methods because the measurements can be collected over a long time period and can be stored for years without losing information. TLDs can also be reused.

Most dosimetry services supply both film and TLD badges. Currently, film badges cost approximately 25% less than TLD badges.

PRACTICAL APPLICATION OF RADIATION SAFETY

Personnel exposure is a result of (1) exposure to the primary beam, (2) exposure from secondary (scatter) radiation caused by interaction of the primary beam with objects in its path, and (3) exposure from "leakage" radiation from the x-ray tube housing.

TABLE 3-2
DOSIMETRY SERVICES MEETING NATIONAL VOLUNTARY LABORATORY ACCREDITATION PROGRAM GUIDELINES*

Radiation Detection Company
162 Wolfe Road
P.O. Box 1414
Sunnyvale, CA 94088
(408) 735-8700

Thermo Analytical, Inc.
TMA/Eberline
5635 Kircher Boulevard NE
P.O. Box 3874
Albuquerque, NM 87109-3874
(505) 345-9931

R.S. Landaurer Jr. & Company
Glenwood Science Park
2 Science Road
Glenwood, IL 60425
(800) 323-8830

Proxtronics, Inc.
Radiation Monitoring Services
P.O. Box 12150
Burke, VA 22009
(800) 435-4811

Teledyne Isotopes
50 Van Buren Avenue
Westwood, NJ 07675
(201) 664-7070

ICN Dosimetry Service
Div. of ICN Biomedicals, Inc.
330 Hyland Avenue
ICN Plaza
Costa Mesa, CA 92626
(800) 251-3331

United States Testing Company
2800 George Washington Way
Richland, WA 99352
(509) 946-8738

*List does not include all organizations that have dosimetry service.

Exposure to the **primary beam** is usually the result of technical error. At no time should personnel have any part of their own body in the primary beam, even with proper shielding such as lead aprons and gloves. Each individual in the radiography suite must ensure his or her own radiation protection at the time of exposure.

Beam-limiting devices, such as a collimator, help reduce scatter radiation exposure to the patient and to those assisting with the radiographic procedure.

Radiation exposure caused by leakage from the x-ray tube housing is another possibility. Current regulations for the manufacturing of x-ray tubes require sufficient shielding to minimize exposure to personnel and patients. Normally, a recently manufactured tube head can be considered safe. Unfortunately, many veterinary clinics in the United States still use extremely old x-ray units that have minimal shielding in the tube housing. Such x-ray tubes require additional shielding to decrease the amount of exposure leakage. If the machine is older or if there is a question of radiation leakage, the x-ray tube should be checked by the state department of health.

All states have one safety code in common; each requires that a minimum of 2.5 mm aluminum filtration of the primary beam be used in any diagnostic x-ray machine that has the capacity greater than 70 kilovoltage (kVp). The filter is located between the window of the x-ray tube and the collimator (Fig. 3-3). This filtration essentially eliminates less-penetrating, or "soft," x-rays. Soft x-rays, when not filtered, add to the skin exposure of the patient and the assisting personnel. Without added filters, the total skin radiation dose of both patient and personnel would be increased approximately four times.

Radiation exposure from **secondary radiation,** or scatter radiation, is produced when the primary beam interacts with objects in its path. Scatter can be produced within the patient, tabletop, floor, or any other object in the path of the primary beam (Fig. 3-4). The amount and direction of scatter depend on the intensity of the beam, the composition of the structure being radiographed, the kVp level, and the thickness of the patient.

Scatter is produced in all directions and travels in straight lines. A large portion of scatter travels in an upward path toward the torso and head of the restrainer. Personnel involved in the radiographic procedure should leave as much distance as possible between them and the primary beam at all times. Looking away from the primary beam during exposure will minimize radiation to the lenses of the eye. At no time should personnel lean over or sit on the x-ray table (Fig. 3-5). Provided that the recommended precautions are observed, most animals can be radiographed without anyone receiving a significant amount of radiation.

Chemical restraint of the animal should be considered whenever possible to minimize exposure to employees in the workplace. (*Note:* Some states forbid humans from restraining animals in veterinary radiography.) Ideally, the animal should be sedated and positioned with supporting devices (Fig. 3-6). The operator is then shielded by the wall of the control booth or behind a leaded screen during exposure.

If chemical restraint is not possible, certain safety measures must be observed. All personnel should wear the appropriate protective apparel such as lead aprons and lead gloves that have a 0.5-mm lead equivalent thickness. Mobile lead screens with a lead glass window or leaded plastic shields that hang from the ceiling are also available. The lead glass window or lead plastic shield permits

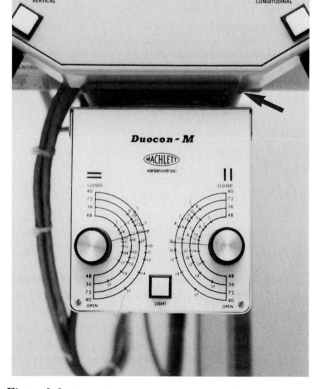

Figure 3-3 *An aluminum filter (arrow) is placed between the x-ray tube and the collimator to absorb "soft" x-rays.*

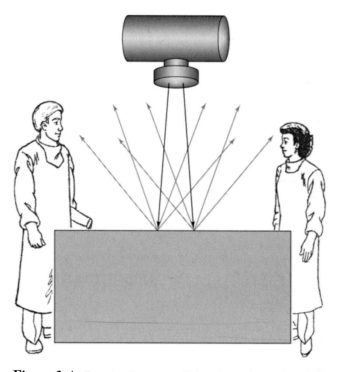

Figure 3-4 *Example of scatter radiation due to interaction of the primary x-ray beam with the table-top.*

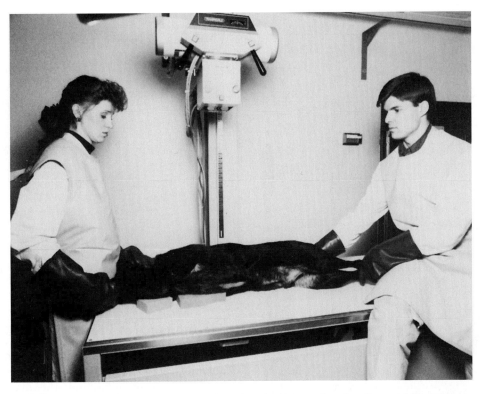

Figure 3-5 *Incorrect posture for manual restraint. At no time should a restrainer sit on the x-ray table during exposure.*

observation of the patient yet provides adequate protection from exposure. Lead walls are useful but are an expensive method of protection (Fig. 3-7).

When restraining an animal on the x-ray table, personnel should stand in an upright position at the end of the table. This increases the distance between the source of scatter radiation and the restrainer (Fig. 3-8). The restrainer should never be exposed to the primary beam of radiation, even if shielded (Fig. 3-9). The lead apparel will usually reduce the dose of scatter radiation significantly; however, only a fraction of the higher energy of the primary beam will be absorbed by the lead apparel.

A common artifact seen on veterinary radiographs is the fingers or entire hands holding an animal in position (Fig. 3-10). This artifact is considered "illegal" and should be avoided.

No individuals other than the operator and necessary restrainers should be present when exposures are being made. If restraint by humans is used, rotate personnel that are required. This practice decreases the possibility of one or two persons exceeding their MPD.

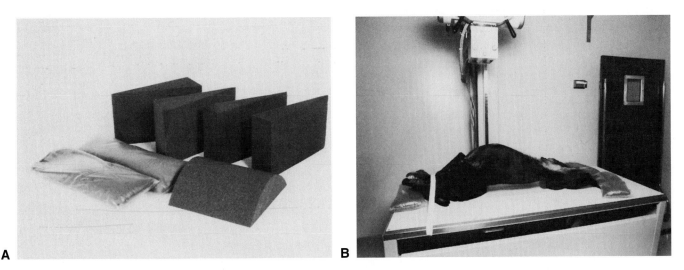

A   **B**

Figure 3-6 *A, Examples of various positioning aids. B, A sedated patient held in place with the assistance of positioning aids.*

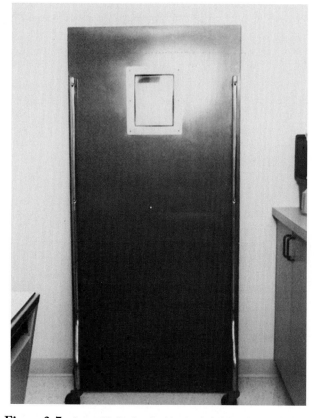

Figure 3-7 *A portable lead wall with a leaded glass window. The lead wall is designed to allow the radiographer to remain in the x-ray room during exposure by providing protection from radiation exposure.*

One of the best ways to minimize radiation exposure in the workplace is to avoid the occurrence of retakes. It should be the radiographer's goal to achieve a quality radiograph on the first attempt. This not only reduces radiation exposure to the patient and restrainers, but it is also cost effective and saves time.

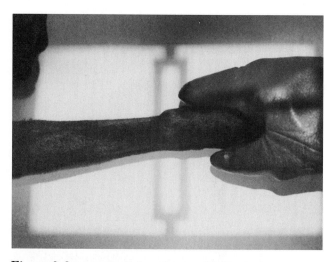

Figure 3-9 *A poor radiation safety practice. Hands should never be positioned within the field of the primary x-ray beam, even with lead gloves on.*

Maintenance of Protective Apparel

Proper care of protective apparel is essential to continued radiation safety. Protective aprons and gloves are made of lead-impregnated rubber and other materials that have an equivalent range of thickness from 0.25 to 1 mm of lead. Regulations in veterinary radiography require 0.5 mm of lead equivalent in the aprons and gloves because the restrainer is often close to the primary beam.

The shielding material is constructed to allow the wearer agility. Therefore cracks can result from improper handling and storage. Aprons should be hung vertically over a round surface (not <3 cm in diameter) or laid flat when not in use. Gloves should be placed on vertical holders that allow air to circulate throughout the inside (Fig. 3-11). Another method that will allow air circulation is to place metal soup cans (with both ends cut out) in the gloves. With the cans in place, the gloves can be

A **B**

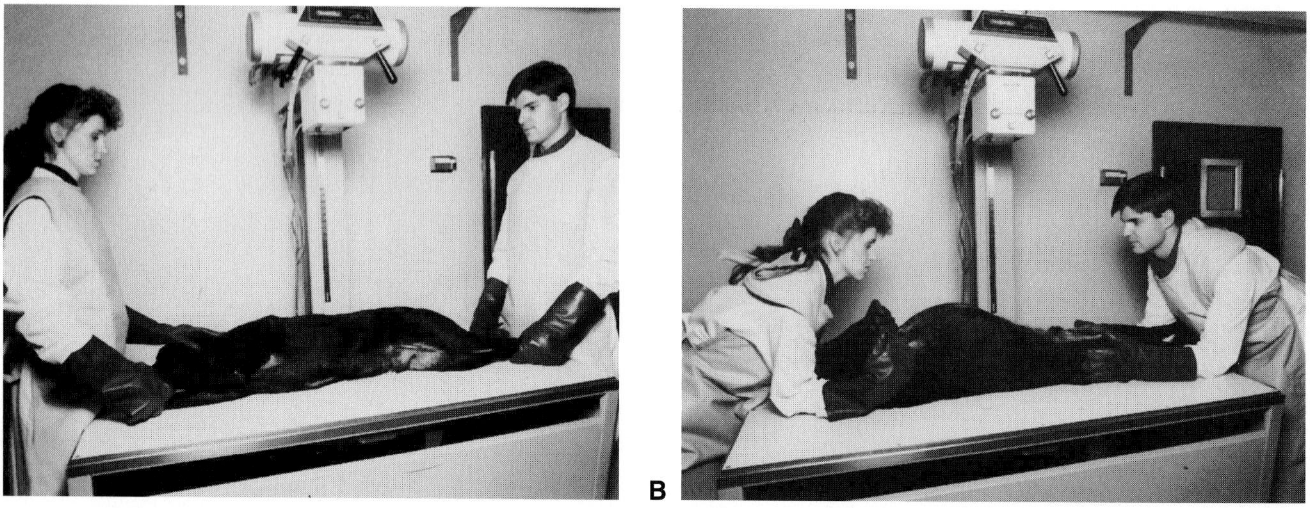

Figure 3-8 **A,** *Appropriate posture for manual restraint during exposure.* **B,** *Improper posture for manual restraint during exposure.*

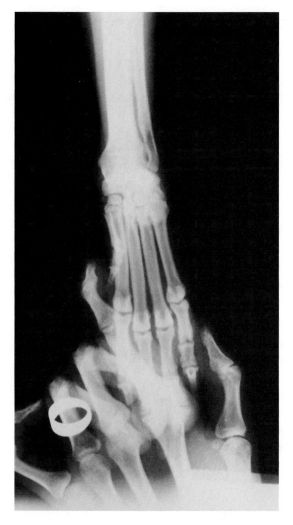

Figure 3-10 *Radiograph of a forelimb of a canine patient with a human hand holding the limb. This type of restraint is inappropriate; human anatomy should never be viewed on a veterinary radiograph.*

laid horizontally on a flat surface. This circulation of air is necessary to eliminate the moisture that can accumulate in the gloves.

Lead aprons and gloves should be inspected periodically for damage. Every time the apparel is worn, a visual inspection should be made. Obvious tears, cracks, or signs of deterioration should be investigated further. The aprons and gloves should be checked manually on a quarterly basis. A manual inspection includes feeling the internal and external surfaces for defects or irregularities. The most conclusive inspection method is taking a radiograph (or a fluoroscopic study, if available) of all protective apparel. If any cracks are present in the lead lining, they will be apparent on a radiograph. After processing, the film should remain relatively clear. If there are any breaks in the lead of the apron or glove, an increase in density (blackness) will appear on the film surface (Fig. 3-12).

If the apron is defective within the main body area, it should be repaired or discarded. If the defect is located near the hem or shoulder area, it can be marked with a permanent marker and checked more frequently. A person

wearing a defective lead apron or glove is potentially being exposed to radiation at the area of the defect. To prevent unnecessary exposure, this safety test should be performed at least annually.

Radiation Safety Rules: A Checklist

- Remove all unnecessary personnel from the radiographic suite during exposure.
- Never permit persons younger than age 18 or pregnant women in the radiographic suite while it is in use.
- Rotate personnel who assist in radiographic procedures to minimize exposure.
- Use mechanical restraints whenever possible (e.g., sandbags).
- Use chemical restraint whenever possible (anesthetize or tranquilize).
- Always wear protective apparel designed to absorb secondary radiation effectively (0.5-mm lead thickness).
- Ensure maximum life of protective apparel through proper use and care.
- Never permit any part of the body to be within the primary beam *whether shielded or not.*
- Use collimation whenever possible to decrease field size and scatter radiation.
- Use a 2.5-mm aluminum filter to remove soft x-rays from the primary beam.
- Do not aim the x-ray beam directly at any personnel or adjacent occupied room.
- Never handhold the x-ray tube.
- Wear film or TLD badges near the collar, outside the lead apron, to monitor radiation exposure to the thyroid gland, face, and eyes.
- Plan the radiographic procedure carefully to avoid unnecessary retakes.
- Maintain darkroom chemicals in good operating condition.
- Have the x-ray machine calibrated annually by a qualified service representative.
- Keep an exposure log that identifies the patient, the type of study performed, and the exposure values.
- Adhere to the radiation safety codes for your state.
- Remember that patience is an important virtue.

Additional Radiation Safety Rules for Fluoroscopy

Fluoroscopy is employed for special radiographic diagnostic studies when a "live view" of the internal anatomy is necessary. The primary x-ray beam of the fluoroscope is directed through the animal onto a view screen (Fig. 3-13). A primary use of fluoroscopy is for evaluation of the alimentary function. This is observed by the passage of barium sulfate (a radiopaque contrast medium) through the stomach and intestines. Because sedation or general anesthesia affects normal bowel activity, manual restraint is usually necessary.

During fluoroscopy, a continuous stream of x-rays is emitted while the machine is activated. Because of the high levels of radiation and the need for manual restraint, the following special safety rules must be obeyed.

Never use fluoroscopy in place of radiography.
Always use protective aprons, gloves, and shields.
Keep the collimator beam as small as possible.
Never palpate the anatomic area that is being viewed while the machine is activated.
Follow all rules that apply to the use of a regular x-ray machine.

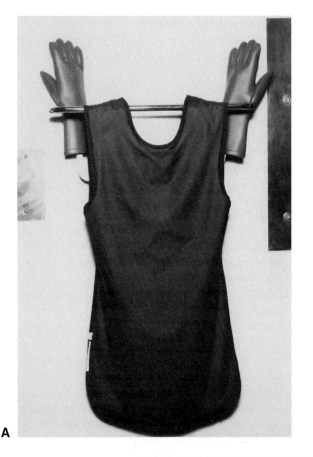

A

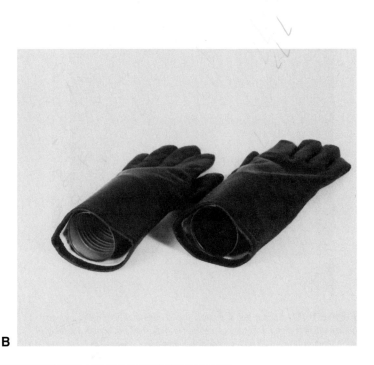

B

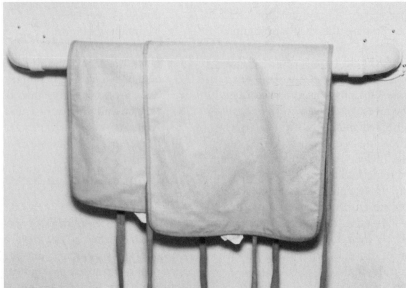

C

Figure 3-11 *A*, Vertical storage of lead aprons and gloves. *B*, Lead gloves stored in a horizontal position with cans placed inside to allow air circulation. *C*, Lead aprons draped over a "homemade" hanger. The hanger consists of a cylindric tube that is 4 inches or greater in diameter.

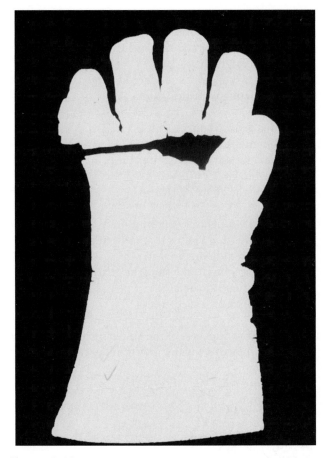

Figure 3-12 *Radiograph of a lead glove showing a crack in the lead lining.*

KEY POINTS

1. Personnel who restrain animals should never sit on or lean over the x-ray table.
2. Radiographers must allow as much distance as possible between themselves and patients.
3. All personnel present in the radiography room when an exposure is made should wear appropriate protective lead apparel.
4. Genetic damage is not detectable until further generations are produced.
5. Damage from radiation is more extensive after a single massive dose than after smaller, cumulatively equivalent repeated doses.
6. Defects in protective lead apparel can occur with improper use or storage; protective lead apparel should be checked regularly.

REVIEW QUESTIONS

1. Which of the following is a type of somatic damage caused by radiation?
   a. Gene mutation
   b. Cataracts
   c. Sterility
   d. None of the above

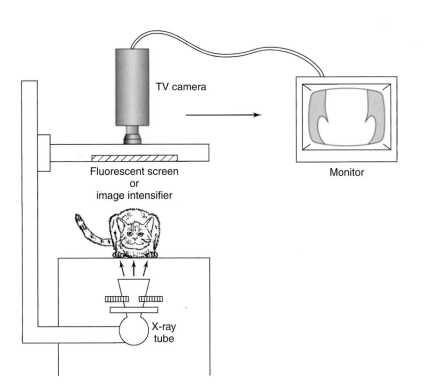

Figure 3-13 *Schematic drawing of a fluoroscopy unit. The x-ray tube is located under the table, with the x-ray beam directed upward, through the patient, toward a fluorescent screen.*

2. Which statement is true?
   a. The body's cells are all approximately equally sensitive to radiation.
   b. Ionizing radiation only damages chromosomal material (DNA) within reproductive cells.
   c. Chemical restraint of veterinary patients is prohibited by NCRP in the United States.
   d. Genetic damage is not detectable until future generations are produced.

3. What is the upper limit of exposure that an occupationally exposed individual may receive according to state and federal regulations?
   a. 0.5 Sv/year
   b. 100 rem/year
   c. 0.05 Sv/year
   d. 0.005 Sv/year

4. All of the following are true except:
   a. animals' cells are not as susceptible to damage from irradiation as human cells.
   b. radiation can affect the body's ability to produce red and white blood cells.
   c. exposure to radiation can affect the lens by causing cataracts.
   d. individuals younger than 18 years of age may not assist with animal restraint while radiographs are taken.

5. A film badge:
   a. is a type of pocket ionization chamber.
   b. is a type of dosimeter designed to monitor the actual amount of radiation received.
   c. must always be worn on the collar.
   d. should always be submitted weekly to determine the level of exposure.

6. What type of dosimeter can be stored for years, maintains its information, and can be reused?
   a. Pocket ionization chamber
   b. Collimator
   c. Thermoluminescent dosimeter
   d. Film badge

7. Which of the following statements is true?
   a. Veterinary personnel who restrain animals for radiographs are often exposed to the primary beam.
   b. Scatter radiation can be reduced by the collimator.
   c. Aluminum filtration helps to increase soft, less-penetrating x-rays, thus increasing the quality of the radiograph.
   d. Scatter radiation is produced by the primary beam interacting with the anode.

8. Scatter depends on:
   a. the intensity of the beam.
   b. the composition of the structure being radiographed.
   c. kilovoltage (kVp) level.
   d. All of the above.

9. The most conclusive method used to inspect lead-lined gloves and aprons for cracks and defects is:
   a. taking a radiograph of it.
   b. holding it up to the sunlight or a bright light.
   c. inspecting it manually.
   d. Both b and c are correct.

10. What is the thickness of the lead-impregnated rubber lining protective apparel in veterinary radiography?
    a. 1 cm
    b. 10 mm
    c. 0.5 mm
    d. 0.5

*S*uggested *R*eadings

Burkhart RL: *A basic quality assurance program for diagnostic radiology facilities*, HEW Publication (FDA) 83-8218, Rockville, Md, 1983, FDA.

Burkhart RL: *Patient radiation exposure in diagnostic radiology examinations: An overview*, HHS Publication (FDA) 83-8217, Rockville, Md, 1983, FDA.

Gray JE et al: *Quality control in diagnostic imaging*, Rockville, Md, 1983, Aspen.

McKinney WE: *Radiographic processing and quality control*, Philadelphia, 1988, JB Lippincott.

Minnesota Department of Health Advisory Work Group: *Rules governing sources of ionizing radiation*, Rochester, Minn, 1996, Mayo Clinic.

NCRP: *Radiation protection in veterinary medicine (#36)*, Bethesda, Md, 1970, NCRP.

NCRP: *Structural shielding design and evaluation or medical use of x-rays and gamma rays of energies up to 10 MeV (#49)*, Bethesda, Md, 1970, NCRP.

chapter 4

Exposure Factors

CHAPTER OUTLINE

Milliamperage and Time
Kilovoltage
Distance

How Radiography Works: A Review
How Radiography Works: A Different Look

OBJECTIVES

Upon completion of this chapter, the reader should be able to do the following:

- State the variable that controls the quality of an x-ray beam
- State the variable that controls the quantity of an x-ray beam
- Define the role of milliamperage in the production of x-rays
- Define the role of time in the production of x-rays
- List the advantages of high milliamperage settings
- State the equation used to determine milliamperage-seconds (mAs)

- Define the role of kilovoltage in the production of x-rays
- List the effects of increased kilovoltage on the x-ray beam
- Define Santes' rule and use the equation, given a measurement in centimeters
- State the effect of distance on the intensity of an x-ray beam
- Define the inverse square law
- Describe how radiography works

GLOSSARY

Caliper: A device used to measure the thickness of anatomic parts.

Contrast: The measurable difference between two adjacent densities.

Density: The degree of blackness on a radiograph.

Exposure time: The period of time during which x-rays are permitted to leave the x-ray tube.

Inverse square law: The intensity of the radiation varies inversely as the square of the distance from the source.

Kilovoltage: Related to thousands of volts. Describes the electrical potential (difference) between the cathode and the anode; it is responsible for accelerating the electrons from the cathode to the anode and relates to the penetrating power of the x-rays.

Kinetic energy: The energy related to motion.

Milliamperage-seconds (mAs): The number of x-rays produced over a given period. Calculated by multiplying the milliamperage by the time.

Milliampere: One thousandth of an ampere. A measure of electron current to the filament, which has a direct relationship to the number of x-rays produced.

Santes' rule: A method of estimating kilovoltage in relation to area thickness: (2 × thickness) + 40 = kVp.

Source-image distance (SID): Formerly called *focal-film distance (FFD)*; the distance between the source of x-rays and the image receptor or film.

Thermionic emission: The process of releasing electrons from their atomic orbits by heat.

INTRODUCTION

For an x-ray tube to produce x-rays, suitable electrical currents must be supplied to both the cathode filament and the field between the cathode and the anode.

The quality of an x-ray beam is determined by its penetrating power. Shorter wavelength radiation has increased penetrating power and is said to have increased penetrating ability.

The *quantity* or intensity of the x-ray beam is defined as the amount of energy flowing per second through a unit area perpendicular to the direction of the beam. Simply stated, it is the number of x-rays traveling from the x-ray tube toward the image receptor in a period of time.

The quantity and quality of the x-ray beam are affected by various factors.

MILLIAMPERAGE AND TIME

Electrons are produced by heating the cathode filament. When a calibrated electrical current is passed through the low-tension circuit of the x-ray machine, the metal of the filament is heated and electrons are released. The process of "boiling off" the electrons from their atomic orbits is known as **thermionic emission.** The "free" electrons form a cloud around the filament. The number of electrons in the electron cloud is directly proportional to the temperature of the filament (Fig. 4-1).

The electrical current that heats the filament is measured in **milliamperes** (one thousandth of an ampere). As the milliamperage (mA) is increased, the number of electrons available is also increased. The number of x-rays produced at the anode depends on the size of the electron cloud. Therefore the mA affects the intensity of the x-ray

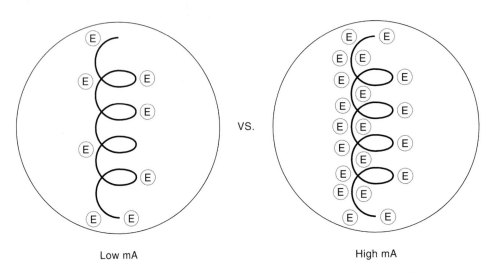

Low mA   vs.   High mA

Figure 4-1 *Drawing showing the effect of mA placed on the filament; the mA setting is proportionate to the number of electrons produced.*

beam and is the measure of quantity of x-radiation produced.

The total quantity of x-rays produced during a given exposure also depends on the length of exposure. That is, there is a direct relationship between mA and the length of exposure (time). The period during which the x-rays are permitted to leave the x-ray tube is termed the **exposure time;** it is measured in fractions of seconds. The number of electrons and the period of time set for their release determine how many x-rays are available. Therefore the quantity of x-rays required for a given exposure is best expressed as the product of the mA, and the time in **milliamperage-seconds (mAs)** can be calculated by the following equation:

$$mA \times time \text{ (in seconds)} \times mAs$$

Examples:

20 mA × 1/2 sec = 10 mAs
100 mA × 1/10 sec = 10 mAs
200 mA × 1/20 sec = 10 mAs
300 mA × 1/30 sec = 10 mAs

Using high mA settings is advantageous. As seen in the examples, a higher mA setting allows for a shorter time setting with the same number of x-rays produced. With a shorter time setting, the possibility of motion occurring on a radiograph is decreased. Motion is considered the most common artifact in veterinary radiography ("Murphy's law" of veterinary radiography states that an animal will move at the moment the exposure is made). A shorter exposure time also decreases the exposure of restraining personnel. Therefore it is advantageous to use the highest mA setting possible.

Another advantage of a higher mA setting is the greater amount of x-rays produced. A suitable mA setting depends on the thickness and type of tissue being radiographed. A machine with high mA capability allows examination of thicker anatomic areas of the patient.

X-ray machines vary according to their mA potential. Machines that have a higher mA capacity are more powerful and have increased diversity of use in practice. Smaller x-ray machines, however, have a constant mA capability with no provision for alteration. Other small units have variable settings in the range of 10 to 30 mA. Larger, more expensive equipment may have a maximum mA value as high as 1600 (Figs. 4-2 and 4-3; see also Fig. 2-4).

KILOVOLTAGE

During an exposure, the anode is maintained at a high positive electrical potential relative to the cathode. Because of this difference in electrical charge, the electron cloud at the filament is formed into a narrow beam and accelerates toward the anode at a high speed. The **kinetic energy** of the electrons when they reach the target is proportional to the potential difference placed between

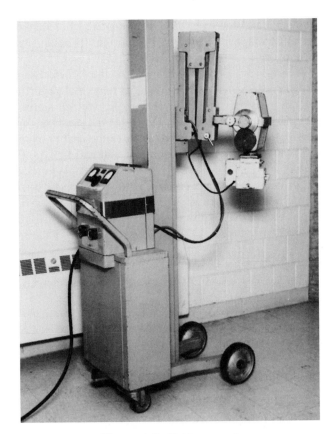

Figure 4-2 *Mobile x-ray unit.*

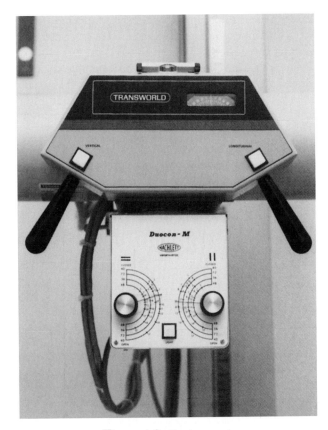

Figure 4-3 *Fixed x-ray unit.*

the anode and the cathode. This potential difference, or the **kilovoltage**, is measured in kilovolts (thousands of volts, or kV).

Another term commonly used for the kilovoltage is *kilovoltage peak* (kVp). The word *peak* indicates the maximum energy available at that kilovoltage setting. The higher the kilovoltage, the faster the electrons are accelerated. This acceleration increases the energy of the x-rays produced at the electron collision with the anode target.

A change in kilovoltage has a number of effects. First, it results in a change in penetrating power of the x-ray beam. When the kVp is raised, new, shorter wavelength x-rays are produced.

The kVp determines the quality of the x-ray beam and thus its ability to penetrate tissue. Higher kVp settings produce more-penetrating beams, with a higher percentage of radiation reaching the film (Fig. 4-4).

Higher kVp settings allow for lower mAs settings, which generally call for shorter exposure time. An inverse relationship exists between kVp and mAs. The following settings would produce radiographs of comparable density if other factors remained constant:

60 kVp and 4 mAs (10 mA × 0.4 sec)
70 kVp and 2 mAs (10 mA × 0.2 sec)
80 kVp and 1 mAs (10 mA × 0.1 sec)
90 kVp and 0.5 mAs (5 mA × 0.1 sec)

(Note: Although the techniques provide a comparable density, the radiographic contrast is affected, which alters the appearance of an image. This is discussed in Chapter 5.)

The kVp can be estimated by an equation known as Santes' rule, which uses the thickness of the area of interest to be radiographed to calculate the kVp necessary. Santes' rule follows:

$$(2 \times \text{thickness}) + 40 = \text{kVp}$$

Measurement of an anatomic area is taken with a **caliper** and is measured in centimeters (Fig. 4-5). The number 40 represents the distance from the x-ray tube's focal spot

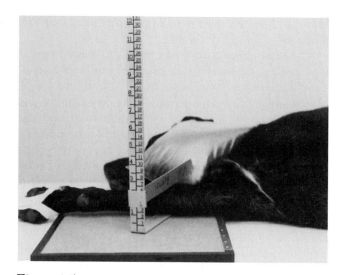

Figure 4-5 *Example of a caliper, the instrument used to measure the thickness of an anatomic area. The measurement is taken in centimeter increments, using the scale on the left side of the caliper. In this case, the measurement is 4 cm.*

(source of x-rays) to the image receptor (x-ray film) in inches and is referred to as the *focal film distance* (FFD). The **source-image distance** (SID) is discussed later.

The sum of Santes' rule is the kVp necessary for an exposure with the film on the tabletop, without the use of a grid or film Bucky tray system. Santes' rule supplies the radiographer with a starting point that can be modified for the grid, cassette tray, or other variable.

Example:

Dr. Smith has requested an abdominal radiograph on a Labrador retriever. The measurement of the lateral view was 16 cm.

$$(2 \times 16) + 40 = 72 \text{ kVp}$$

DISTANCE

The distance between the source of x-rays (focal spot of the x-ray tube) and the image receptor (x-ray film) also affects the intensity of the image produced. As the SID is decreased, the intensity of the x-rays is increased.

To demonstrate this phenomenon, take a flashlight into a room with little or no light. Stand approximately 3 m away from a wall, and shine the light at the wall. Keeping the light aimed at the same point, walk toward the wall. Notice how the light intensity increases as the distance between the light and the wall decreases. Exactly the same thing happens with x-rays.

In the same respect, as the SID is increased, the intensity of the x-radiation is decreased. Increasing the distance from the radiation source reduces the intensity of the beam according to the **inverse square law**.

X-rays obey the laws of light in that they diverge from the point source. The intensity of the beam varies inversely according to the square of the distance (Fig. 4-6). A change in distance is similar to a change in mA in its effect on

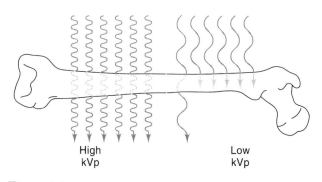

High   Low
kVp   kVp

Figure 4-4 *Drawing showing the effect of the kVp level on penetration. High kVp settings produce a more-penetrating x-ray beam, with a higher percentage of x-rays reaching the film.*

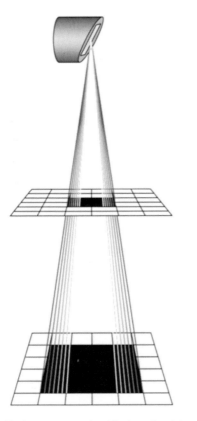

Figure 4-6 *The inverse square law. The intensity of the primary x-ray beam is inversely proportionate to the source-image distance. The intensity of the primary beam projected on a given perpendicular plane is reduced to one quarter by doubling the distance from the point source.*

the overall intensity of the beam. In other words, radiographic density is affected by a change in distance.

When the SID is changed, the total amount of x-rays must be increased or decreased in order to make a comparable exposure using the new distance. This can be done by changing the mAs, which governs the rate in which the x-ray tube produces x-radiation. When a different distance is used, the adjustment of the mAs can be calculated as follows:

$$\text{old mAs} \times \frac{(\text{new SID})^2}{(\text{old SID})^2} = \text{new mAs}$$

$$10\,\text{mAs} \times \frac{(150\,\text{cm})^2}{(75\,\text{cm})^2} = \frac{40}{1} = 40\,\text{mAs}$$

When the SID is changed, image detail is changed. As any SID is decreased, image sharpness is decreased. This topic is discussed later.

The SID is an important exposure factor. Whenever possible, the SID should be kept constant. The most common SID in veterinary practice ranges from 36 to 40 inches (90 to 100 cm). The distance is usually noted on the x-ray tube stand or is measured with the tape mounted on the side of the tube housing. Verifying the correct SID before every radiograph is important because of the effect of the SID on radiographic film density.

HOW RADIOGRAPHY WORKS: A REVIEW

X-rays are generated in an x-ray tube. The tube consists of a cathode side (with a negative electrical charge) and an anode side (with a positive charge). In the tube, a stream of fast-moving electrons is attracted and directed from the cathode to the anode. As the electrons collide and interact with the atoms on the anode target, a great amount of energy is produced; 1% of this energy is in the form of x-radiation.

The cathode consists of a wire filament that emits electrons when heated. The filament temperature is controlled by the mA setting on the console of the machine. As the mA is increased, the temperature of the filament is increased and the filament produces more electrons. The period of time during which the electrons (x-rays) are permitted to leave the x-ray tube is measured in fractions of seconds. The number of electrons available and the time period set for their release determine how many x-rays are available. The mAs thus control the total number of x-rays produced.

The anode, which attracts negatively charged electrons, is angled so that the x-rays produced are directed downward (toward the film) through a window in the metal housing of the x-ray tube.

The electron speed necessary to create a high-energy impact is achieved by applying thousands of volts (kVp) across the anode and cathode field. High voltage produces x-rays with greater penetrating power and intensity. The kVp thus controls the penetrating power of the x-rays.

This version of how radiography works is abridged, and some confusion may remain. The following section is intended to demonstrate a simplified version of how the variables work together to form a radiograph of good quality.

HOW RADIOGRAPHY WORKS: A DIFFERENT LOOK

Imagine yourself in a grocery store, with a grocery cart and ready to go. Your purpose, however, is not to shop for the week's food but to knock down a large pile of tomato juice cans stacked in a pyramid. The pyramid is located in the center of the store and stands 10 feet tall. To accomplish your goal, you have only the cart and all the muscle you can muster.

With a running start, you head for the pyramid. Despite your running speed and strength, you are unable to knock down all of the cans of tomato juice—only a few are displaced. The grocery cart is stopped in its tracks, and you are thrown into the produce aisle. Among the canned goods, you decide to put something inside the cart to increase its weight. Perhaps the momentum of a heavy cart pushed with great force will knock down the pyramid. You fill the cart with cans of beans (Fig. 4-7). Straining with effort, you slowly push the cart toward

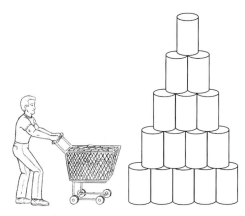

Figure 4-7 *Bean scenario illustrated (see text).*

the stack of juice cans. Because of the extreme weight in the cart, your strength is insufficient to break through the pyramid.

Feeling a bit dismayed, you sit once again. But with sudden inspiration, you remove half the beans from the cart and again race toward the stack of juice cans. The sufficient weight and your adequate strength enable you to topple the entire pyramid.

To apply this parable, it is necessary to examine the facts. To topple the pyramid, you needed a certain number of cans of beans in the cart and sufficient strength to push the cart. The beans represent the amount of electrons (number of x-rays) or mAs, the muscle power pushing the cart represents the kVp, and the pyramid represents the patient. If there are insufficient mAs (beans), it is impossible to produce a good-quality radiograph, regardless of the amount of kVp (pushing power).

Similarly, regardless of the amount of weight in the cart, it is impossible to penetrate the pyramid if there is inadequate strength (kVp). The necessary amount of muscle and beans always depends on the size of the pyramid. The amount of mAs and kVp required for a given patient depends on the density of the anatomic part being radiographed.

KEY POINTS

1. In general terms, the kVp controls the wavelength and penetrating power of x-radiation and the mAs controls the number of x-rays produced.
2. The most common artifact in veterinary radiography is motion.
3. Radiation of a shorter wavelength has better penetrating ability and therefore produces a higher-quality radiograph.

REVIEW QUESTIONS

1. Ways to decrease the number of personnel in the radiology suite include:
   a. using higher kVp setting.
   b. using longer time setting with a higher mA setting.
   c. sedating patients.
   d. none of the above.

2. Ways to increase penetrating power of x-rays include:
   a. increasing kVp.
   b. increasing the time setting.
   c. increasing thermionic emission.
   d. increasing mAs.

3. The milliamperage-seconds (mAs) for 1000 mA and 1/10 sec is:
   a. 10 mAs.
   b. 10,000 mAs.
   c. 100 mAs.
   d. 1 mAs.

4. According to Santes' rule, if a cat's abdomen measures 12 cm, kVp is:
   a. 72.
   b. 64.
   c. 66.
   d. 52.

5. The source-image distance:
   a. is directly proportional to the intensity of the x-radiation.
   b. must be considered each time the control panel is set.
   c. changes only a few inches between patients and is negligible.
   d. most commonly ranges from 36 to 40 cm in veterinary practices.

6. One percent of the energy produced at the anode is in the form of:
   a. heat.
   b. x-rays.
   c. sound.
   d. none of the above.

7. The temperature of the filament within the cathode is controlled by:
   a. time setting.
   b. the source-image distance.
   c. kVp setting.
   d. mA setting.

8. Which is a characteristic of x-rays?
   a. Their total number produced is determined by kVp.
   b. Longer wavelengths have more penetrating power.
   c. Their intensity increases as SID decreases.
   d. They diverge from a light source.

9. The potential difference between the anode and cathode is measured in:
   a. kilovolts.
   b. calipers.
   c. milliamperes.
   d. centimeters.

10. A higher kVp setting allows for a _____ mAs and _____ exposure time.
    a. higher; lower
    b. lower; higher
    c. lower; lower
    d. higher; higher

Suggested Readings

Ball JL, Moore AD: *Essential physics for radiographers,* Boston, 1980, Blackwell Scientific.

Cunliffe-Lavin LM: Radiographic technique: a ray of hope, *Vet Tech J* 12:444, 1991.

Curry TS, Dowdy JE, Murry RC: *Christensen's physics of diagnostic radiology,* ed 4, Philadelphia, 1990, Lea & Febiger.

Douglas SW, Herrtage ME, Williamson HD: *Principles of veterinary radiography,* ed 4, Philadelphia, 1987, Bailliere Tindall.

Eastman Kodak Company: *Kodak: the fundamentals of radiography,* ed 12, Rochester, NY, 1980, Kodak.

Morgan JP, Silverman S: *Techniques of veterinary radiography,* ed 4, Ames, Iowa, 1987, Iowa State University Press.

chapter 5

Radiographic Quality

CHAPTER OUTLINE

Radiographic Density
Contrast
Exposure Factors

Scatter Radiation
Grid
Radiographic Detail and Definition

OBJECTIVES

Upon completion of this chapter, the reader should be able to do the following:

- Define radiographic density
- List the factors that affect radiographic density
- Define contrast, radiographic contrast, and subject contrast
- List and describe the exposure factors that affect contrast and density
- Define scatter radiation and its effect on the radiographic image
- Describe a grid and its purpose in radiography
- Define grid focus and its significance

- Describe grid cutoff, its radiographic appearance, and the various ways it is produced
- State the variables that contribute to grid efficiency
- List and describe the various grid types and their advantages and disadvantages
- Describe the correct care of a grid
- Define radiographic detail
- List and describe the factors that affect radiographic detail

GLOSSARY

Backscatter: Process of scattering or reflecting radiation in the opposite direction from that intended. Radiation that is reflected from behind the image plane back to the image.

Contrast: The measurable difference between two adjacent densities.

Crossed grid: Two parallel or two focused grids that are set at right angles. Also called *crisscross grid.*

Elongation: Distortion of anatomic structures so that the image appears longer than actual size, owing to the x-ray beam not being directed perpendicular to the film surface.

Focused grid: A grid with a parallel center lead strip and inclined strips on either side that radiate at progressively greater angles.

Foreshortening: Distortion of anatomic structures when the image appears shorter than actual size due to the plane of interest not being parallel to the film surface.

Geometric distortion: Variation in normal size and shape of anatomic structures due to their position in relation to the x-ray source and film.

Geometric unsharpness: Loss of detail due to geometric distortion.

Grid: A device made of lead strips embedded in a spacing material, placed between the patient and the film, designed to absorb non–image-forming radiation.

Grid cutoff: A progressive decrease in transmitted x-ray intensity caused by absorption of primary x-rays by the grid lines.

Grid efficiency: The ability of a grid to absorb non–image-forming radiation in the production of a quality radiograph.

Grid factor: The amount the exposure needs to be increased to compensate for the grid's absorption of a portion of the primary beam.

Grid focus: The distance between the source of x-rays and the grid in which the grid is effective without grid cutoff.

Grid ratio: The relation of the height of the lead strips to the distance between them.

Linear grid: Grid in which the lead strips are parallel.

Lines per centimeter: The number of lead strips per centimeter area of a grid.

Magnification: Distortion of anatomic structures when the image appears larger than actual size.

Potter-Bucky diaphragm: A mechanical device that consists of a focused grid within a diaphragm, which moves the grid across the x-ray beam during the exposure.

Pseudofocused grid: A grid with parallel lead strips that are progressively reduced in height toward the edges of the grid.

Radiographic contrast: The density difference between two adjacent areas on a radiograph.

Radiographic density: The degree of blackness or "darkness" on a radiograph.

Radiographic detail: The definition of the edge of an anatomic structure on a radiograph.

Radiographic quality: The ease with which details can be perceived on a radiograph.

Scatter radiation: Non–image-forming radiation that is scattered in all directions because of objects in the path of the x-ray beam.

Subject contrast: The difference in density and mass of two adjacent anatomic structures.

Unfocused grid: A grid with lead strips that are parallel and at right angles to the film. Also called *parallel grid.*

INTRODUCTION

A radiograph without quality is similar to a story without meaning. To produce a quality radiograph, the radiographer must understand predetermined aspects of quality. Comprehension of the aspects of quality is essential to a complete understanding of how radiography works.

Radiographic quality refers to how easily details can be perceived on a radiograph. We must obtain as much diagnostic information as possible about the internal structures of the patient. Radiographic quality depends on radiographic density, contrast, and geometric factors that affect detail. This chapter will define diagnostic image characteristics and explain how to obtain them (Fig. 5-1).

RADIOGRAPHIC DENSITY

Radiographic density is defined as the degree of blackness, or "darkness," on a radiograph. Black areas on a developed radiograph are produced by deposits of metallic silver in the film emulsion that result from exposure to x-rays and their subsequent processing. A radiograph that has many black areas and is dark when viewed has high density.

An important concept to remember is that *x-rays make radiographic film black.* The degree of blackness on a radiograph depends on the amount of x-rays reaching the film. Density is influenced by the quantity and quality of the x-ray beam, as well as the type and thickness of the tissue under examination.

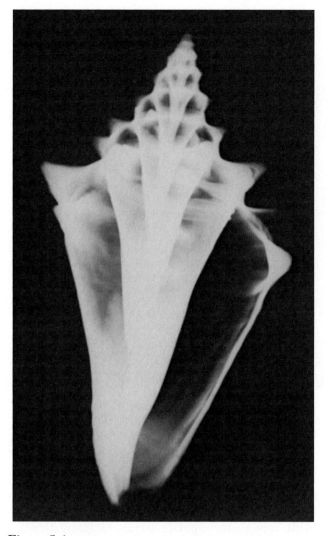

Figure 5-1 *Radiograph of a seashell showing contrast, density, and detail characteristics.*

is inversely proportional to tissue density. In other words, if the density or thickness of tissue doubles, the number of x-rays reaching the film is approximately halved. For example, the body of a 150-lb Saint Bernard will absorb many more x-rays than the body of a 75-lb Labrador retriever. Assuming that the same amount of x-rays was used for the Saint Bernard as required for the Labrador, the area of the film where the body of the Saint Bernard was located would be too white and would lack sufficient radiographic density to be diagnostic. In comparison, the radiograph of the Labrador would have adequate density because the correct exposure levels were selected for its body thickness (Fig. 5-2).

The body of an animal has many different types of tissues as well. Compare an animal's bone with the surrounding muscle. Because the bone has higher tissue density than the muscle, more x-rays will be absorbed by the bone. The area of film under an anatomic area with high tissue density will be lighter (have less radiographic density). In other words, the area of the film where the bone was located will remain relatively white compared with the surrounding muscle tissue. Because x-rays have varied penetrability, the total number of x-rays reaching the film is partially dependent on the tissue density. Simply stated, the higher the tissue density, the lower the radiographic density (Fig. 5-3).

CONTRAST

Contrast is defined as the visible difference between two adjacent radiographic densities. Contrast is divided into two separate categories: radiographic contrast and subject contrast. To avoid confusion, we will define each contrast-associated term and explain how both influence the outcome of a radiograph.

Radiographic Contrast

Radiographic contrast is the density difference between two adjacent areas on a radiograph. When the density difference is great, the radiograph is said to have high contrast or a short scale of contrast. That is, a radiograph with high contrast exhibits many black and white tones. For example, a radiograph with white bone and a black background has high contrast (Fig. 5-4, *A*).

A radiograph that exhibits many grays and a small density difference between two adjacent areas has low contrast, or a long scale of contrast. An increased number of gray tones between the white and black tones on a radiograph constitute a long scale of contrast. In other words, it takes a *long* time to get from black to white on the radiograph. The type of contrast desired for each radiograph depends on the anatomic area (Fig. 5-4, *B*). General guidelines for desired contrast are listed in Table 5-1.

Of course, there are extremes in contrast. It is not desirable to have a radiograph with too high or too low

Factors Affecting Radiographic Density

Greater radiographic density may be produced by increasing (1) the total number of x-rays that reach the film, (2) the penetrating power of the x-rays, (3) the developing time, or (4) the temperature of the developer. (Film development is discussed in Chapter 7.)

As described in Chapter 3, the number of x-rays leaving the x-ray tube is determined by the milliamperage-seconds (mAs). As the mAs is increased, more x-rays reach the patient and film and radiographic density is increased. In the same respect, raising the kilovoltage (or kVp) of the x-ray beam increases radiographic density. As the kVp is increased, the penetrating power of the x-rays is increased, resulting in more x-rays reaching the film. The radiograph becomes darker as more x-rays reach the film.

Radiographic density is also influenced by the thickness and type of tissue being radiographed. Body parts that have greater thickness absorb more x-rays, resulting in a lighter image on the radiograph. Radiographic density

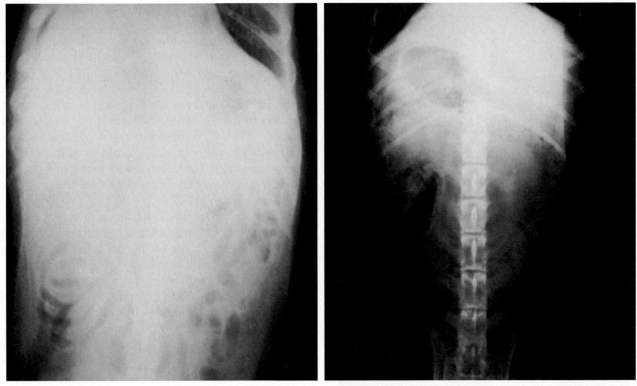

Figure 5-2 *These two radiographs have been exposed with the same exposure factors. **A** is a ventrodorsal view of the abdomen of a Saint Bernard. **B** is a ventrodorsal view of the abdomen of a Labrador retriever. Because of the great difference in size of the Saint Bernard and the Labrador retriever, there is a marked difference in radiographic density. **A** exhibits much less radiographic density than **B**.*

of contrast (Fig. 5-5). A good radiograph should have a suitable range of differentiated radiographic densities (blacks, whites, and grays) so that the eye can easily see the detail.

Radiographic contrast is influenced by (1) subject contrast, (2) kVp level, (3) scatter radiation, (4) film type, and (5) film fog.

Subject Contrast

Subject contrast is defined as the difference in density and mass between two adjacent anatomic structures. Subject contrast depends on the thickness and density of the anatomic part.

As discussed earlier, the body has various tissue densities. Because x-rays cannot penetrate bone tissue as easily as soft tissue, fewer x-rays will reach the film where

the bone is located. Bone will absorb many more x-rays than muscle or fat, assuming both have equal thickness. With appropriate exposure factors, anatomy that has high tissue density can increase the amount of whites and blacks on the radiograph; therefore high subject contrast increases radiographic contrast (Table 5-2).

EXPOSURE FACTORS

The most common cause of poor contrast on a radiograph is inappropriate exposure factors.

TABLE 5-1

GENERAL GUIDELINES FOR DESIRED CONTRAST

TISSUE	CONTRAST	EXPOSURE FACTOR (KVP)
Bone	High	Low
Soft tissue	Low	High

TABLE 5-2

SUBJECT CONTRAST

	LEAST DENSE	HIGH PENETRATION	APPEARS BLACK
1. Gas	↑	↑	↑
2. Fat			
3. Water			
4. Bone			
5. Metal	↓	↓	↓
	MOST DENSE	LOW PENETRATION	APPEARS WHITE

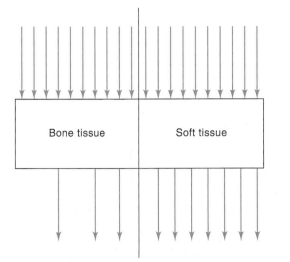

Figure 5-3 *Drawing illustrating the influence of tissue density on radiographic density. Bone tissue is almost twice as dense as soft tissue.*

Milliamperage-Seconds

The mAs may affect contrast only when insufficient or excessive mAs is used. Remember, the mAs is the quantity of the x-rays and is the primary factor that affects density. When a correct mAs setting is used, contrast depends primarily on the kVp setting. However, when the mAs factor is insufficient, the contrast is reduced because the overall density of the radiograph is reduced. If the quantity of x-rays reaching the film is too low, the film will be pale. Close inspection reveals that dense structures have been penetrated and that the anatomic silhouettes are visible, but the images lack density (Fig. 5-6). Overexposure, caused by too much mAs, will result in increased overall density (overall black appearance) but has less effect on radiographic contrast (Fig. 5-7).

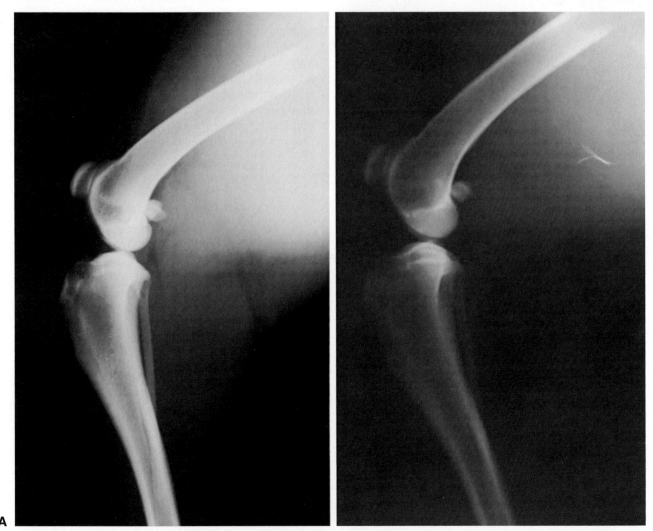

A

B

Figure 5-4 *A, Radiograph of a lateral view of a canine stifle joint showing a short scale of contrast. The bone tissue of the leg is relatively white compared with the surrounding tissue. B, Radiograph of a lateral view of a canine stifle joint showing a long scale of contrast. The entire radiograph—bone and soft tissue—has an overall gray appearance.*

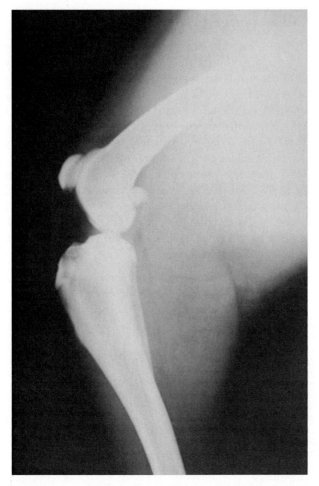

Figure 5-5 *Radiograph of a lateral view of a canine stifle joint showing extremely high contrast.*

Kilovoltage

Both contrast and density are affected by kVp. The correct amount of kVp will produce differential x-ray absorption of soft and dense anatomic structures. A change in kVp has a number of effects. An increase in kVp results in an increase in penetrating power of the x-ray beam. When the kVp is raised, shorter-wavelength x-rays are produced, which raises penetration power. As the penetration is increased, scatter radiation alters radiographic contrast. Scatter radiation is covered in more detail later.

If the kVp is too low, the resulting radiograph will have a "soot and whitewash" (gray-and-white) appearance and the anatomic image will be imperceptible. The image lacks adequate density because the x-rays are unable to penetrate the patient. Therefore the area on the radiograph where the patient was positioned remains white because insufficient x-rays reached the film. This results in a white image against a black background. The contrast within the radiographic image lacks contrast; there is no distinct difference between the anatomic organs (Fig. 5-8).

Increased kVp causes excessive scatter radiation. As a result of the increased penetrating power of the x-rays with high kVp, more x-rays will reach the film. As the x-rays with high kVp travel through the patient, fewer x-rays are absorbed or scattered and a higher percentage of them reach the film. If the x-rays have sufficient penetrating power, the radiographic cassette and its components do not stop them and scatter radiation results (Fig. 5-9).

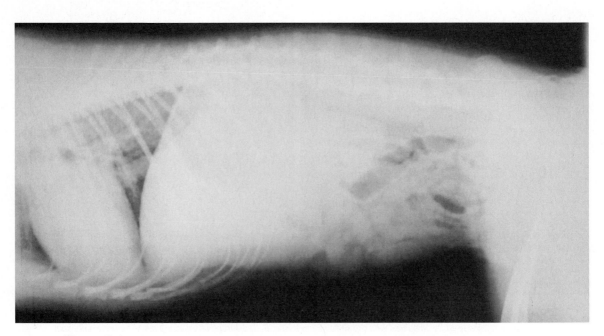

Figure 5-6 *Radiograph of a lateral view of the abdomen that was exposed with an insufficient amount of mAs.*

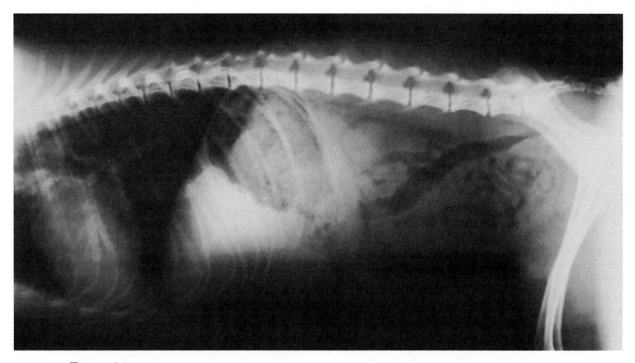

Figure 5-7 *Radiograph of a lateral view of the abdomen that was exposed with too much mAs. Note that the radiograph is too dark, yet the contrast is not altered drastically.*

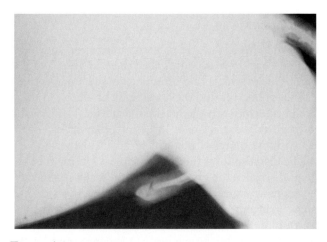

Figure 5-8 *Radiograph of a lateral view of the abdomen that has been exposed with an insufficient amount of kVp. The radiograph has little contrast within the abdominal cavity because of the lack of x-ray penetration. This lack of penetration resulted in a lack of radiographic density.*

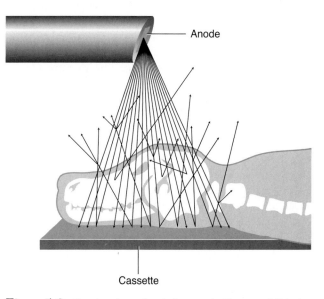

Figure 5-9 *Drawing of a canine skull exposed with too much kVp. As a result of the excessive kVp, a large amount of scatter radiation is produced.*

SCATTER RADIATION

Non–image-forming radiation that is scattered in all directions as a result of objects in the path of the beam is called **scatter radiation.** Scatter radiation is undesirable for a number of reasons. Because inappropriate areas of the film are being exposed, contrast is decreased.

Scatter radiation primarily originates from the patient, but there are other sources as well. Materials such as the table and film tray also act as sources of scatter. Radiation arising from such sources behind the image plane may be scattered back to the image. This phenomenon is referred to as **backscatter.** Limiting the size of the x-ray beam so that the field does not exceed the image receptor is the most effective way to reduce backscatter. In addition, many cassettes contain lead-foil backing to prevent backscatter from reaching the film.

Because kVp controls penetration and, to a degree, the amount of scatter radiation, the primary exposure factor controls contrast. Radiographic examinations rely on correct kVp levels to produce desired contrast. How, then, is it possible to radiograph thick body parts without excessive scatter radiation? A mechanism known as a *grid* reduces the scatter radiation when the high kVp necessary for thick body parts is used.

GRID

A **grid** is a device placed between the patient and the radiographic film that is designed to absorb non–image-forming x-rays (scatter radiation). A grid is composed of alternating strips of lead and spacer material. The lead strips are approximately 0.5 mm in thickness and number between 500 and 1500 on edge. The spacer material usually consists of fiber, aluminum, or plastic because these materials have low x-ray absorption ability. The strips are encased in a protective cover (usually aluminum) to provide strength and durability (Fig. 5-10). The lead strips are aligned with the primary x-ray beam in a way that allows the desirable x-rays to reach the film. The lead absorbs a considerable amount of the x-rays not traveling in the direction of the primary beam. The spacer material permits most of the primary x-rays (desirable x-rays) to pass through to the film (Fig. 5-11).

A grid may be (1) placed directly on top of a cassette, (2) built into a cassette, or (3) placed directly under the x-ray table between the patient and the cassette. Some grids are designed to be placed underneath the x-ray tabletop, above the cassette tray, so that the lead strips run parallel to the length of the table. The cassette tray is discussed later.

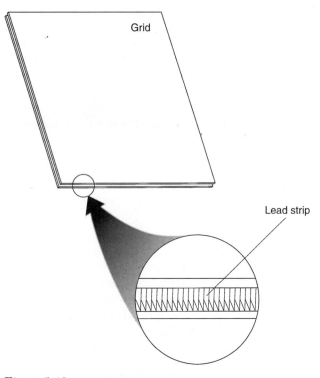

Figure 5-10 *Drawing of grid construction showing the structure of the lead strips and radiolucent interspacers.*

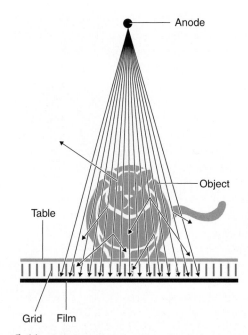

Figure 5-11 *Grid device being used to absorb the scatter radiation caused by an interaction of the x-ray beam with an object in its path. Notice that the lead strips are placed parallel to the primary x-ray beam to allow the desirable x-rays to reach the film.*

Grid Focus

The lead strips of the grid may vary in size and angle, but each grid has a center point, called the *focal point* (or focal line in linear grids). The central x-ray must be centered on this point. Ideally, the focal spot of the x-ray tube should coincide with the focal point (or focal line) of the grid, and the central ray of the x-ray beam should intersect with the center of the grid perpendicularly.

The distance from the source of x-rays (x-ray tube) to the grid is called the **grid focus** and is usually specified by the manufacturer. If the grid is used outside this specified range, **grid cutoff** may occur. Cutoff is a progressive decrease in transmitted x-ray intensity near the edge of the grid caused by absorption of primary x-rays by the grid lines. Radiographically, the image appears lighter, with distinct white lines over the underexposed areas of the film (Fig. 5-12). Cutoff is caused by the misalignment of the grid lines and the x-ray beam. This cutoff can occur for many reasons, ranging from improper centering of the x-ray tube over the grid, to tilting the tube laterally or tilting the grid itself, to having a focused grid upside down.

Grid Efficiency

A grid is used to reduce the amount of scatter radiation and increase the quality of the radiographic image. It is important that the lead lines be barely detectable on the finished radiograph, but this is not always possible. Thick lead strips break up a radiographic image more readily than thin lead strips. The thicker the lead strips, the more radiation is absorbed before reaching the film. As the

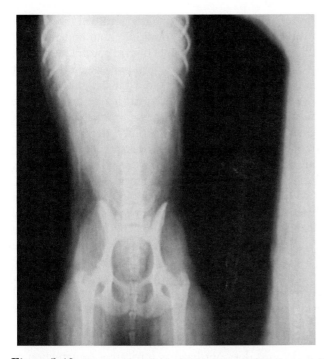

Figure 5-12 *Example of a radiograph with grid cutoff. Note the area of the film is off-center, the prominent vertical (x-ray absorption) lines, and the overall lack of radiographic density. All of these characteristics are signs of a good cast-off.*

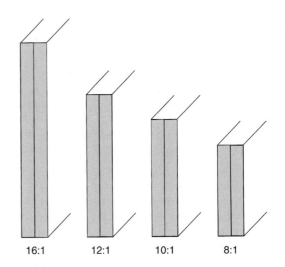

Figure 5-13 *Drawing illustrating various grid ratios. The high-ratio grids absorb more scatter radiation as a result of the smaller angle allowed for the x-rays to pass toward the film.*

strips become thinner and closer together within a grid, they are less perceptible on a radiographic image. However, less radiation is absorbed because of the decreased lead content per lead strip.

Grids vary in size and efficiency. Grid dimensions are usually 2 cm larger than the radiographic film sizes. The height, thickness, and number of lead strips determine the **grid efficiency.** The relation of the height of the lead strips to the distance between them is the **grid ratio.** For example, if the height of the lead strip is six times the width of the interspace, the grid ratio is 6:1. As the grid ratio increases, the efficiency of the grid increases. A 12:1 grid can absorb more scatter radiation than a 6:1 grid because of the greater size of the lead strips (Fig. 5-13).

Grids are also produced with a varying number of lead strips per centimeter. A grid is identified not only by its ratio but also by its **lines per centimeter.** More lines per centimeter mean that the lines are narrower. This is an

important consideration for several reasons. If a grid is used in a stationary manner, narrow grid lines would be less objectionable, as they appear on a radiograph. As the lead lines decrease in width, however, the grid is less efficient in the absorption of higher energy scatter radiation. Very fine grids are made with 40 lines per centimeter (60 to 100 lines per inch).

Grid Factor

It is inevitable that the lead strips of the grid will absorb a portion of the primary x-ray beam. In order to compensate, the exposure must be increased with the use of a **grid factor.** See Chapter 9 for the radiographic techniques used to compensate for the variable grids.

Grid Pattern

Grid pattern refers to the orientation of the lead strips in their longitudinal axis. This grid pattern is what we see from the top view. The two basic patterns are linear and crossed (Fig. 5-14, *A* and *D*).

Linear grid. The **linear grid** is patterned with the lead strips parallel in their longitudinal axis. The parallel grid

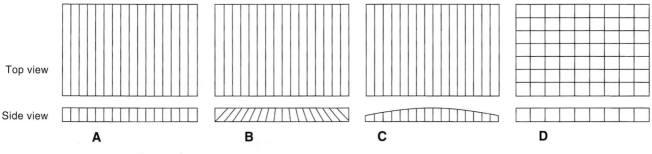

Figure 5-14 *A, Parallel grid. B, Focused grid. C, Pseudofocused grid. D, Crisscross grid.*

lines allow primary x-rays through to the film but absorb x-rays not traveling in a perpendicular path to the film. Most table-type x-ray units are equipped with linear grids. The advantage of a linear grid is that it allows the radiographer to angle the x-ray tube along the length of the grid without loss of primary radiation from grid cutoff.

Crossed grid. A **crossed** (or crisscross) **grid** consists of two superimposed linear grids. The grid ratio of crossed grids is equal to the sum of the ratios of the two linear grids. For example, a crossed grid made up of two 5:1 linear grids has a ratio of 10:1. The advantage of this grid is that the maximum amount of scatter radiation is absorbed. The grid absorbs scatter traveling not only "east and west" but "north and south" as well. The biggest disadvantage of a crossed grid is that it cannot be used with oblique techniques requiring angulation of the x-ray tube.

Focused versus Unfocused Grids

Both linear and crossed grid patterns are designed to be either focused or unfocused. A **focused grid** is made up of lead strips that are angled slightly so that they focus at the central point of the grid (Fig. 5-14, *B*). The lead strips of a focused grid radiate from the center strip, which is parallel to the central x-ray. In other words, beginning from the center lead strip, the slats on either side are progressively inclined at a greater angle. This angling of the grid lines allows for the diverging peripheral x-rays to pass through the grid (Fig. 5-15). Such grids are to be used at a specified source-image distance (SID), with some allowance for variation in distance from the manufacturer's recommendations.

Positioning of the focused grid is extremely important. The grid must not be placed upside down. If the grid is displaced this way, the radiating lead slats will absorb most of the primary x-ray beam, resulting in an underexposed radiograph. This is an example of grid cutoff (Fig. 5-16). The construction of a focused grid must be precise, and it tends to be more expensive than a parallel grid.

An **unfocused** (or parallel) **grid** is one in which the lead strips are parallel when viewed from a cross section. Because they are focused at infinity, they do not have a convergent line. These grids can be used effectively only with very small x-ray fields or with long focal-grid distances (focal spot–to-grid distance).

When a parallel grid is used with a short focal-grid distance, the outer, diverging portion of the primary beam tends to hit the lead slats. The x-rays hitting the lead slats are absorbed rather than passing between them. This is likely to result in an underexposure of the edge of the radiograph, as a result of grid cutoff (Fig. 5-17). Grid cutoff will occur to a certain extent with a parallel grid at any focal-grid distance. But this artifact can be minimized by using the grid according to the manufacturer's recommended focal-grid distance. Because the parallel grid does not have as intricate a construction as other types of grids, the cost is slightly less.

Pseudofocused Grid

The **pseudofocused grid** is a combination of the parallel and focused grids. It was produced to obtain a perfectly uniform parallel grid yet alleviate the absorption of the primary radiation at the edge of the x-ray beam. This was achieved by a progressive reduction in the height of the lead strips toward the edge of the grid (see Fig. 5-14, *C*).

Potter-Bucky Diaphragm

The previous discussion of grids is limited to stationary grids that are permanently fixed under the x-ray table or

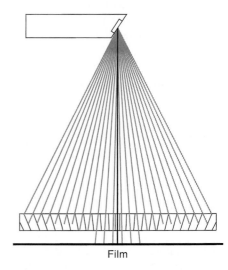

Film

Figure 5-15 *The diverging lead strips of a focused grid allow the diverging x-ray beam to pass through to the x-ray film.*

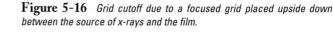

Film

Figure 5-16 *Grid cutoff due to a focused grid placed upside down between the source of x-rays and the film.*

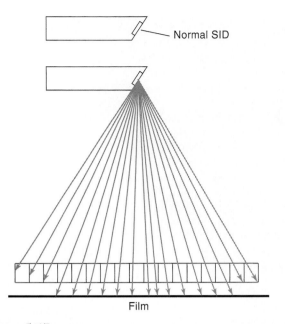

Figure 5-17 *Grid cutoff due to a decreased distance between the anode and the grid (source-image distance). A portion of the primary x-ray beam toward the edges of the film is being "cut off" or absorbed by the grid.*

mounted to a cassette. There is a mechanism, however, that can mechanically move the grid across the x-ray beam at a uniform speed. The device consists of a focused grid within a diaphragm that travels back and forth during exposure. The value of a moving grid lies in filtering scatter radiation while eliminating the grid lines from the finished radiograph.

The **Potter-Bucky diaphragm** ("Bucky") is normally placed directly under the x-ray table or in a vertical well-mounted unit (Fig. 5-18). The grid is positioned so that the lead strips run parallel to the length of the table or wall unit. This device is used extensively in human radiography, and its use is recommended in specialized large-animal facilities that are equipped to radiograph a horse or cow.

Bucky systems are not recommended for portable x-ray equipment, as they lack suitable connections and power. Because the Bucky apparatus is mechanical, it can also break down. Judgment is required to determine if a Bucky system is necessary in a new veterinary installation for small animal use.

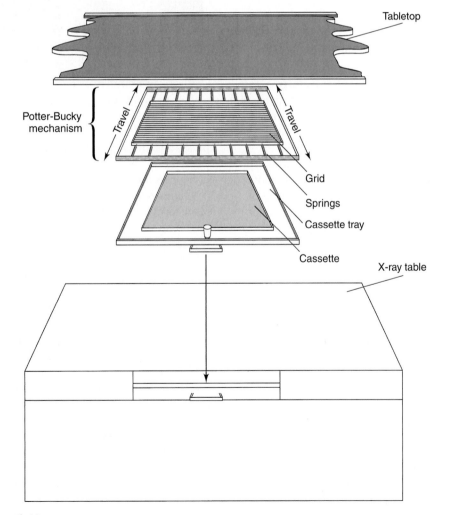

Figure 5-18 *Diagram of the x-ray table, grid, Potter-Bucky diaphragm, and cassette tray with cassette. Note that the direction of the grid lines runs with the length of the table and that the travel of the grid is in a transverse direction during exposure.*

Care of Grids

Grids are delicate and expensive. If a grid is dropped on its edge, it can be damaged permanently. Once the lead strips become bent or warped, a permanent artifact will appear on all radiographs taken with that grid. Grids attached to cassettes are more prone to this type of injury. The grids installed in a Potter-Bucky diaphragm system are well protected under the tabletop and generally need little care.

RADIOGRAPHIC DETAIL AND DEFINITION

Radiographic detail and **definition** are terms used to describe image sharpness, clarity, distinctness, and perceptibility. Detail describes the definition of the edge of an anatomic structure on a radiograph. The radiographer tries to obtain as much diagnostic information as possible about the internal structures of the patient. To achieve this goal, image clarity is essential. Lack of detail can result from several different factors.

Geometric Unsharpness

Geometric unsharpness can be attributed to many factors. To prevent confusion, each is discussed individually.

Loss of detail due to some geometric distortion can result from a large focal spot size or a decreased SID, as discussed in Chapter 3. As the focal spot size increases, the "shadow sharpness" decreases. In the same respect, as the SID increases, the image sharpness increases.

Motion is another possible cause of geometric unsharpness. When an animal, x-ray tube, or x-ray film moves during exposure, blurring of the image results (Fig. 5-19). Patient motion is the most common artifact in veterinary radiography (remember another "Murphy's Law" of veterinary radiography: The animal will move at the least opportune time). Sedation sometimes helps to decrease the chance of motion on a radiograph.

Geometric unsharpness due to the screens and film is another possibility. The screens are located inside the cassette to transform x-rays into light. Certain screen-film combinations are designed to produce radiographs with high detail and some with low detail. Screens and film are discussed in Chapter 6.

Geometric Distortion and Magnification

X-rays, like visible light, travel in straight lines that diverge from a central projection. All geometric anomalies that occur with visible light also occur with x-rays and can be explained using visible light as an analogy.

The best way to describe **geometric distortion** is to use the example of your shadow on a sunny day. At 12 o'clock noon, when the sun is directly overhead, your shadow will be directly underneath your body. As time

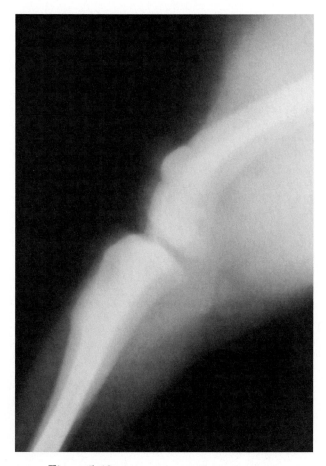

Figure 5-19 *Radiograph illustrating patient motion.*

passes and the sun begins to set, the shadow projected by your body will be elongated and distorted. This phenomenon is called *geometric distortion.*

Geometric distortion of a radiographic image may result in difficulty during interpretation. To alleviate the possibility of any geometric distortion on a radiograph, the radiographer needs a basic understanding of the geometric projection of a subject onto the image receptor.

To maintain an accurate geometric projection, the subject under examination must be parallel to the image receptor (Fig. 5-20). If the anatomic part under examination is not parallel to the image receptor, geometric distortion results. The simplest way to demonstrate this phenomenon is with a flashlight and the image of a subject (an object) projected on a wall. With the flashlight approximately 1 m from the wall, interpose an object into the path of the light. The shadow of the subject will appear on the wall. When the object is close to the wall, the projected shadow appears approximately the same size as the subject, and the edges of the image are distinct. As the subject is moved away from the wall, closer to the flashlight, the image becomes progressively larger and more diffuse (**magnification**). The edges of the magnified image become blurred, and the subject becomes almost unrecognizable. Now move one side of the object farther from the wall. Note that the edge

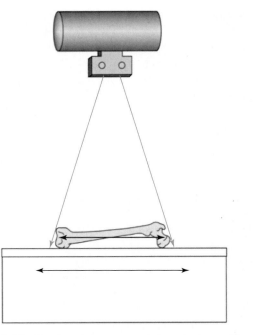

Figure 5-20 *Drawing of correct geometric projection position. The subject should remain parallel to the image receptor (film).*

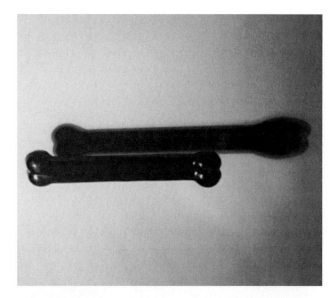

Figure 5-22 *With use of a small light source and a bone, this photograph illustrates the distortion known as* elongation. *The light source should remain perpendicular to the wall to achieve accurate image projection. In this case the light source was not directly above the bone, and the image of the bone was elongated.*

farthest from the wall is distorted and magnified. When the subject is not parallel to the wall, the entire image is distorted (Fig. 5-21). This experiment proves two points. When the subject of interest is not close and parallel to the image receptor, the image is distorted and lacks detail.

In the same manner, the focal spot of the x-ray beam must be directly above the object and centered on the point of interest, or geometric distortion will result. To illustrate this point, another experiment can be performed with a flashlight and an object projected in its path. This

time, instead of moving the subject toward the light source, follow the parallel plane of the wall and move the subject to the left or right. Notice that the shadow image, when not directly under the source of light, becomes elongated and diffuse on one edge of the projected image (Fig. 5-22). This is called **elongation** distortion.

With the same object and light source, perform one more experiment. This time, assume the correct position in the path of the light source with the subject directly

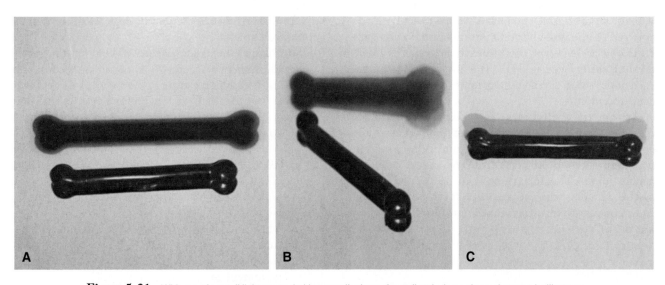

Figure 5-21 *With use of a small light source held perpendicular to the wall and a bone, these photographs illustrate the importance of keeping the subject under radiographic investigation close and parallel to the image receptor.* **A,** *The bone is parallel but far away from the wall, and the image projected on the wall is magnified.* **B,** *This distortion is known as* foreshortening, *which is a result of the object not being parallel to the wall.* **C,** *The bone is close and parallel to the wall, and the image projected is relatively accurate.*

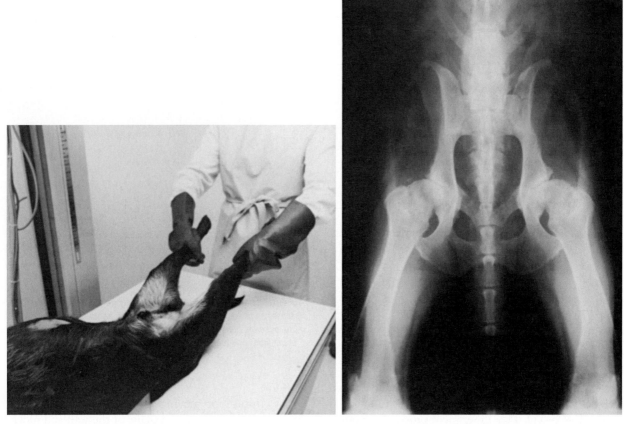

A

B

Figure 5-23 *A, Dogs with severe hip dysplasia may be difficult to position correctly. The most common problem is the inability to extend the rear limbs properly for the radiograph, which can result in distortion of the image. **B**, As a result, the radiograph shows the distortion known as* foreshortening. *Note that the femurs appear shorter and the distal femurs are enlarged.*

centered in the beam of light and the subject positioned parallel and relatively close to the wall. In this experiment, move only one side of the subject away from the wall, keeping the other side stationary. Notice that the image projected on the wall appears shorter than the actual size of the object. This type of geometric distortion is called **foreshortening** (see Fig. 5-21, *B*). This proves the importance of the subject remaining parallel to the plane of the image receptor.

Foreshortening distortion is a common occurrence when radiographing a dog with severe hip dysplasia. The hips of a dog with severe dysplasia are difficult to position because of the bone changes that have occurred within the hip joints. The femurs need to be parallel to the cassette. In a dog with hip dysplasia, it can be difficult, if not impossible, to maneuver the femurs into this position (Fig. 5-23).

KEY POINTS

1. The purpose of a grid is to reduce the amount of scatter radiation and increase the quality of the radiographic image.

2. The most effective way to reduce backscatter is to limit the size of the x-ray beam to include only the image receptor.

3. Exposure of a radiographic film to x-rays makes the film black.

4. The higher the tissue density, the lower the radiographic density.

5. The most common cause of poor radiographic contrast is inappropriate exposure factors (kVp, mAs, exposure time).

REVIEW QUESTIONS

1. Which of the following increases radiographic density?
   a. Thicker body parts
   b. Increased mAs
   c. Increased density of the body part being radiographed
   d. Decreased kVp

2. Which of the following radiographs should have the shortest scale of contrast?

a. Abdomen
b. Thorax
c. Femur
d. All are approximately equal

3. High subject contrast _____ radiographic contrast.
   a. increases
   b. decreases

4. If kVp is too low for an abdominal radiograph, which of the following will be evident on a radiograph?
   a. No distinct difference exists among anatomic organs.
   b. The penetrating power is weak, and x-rays cannot penetrate the patient.
   c. The radiograph will have a "soot and white-washed" appearance (gray and white).
   d. All of the above.

5. The primary exposure factor that controls scatter radiation is:
   a. KVp
   b. mAs
   c. increased exposure time.
   d. the collimator setting.

6. What do grids contain that controls scatter radiation?
   a. Molybdenum
   b. Aluminum
   c. Silver
   d. Lead

7. Where is a grid located?
   a. Between the patient and the cassette
   b. In the anode
   c. In the cathode
   d. The radiographer wears it on the hand or collar.

8. Which grid ratio can absorb more scatter radiation?
   a. 6:1
   b. 8:1
   c. 1:6
   d. 2:1

9. To prevent magnification and distortion of the object being radiographed, the patient must:
   a. be as parallel to the film as possible.
   b. be as close to the film as possible.
   c. be as close to the x-ray tube as possible.
   d. Both a and b are correct.

10. If a dog is being radiographed for hip dysplasia, what phenomenon will occur if the femurs are not parallel to the film?
    a. Foreshortening
    b. Elongation
    c. Grid cutoff
    d. Contrast

Suggested Readings

Curry TS, Dowdy JE, Murry RC: *Christensen's physics of diagnostic radiology,* ed 4, Philadelphia, 1990, Lea & Febiger.

Douglas SW, Herrtage ME, Williamson HD: *Principles of veterinary radiography,* ed 4, Philadelphia, 1987, Bailliere Tindall.

Eastman Kodak Company: *Kodak: the fundamentals of radiography,* ed 12, Rochester, NY, 1980, Kodak.

Gray JE et al: *Quality control in diagnostic imaging,* Rockville, Md, 1983, Aspen.

Morgan JP, Silverman S: *Techniques in veterinary radiography,* ed 4, Ames, Iowa, 1987, Iowa State University Press.

Sweeney RJ: *Radiographic artifacts: their cause and control,* New York, 1983, JB Lippincott.

Ticer JW: *Radiographic techniques in small animal practice,* ed 2, Philadelphia, 1984, WB Saunders.

chapter 6

Image Receptors

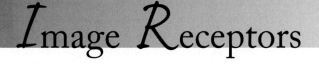

CHAPTER OUTLINE

The Cassette
Intensifying Screens

X-Ray Film
Film-Screen Systems

OBJECTIVES

Upon completion of this chapter, the reader should be able to do the following:

- Describe a cassette
- State the proper care of a cassette
- List the three properties that determine efficiency of a screen
- Describe intensifying screen construction
- List the common phosphor types used in diagnostic intensifying screens
- List and describe the factors that govern screen speed
- Explain how screen speeds are rated
- Define quantum mottle
- Describe the correct method of mounting a screen inside the cassette

- Define and describe fluoroscopy
- Describe proper screen care
- State the purpose of x-ray film
- Describe the composition of x-ray film
- Define a latent image
- List the two general categories (types) of x-ray film
- Describe how film speed is determined
- Define film latitude
- Describe proper film care
- State the significance of film-screen system comprehension

Afterglow: The tendency of a luminescent compound to continue to give off light after x-radiation has stopped.

Base: A transparent flexible polyester support layer of radiographic film.

Cassette: A lightproof encasement designed to hold x-ray film and intensifying screens in close contact.

Emulsion: A layer of radiographic film made of gelatin containing suspended silver halide crystals.

Film latitude: The exposure range of a film that will produce acceptable densities.

Fluoroscopy: A special radiographic diagnostic method by which a "live view" of the internal anatomy is possible.

Intensifying screens: Sheets of luminescent phosphor crystals bound together and mounted on a cardboard or plastic base.

Latent image: An invisible image on the x-ray film after it is exposed to ionizing radiation or light before processing.

Nonscreen film: Film that is more sensitive to ionizing radiation than to fluorescent light.

Quantum mottle: An artifact of faster screens that results in density variation due to random spatial distribution of the phosphor crystals within the screen.

Reflective layer: A layer of an intensifying screen that reflects the light from the phosphor layer toward the film.

Screen film: Film with silver crystals that is more sensitive to fluorescent light emitted from intensifying screens than to ionizing radiation.

Silver halide: A compound of silver and bromine, chlorine, or iodine, all of which are in the halogen group of elements.

Supercoat: A clear protective layer on radiographic film.

INTRODUCTION

In previous chapters, discussions were limited to the production and action of x-rays. To further understand radiography, we need to discuss how a permanent record is produced using x-rays.

Essentially, a radiograph is formed with light-sensitive film contained in a lightproof encasement. In radiography, the lightproof encasement used most often is called a *cassette* (Fig. 6-1). The general-use cassette is designed to hold a piece of double-emulsion x-ray film sandwiched between two fluorescent sheets of plastic called *intensifying screens.* The intensifying screens are responsible for converting the x-ray radiation into visible light, which creates a *latent image* on the x-ray film. The film is then processed to convert the latent image into a visible image. Remarkably, more than 95% of the exposure recorded on the film is due to the light emitted from the intensifying screens. Only 5% of the exposure of the film results from the ionization of x-rays.

Many different types of image receptors and detectors convert invisible ionizing radiation into a visible image. These detectors and receptors can take many forms and, in turn, assist a number of diagnostic procedures that use radiant energy including the following:

1. The exposure of fluorescent materials that converts x-ray radiation into visible light, which can be used to expose special film containing silver halide/bromide crystals (radiography).
2. The interaction of x-rays with charged selenium plates. When exposed, the distribution of the electrical charge is altered, producing a negative image on the plate (xeroradiography).
3. The absorption of x-rays by ionizing chambers to produce voltage pulses, which can be displayed on cathode ray tubes (computed tomography).
4. The injection of a radiopharmaceutical followed by imaging distribution of the radioactivity with a sodium iodide crystal gamma camera (nuclear scintigraphy).

This list is only a sample of the imaging techniques that use radiant energy. We will redirect our attention to fluorescent intensifying screens and silver halide films as image receptors.

THE CASSETTE

In radiography, the **cassette** is a rigid film holder designed to hold the x-ray film and intensifying screens in close contact. The cassette must be constructed with materials that are light-tight to prevent any unwanted exposure to the film yet that allow penetration of the x-rays.

The first cassettes were constructed with cardboard. This material could not be reused and thus did not pass the test of time. Over the years, cassettes made of aluminum became standard. Aluminum cassettes are still common today; however, improvements have been made to cassette fronts. As mentioned, the front of the cassette must be strong and opaque to light yet radiolucent to x-rays. Examples of available cassette fronts are those made of (1) polycarbonate (Bakelite), (2) aluminum, (3) magnesium, and (4) carbon fiber.

Some cassette fronts are color coded or have a colored dot on the edge to indicate the screen type inside. Color coding allows easy identification when choosing a cassette for each clinical situation. The front may also be marked

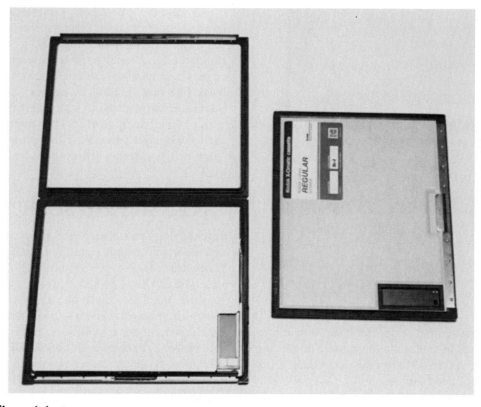

Figure 6-1 *Two cassettes, one open and one closed. Inside the cassette are two fluorescent screens that sandwich the radiographic film. When closed, the cassette provides a lightproof environment for the film.*

into four quadrants to assist more than one exposure per film. Taking a number of exposures on one film is accomplished by exposing one quadrant while shielding the others with lead rubber strips (Fig. 6-2). An area approximately 3 × 7 cm may also be marked in the corner of the cassette front to indicate the presence of a lead blocker (Fig. 6-3). This lead blocker is present to prevent irradiation of the part of the film necessary for identification. (Film identification is discussed in Chapter 7.) Care must be taken not to superimpose any vital areas of the patient over this blocker.

The cassette front is attached to the back with hinges and catches. Several types of hinges and catches that provide a tight seal between the front and the back of the cassette are available. The closure styles range from hinges with slide catches to crossbars that pivot on a shoulder rivet in the middle of the back of the cassette. The back of the cassette is constructed with heavier material than that for the front and is normally lined with lead to absorb backscatter radiation that would cause fogging of the film.

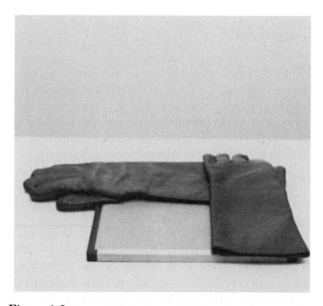

Figure 6-2 *The cassette has been divided into four quadrants so that a number of views can be exposed. Three of the sections are being shielded with lead to prevent exposure until desired. In this case the quadrants are being shielded with lead gloves. Commercially available lead sheets can be purchased for this purpose as well.*

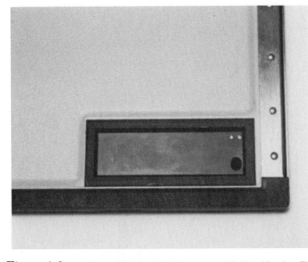

Figure 6-3 *A 3 × 7 cm lead blocker for photographic identification. The blocker prevents exposure to x-rays to this area so that information can be exposed on the film in the darkroom with the use of a photoimprinter.*

Inside the cassette, both sides are lined with felt or foam pressure pads that ensure close contact of the film and screens. The choice of felt versus foam pads varies with each cassette manufacturer.

Cassette sizes also vary and correspond to screen and film sizes (in both metric and English). Their cost varies according to size and quality. (Note: The price quotes in most catalogs are for the cassettes only and do not include the screens.)

Cassette choice is an important aspect of veterinary radiography. The purchase of a certain cassette may help or hinder the production of quality radiographs. A cassette should have sturdy construction, maintain screen-film contact, and be user friendly in the darkroom.

Cassette Care

As with any expensive piece of equipment, the cassette should be handled with care. In veterinary medicine, cassettes tend to be exposed to some physical abuse. This is especially true in a large-animal practice. The most common causes of physical damage are (1) dropping the cassette on a hard surface and (2) leakage of fluid such as blood or urine into the cassette.

Dropping a cassette on a hard surface can result in a loss of contact between the screens and film, which results in a blurred radiographic image. (See Chapter 10 for the test procedure for screen-film contact.)

Keeping a cassette clean when working with animals is always a challenge. Precautions such as placing the cassette in a plastic bag when a "messy" situation is expected will prevent damage to the cassette's exterior and interior. A cassette should be cleaned on a regular basis with mild soap and water. Cleaning the exterior of the cassette when the screens are cleaned (monthly) is usually adequate unless circumstances necessitate a more frequent schedule.

All cassettes should be numbered. This way, any noticeable defects on a radiograph can be traced to the "problem" cassette. Most intensifying screens within the cassette have a serial number imprinted on the screen edge. These numbers are small, however, and difficult to read. The best method of cassette identification is to number each intensifying screen near the edge or corner with a black felt-tip marker. This number will appear on each radiograph taken with that cassette. The exterior (back of the cassette) should be marked with the same number.

INTENSIFYING SCREENS

Intensifying screens are sheets of luminescent phosphor crystals bound together and mounted on a cardboard or plastic base. Two screens are normally inside the cassette to sandwich the x-ray film, which has a coating of light-sensitive emulsion on both sides (double emulsion). When the phosphor crystals in the screen are struck by x-radiation, the crystals fluoresce, and x-rays are converted into visible light (Fig. 6-4). This visible light exposes the x-ray film. As stated earlier, more than 95% of the exposure to the film is due to light emitted from the intensifying screens.

The primary purpose of the intensifying screen is to reduce the amount of radiation exposure required to produce a diagnostic radiograph. The use of screens results in lower milliamperage-seconds (mAs), thus decreasing the dose of radiation to the patient and the chance of motion on the radiograph.

Three properties determine the efficiency of the screen materials:

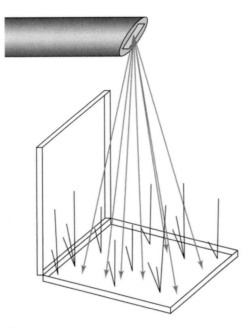

Figure 6-4 *Fluorescent screens emit light when x-rays strike them. This drawing illustrates how the screens "glow" during exposure.*

1. They must have a high level of x-ray absorption.
2. They must have high x-ray–to-light conversion with suitable energy and color.
3. There must be little or no "afterglow" once radiation has ceased.

Screen Construction

An intensifying screen has four integral layers: (1) a base or support, (2) a reflective layer, (3) a phosphor crystal layer, and (4) a protective coat (Fig. 6-5).

The base serves as a flexible support to attach the phosphor layer to the cassette. The base must have a tough, moisture-resistant surface and not become brittle with extended use.

The reflective layer, which is attached to the base, is made of a white substance such as titanium dioxide. The purpose of the reflective layer is to reflect the light emitted by the phosphor layer back toward the x-ray film. The reflective layer increases the efficiency of the screen so that none of the light photons are lost through the base layer.

The phosphor crystal layer consists of uniformly distributed phosphor crystals held in place with a binder material. It is extremely important that this layer not change in thickness, crack, or discolor with age. Any variance in screen uniformity would alter the amount of light produced when irradiated and would alter the uniform exposure of the film (Fig. 6-6).

The protective coat is a clear coating placed on the outer surface of the screen; it provides the necessary protection to the phosphor layer. This layer must be strong enough to resist marks and abrasions and easy to clean. Veterinary radiography has many pitfalls, one of which is animal hair. Any foreign material caught in the cassette between the intensifying screen and the film will alter the exposure to the film. The debris on the screen will result in radiographic artifacts (Fig. 6-7). Because of the likelihood of artifacts and the need for subsequent screen cleaning, the protective surface must be durable and resistant to deterioration.

Phosphor types. As discussed previously, x-rays can cause phosphors to emit light. The phosphor chosen for an intensifying screen must absorb x-rays efficiently, have a minimum afterglow, and emit sufficient light of the desired color.

Afterglow is the tendency of a phosphor to still give off light after the x-radiation has stopped. This continued phosphorescence can interfere with rapid-succession serial film changers. A serial film changer is used when a number of films are necessary per second. For example, a rapid serial film changer is necessary for angiography to view the action of the heart. With a radiopaque liquid contrast medium injected intravenously, the movement of the fluid through the chambers of the heart can be

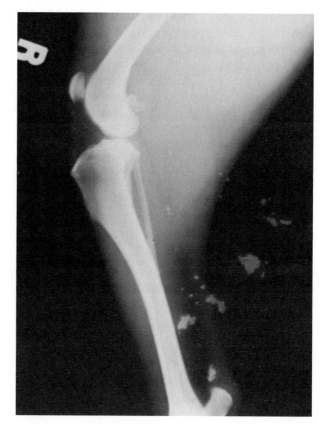

Figure 6-7 *Radiographic artifact that is the result of dirt within the cassette.*

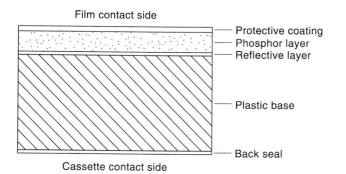

Film contact side
— Protective coating
— Phosphor layer
— Reflective layer
— Plastic base
— Back seal
Cassette contact side

Figure 6-5 *Cross section of an intensifying screen.*

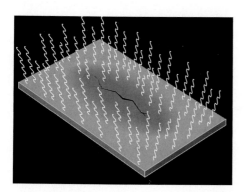

Figure 6-6 *A crack in an intensifying screen. During exposure to x-rays, an irregular light emission results where the screen is damaged.*

recorded. A serial film changer can expose many films per second. If any afterglow from the intensifying screen were present, it would interfere with the exposure of each successive film.

The absorption rate of the phosphor refers to the extraction of x-ray photons from the beam. The absorption of one x-ray quantum (unit of radiant energy) results in the emission of hundreds of light quanta from the screen. These light photons are more readily absorbed by the x-ray film than are x-ray photons. The more x-ray quanta absorbed, the greater the amount of light produced.

The first phosphor intensifying screen, introduced in 1896 by Thomas Edison, was made of calcium tungstate, which was chosen because its emission of light is in the blue regions of the ultraviolet spectrum. This was important because of the high sensitivity of silver halide to this spectrum of light. Calcium tungstate has a relatively high x-ray absorption ability and is physically strong, but it is lacking in light conversion efficiency. Despite this weakness, calcium tungstate screens are still widely used today.

GENERAL RULES

> Large crystals: Faster screens • Less detail • High grain
> Small crystals: Slower screens • More detail • Low grain

New phosphor technology has led to the introduction of phosphors with greater speed. In 1972 a class of phosphors known as the *rare-earth elements* was developed. The term *rare earth* is used because these elements are difficult and expensive to separate from the earth and from each other, not because they are scarce. The rare-earth group is also known as the lanthanide series because it consists of elements with atomic numbers 57 (lanthanum) through 71 (lutetium).

The x-ray–to-light conversion efficiency of rare-earth phosphors is significantly greater than that of calcium tungstate. The light conversion of a rare-earth screen is four times as great as that of a calcium tungstate screen. The spectral emission of rare-earth phosphors is in the green light part of the spectrum. Because standard x-ray silver halide film will not absorb (i.e., is not sensitive to) light in the green area, a special film that is sensitive to the green spectrum of light must be employed with this type of screen.

Screen Speed

Factors other than phosphor type affect the speed and efficiency of a screen. Many types of screens are available today, all of which are graded by their speed and efficiency. Screen speed is governed by crystal size, phosphor layer thickness, reflective layer efficiency, and dyes in the phosphor layer.

Crystal size. Within certain limits, the larger the crystal, the greater its light emission. An x-ray striking any part of a phosphor crystal causes the entire crystal to fluoresce. Because of the larger flashes of light with larger crystals, less x-radiation is necessary to expose the x-ray film (Fig. 6-8). Another way to consider this concept is illustrated in the following scenario.

Imagine that you are standing 10 feet away from a wall that has two mirrors hanging on it. One mirror is 2 inches in diameter, and the other is much larger with a 10-inch diameter. Facing the wall, you shine a flashlight beam at the mirrors. As you examine the light being reflected, you notice that the amount of light from each mirror is not equal. What is reflected from the smaller mirror is significantly less than that from the larger mirror.

The same principle applies to phosphor crystal size. Unfortunately, as the crystal size increases, the detail of

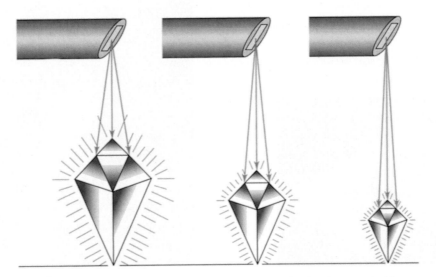

Figure 6-8 *One factor that influences the speed of screens is the size of the phosphor crystals. A large crystal emits a larger amount of light than a smaller crystal.*

the image decreases. The result of increasing the speed of the screen by increasing the crystal size is a grainy image. Within certain limits, an increase in crystal size is acceptable and will not compromise radiographic detail excessively. In comparison, smaller crystals produce a film with increased detail but larger amounts of radiation are required.

Phosphor layer thickness. The thickness of the phosphor layer is another factor that influences both screen speed and image detail. When the thickness is increased, the x-ray absorption and light emission are increased. Screen thickness has limits, however. An increase in the thickness of the phosphor layer results in a decrease in image detail. The image is blurred as a result of the diffusion, or "spreading out," of the light as it travels through the screen from the phosphor crystal, where the light originated. Recall that light leaves a central point and diverges outward. Lateral spreading of light is a result of this light divergence (Fig. 6-9).

Reflective layer efficiency. As mentioned earlier, the **reflective layer** is positioned between the base and the phosphor layer. The purpose of the reflective layer is to reflect all light emission from the phosphor layer toward the x-ray film. If the reflective layer contains a light-absorbing material, however, a portion of the light produced by the phosphors will be lost. More x-radiation is necessary to produce an adequate exposure on the x-ray film. Therefore it is important that the reflective layer material has a high reflective capability and a low absorption capacity.

Dyes in the phosphor layer. A light-absorbing dye (pigment) may be incorporated into the binder material of the phosphor layer of some screens. The primary purpose of the dye is to decrease lateral spreading of the light emitted from the phosphor crystals. When the lateral spread is reduced, blurring of the radiographic image is decreased. Unfortunately, the light intensity emitted by the screen is also reduced and the speed of the screen is decreased. Common pigments used are yellow, gray, and pink.

Screen Speed Ratings

Because many factors affect screen speed, it is natural to assume that there are many screens from which to choose. It might also be assumed that screen speeds can be accurately measured and that screen speed categories are clearly defined. Unfortunately, this is not the case; screen speed categories are broad and general. Most manufacturers divide screen speeds into three basic categories relative to the screen's light output:

1. *Slow* (also referred to as *high definition, ultradetail, or fine grain*): This group of screens is specifically designed for radiographic examinations that require optimal detail and in which exposure time is not critical.
2. *Medium* (also referred to as regular, midspeed, normal, or par speed): This category is the most common in private veterinary practice. Medium-speed screens provide good resolution with relatively low exposures.

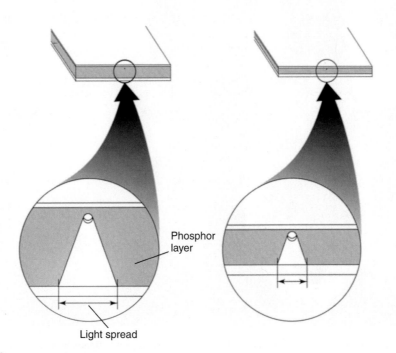

Phosphor layer

Light spread

Figure 6-9 *A cross section of two screens. Because one screen is much thicker than the other, the light spread is much greater with the thicker screen.*

3. *Fast* (also referred to as high speed): High-speed screens reduce exposure time or patient exposure or penetrate extremely thick tissue areas where more exposure is necessary.

One manufacturer's screen speed categories may not correlate precisely with another's. For example, manufacturer A may produce a par speed screen that is 10% faster than the par speed screen produced by manufacturer B.

Increased screen speed has led to a radiographic artifact known as **quantum mottle.** This artifact gives a radiograph a spotty or mottled appearance. Quantum mottle occurs because the new, faster screens are so sensitive that only a few x-ray quanta are necessary to produce the desired density on the x-ray film. As the small number of quanta strike the intensifying screen, not all of the phosphor crystals are struck and therefore not all of them fluoresce. Inconsistent fluorescence from the phosphors results in a density variation (mottling) on a uniformly exposed radiograph. Quantum mottle is a disadvantage of rare-earth screens for brief exposures, but its effects are greatly reduced with correct film-screen combinations.

Screen Speed Summary

In radiography, screen speed is inversely proportional to the exposure required to produce a given effect. That is, a fast screen requires a small exposure, and a slow screen requires a larger exposure. A fast screen has the physical capability to emit more light when struck by x-radiation than does a slow screen, given the same exposure (Fig. 6-10).

In the same respect, radiographic detail is inversely proportional to the speed of the screen. A screen that is manufactured to be fast will inherently produce a radiograph with less detail. The disadvantage of fast screens is increased graininess. Although slow screens require more x-radiation, the detail is greatly increased.

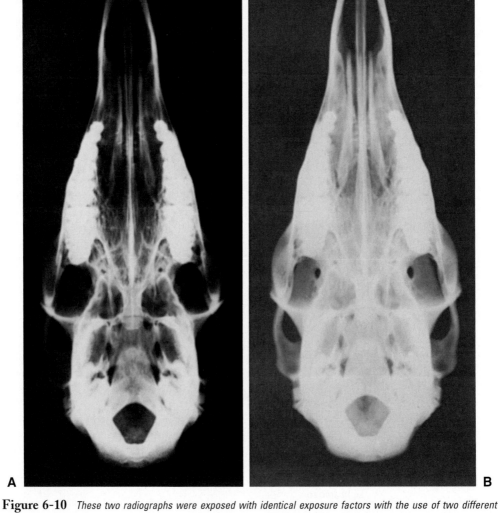

A   B

Figure 6-10 *These two radiographs were exposed with identical exposure factors with the use of two different screen types. **A** was exposed with fast screens, and **B** was exposed with slow screens. Note that **A** is properly exposed, whereas **B** is too light. Slow screens need a greater amount of exposure compared with fast screens.*

Mounting Screens in the Cassette

Intensifying screens are usually mounted in pairs in the cassette. Most screens are labeled FRONT and BACK and should be placed in the cassette appropriately. The screen on the front side is slightly thinner than that on the back so that the front does not absorb an excessive amount of the x-ray beam and the exposure of light to both sides of the film is even.

Securing the screens in the cassette is vital. Screens should never be loose inside the cassette. Double-sided tape, provided by the manufacturer, should be applied to secure the screens. Commercial liquid adhesives should be avoided because certain chemicals can interact with the screens.

Some screens are used singly in a cassette. The use of only one screen increases the image resolution but tends to be slower and to need more exposure to achieve a desired product. Single-screen cassettes are used primarily for extremity radiography, in which image detail is critical, and must be paired with single-emulsion film.

Specialized Screens: Fluoroscopy

Fluoroscopy is essentially the visualization of a "live" or "real-time" radiographic image. Fluoroscopy is used for a number of purposes including the following:

1. To evaluate the esophagus and upper and lower gastrointestinal tract configuration and function
2. To assist in surgical procedures (e.g., foreign body removal, cardiac catheterization)
3. To evaluate ventilation mechanics (e.g., trachea, lungs, diaphragm)
4. To evaluate cardiac function

The main feature of a fluoroscopy unit is its screen. Special crystals such as cadmium sulfide or caesium iodide are in the screen because they emit green light, to which the human eye is most sensitive. The screen is substituted for conventional x-ray film and is placed in the path of the x-ray beam after it has passed through the patient. The fluoroscopic screen enables the radiographer to visualize the fluorescent image created by the interaction of x-rays and phosphor crystals as it occurs.

The image viewed is the opposite of an x-ray seen on a view box, or a "positive" image. The black-and-white areas on the screen are reversed compared with a normal radiograph. The intensity of the light emitted by each part of the screen is proportional to the intensity of the x-rays striking that part of the screen. The visible light pattern corresponds precisely with the x-ray pattern.

Fluoroscopy equipment is installed opposite to conventional x-ray equipment. The fluoroscopic screen is suspended above the x-ray table, and the x-ray tube, coupled to the screen, is under the table directed toward the screen (Fig. 6-11). Leaded glass is positioned over the

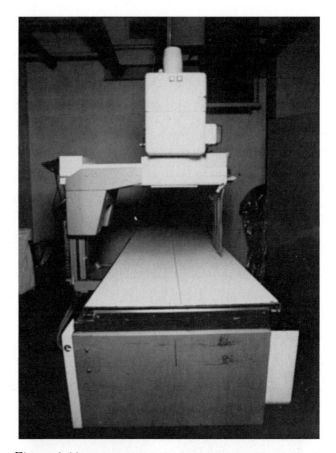

Figure 6-11 *Fluoroscopy unit. The x-rays are emitted from under the table and projected on a fluorescent screen above the table. The image is then transferred to a television monitor.*

screen so that the image can be viewed without exposing the operator's eyes to radiation.

Today, technology has replaced this type of fluoroscopy unit with an image-intensifying unit. An image intensifier essentially converts and transfers the image on the intensifying screen to a photoelectric surface. Image-intensified fluoroscopy can be observed through an optical lens and mirrors (mirror optics system) or on a television monitor.

At no time should fluoroscopy replace radiography. Not only is there more risk of radiation exposure, but the image created by the fluoroscope has far less resolution. In the past, some veterinary practices used handheld fluoroscopy units exclusively to save the time and expense of exposing and developing x-ray film. This practice is deemed illegal in most states in the United States.

Screen Care

Because of the cost of screens and their sensitivity to damage, the importance of screen care cannot be minimized. Screens should be inspected and cleaned on a regular basis to keep them free of dirt and foreign material. Dust and animal hair are common artifacts in veterinary radiography (Fig. 6-12). Any abrasion, chemical spill, or artifact will be noticeable on all films taken in conjunction

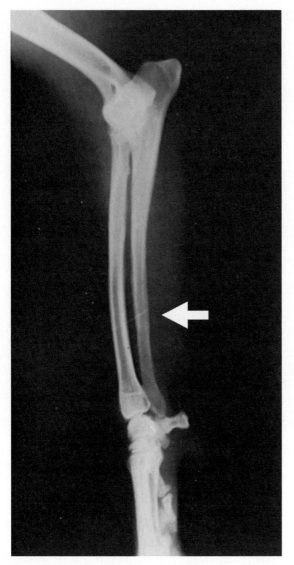

Figure 6-12 *Radiograph showing a hair artifact. The hair was trapped inside the cassette during exposure.*

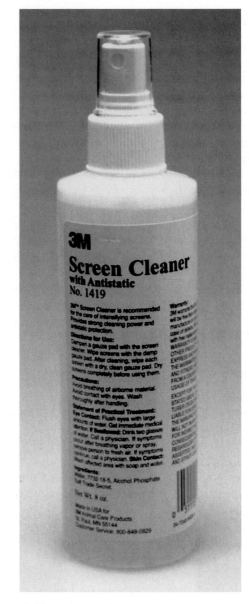

Figure 6-13 *Use commercial screen cleaner to clean the surface.*

with that screen. Incorrect diagnoses have occurred as a result of unsuspected screen artifacts.

Screens should be cleaned according to the manufacturer's instructions to avoid damage to the screen surfaces. For example, a soft brush or pressurized air can remove loose foreign material. The surface protective coat can be cleaned by careful swabbing with dampened gauze pads and cleaning solution. Commercial screen cleaning solutions (Fig. 6-13), mild soap and water, or dilute ethyl alcohol are recommended. Commercial solutions have the advantage of possessing antistatic properties.

After cleaning, the cassette should be left open and propped in a vertical position to dry completely before reloading. The vertical position prevents any dust or foreign material from settling inside the cassette. At all other times, the cassette should be kept closed to prevent accidental damage and artifacts. Take care when loading and unloading film from the cassette to avoid "digs" and scratches on the screen surface. Touching the screens and

writing on film that is still in the cassette should also be avoided. Damage to the screen surface is permanent and cannot be repaired.

X-RAY FILM

The purpose of x-ray film is to provide a permanent record containing essential diagnostic information. X-ray film provides information not only for present use but for later evaluation as well.

X-ray film consists of a polyester base coated on both sides with a light-sensitive emulsion containing silver halide crystals. When visible light or ionizing radiation (x-rays) interacts with the silver halide crystals, an invisible (latent) image is formed. Through processing, this invisible image is converted into a visible image. The final product is a radiograph.

Film Composition

X-ray film has a number of layers, each with individual characteristics and purposes (Fig. 6-14). The transparent polyester **base** provides a flexible support with a thin adhesive subcoating on each side. The adhesive serves to bind the next layer, the emulsion, to the base. **Emulsion** consists of gelatin that contains silver halide microcrystals suspended and dispersed evenly throughout the layer. Gelatin provides reasonable permanence and allows rapid processing because it is easily penetrated by developing solutions.

Silver halide is a compound of silver and bromine, chlorine, or iodine, which are members of the halogen family. (Silver bromide crystals are common in diagnostic x-ray film.) Viewed through a microscope, the emulsion appears to be filled with tiny grains of sand. These tiny grains are the silver microcrystals suspended in the gelatin—there are billions of crystals per cubic centimeter of emulsion. Over the emulsion is a clear **supercoat** of protective material to decrease the possibility of damage to the fragile emulsion.

Latent Image

As the silver halide crystals absorb energy from visible light or x-rays, a physical change occurs and a latent image is formed. By definition, a **latent image** is an invisible image on the x-ray film after it is exposed to ionizing radiation or visible light before processing. After processing with a special chemical developer solution, the latent image is converted into a visible image.

The latent image is formed on a screen-type film by the absorption of a light photon by a grain of silver halide. When exposed, the silver halide is converted to metallic silver. The greater the number of silver halide crystals that are converted to metallic silver, the blacker the film will be once developed. The unexposed silver halide crystals are cleared off the film during the fixing portion of the processing procedure. A film that has not been exposed to any ionizing radiation or visible light will be clear after processing because none of the silver halide crystals were converted to metallic silver (Fig. 6-15).

Film Types

The two general categories of film used in diagnostic radiography are screen and nonscreen.

Screen film. Screen film is manufactured with silver crystals that are sensitive to fluorescent light emitted from intensifying screens and less sensitive to ionizing radiation. This type of film requires less exposure of x-rays to produce a quality image because of its high sensitivity to fluorescent light.

For many years, screen film has primarily been "blue-sensitive," that is, highly responsive to the ultraviolet,

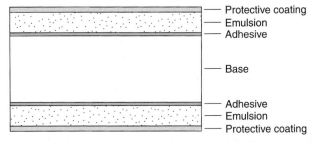

Figure 6-14 *Cross section of x-ray film.*

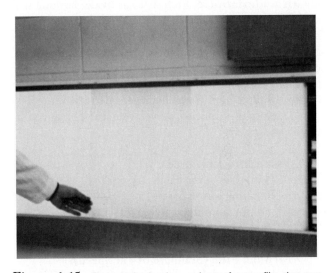

Figure 6-15 *Photograph showing a sheet of x-ray film that was unexposed and processed. Because the silver crystals in the film emulsion were never exposed to light or x-rays, all of the unexposed silver crystals were cleared off the film during the processing procedure.*

violet, and blue spectrum of light. Today, newer films have been developed that are sensitive to green light as well. The importance of this is linked to the new generation of intensifying screens known as rare-earth screens. Some rare-earth screens emit primarily a green spectrum of light, whereas calcium tungstate uses phosphors that convert the energy of x-rays into blue light. Because of this variation, it is important to match a suitable film to an appropriate screen.

Nonscreen film. Nonscreen film is exposed by the direct action of x-radiation. This type of film is manufactured to be more sensitive to ionizing radiation. Because there is no intensification of the x-ray beam, greater exposures are required. However, because intensifying screens are not used, there is no loss of detail due to the screens. The resulting radiographs have greater detail. This film is of particular value in bone or dental radiography, but because of the necessity for greater exposure, nonscreen film should be used only for areas where tissue thickness is minimal.

One problem with nonscreen film is the absence of a strong protective cover. The film is normally packaged in a light-tight envelope made of heavy paper. Because this paper offers little protection, the film is highly sensitive to pressure (e.g., from a dog's nails when extremities are being radiographed).

Film Speed

Film is manufactured with various speeds through the use of different-sized silver halide crystals. Speeds of radiographic films are determined from the exposures required to produce an image with adequate density. The exposure range over which acceptable densities are produced is known as **film latitude.** Film that has "wide" latitude will accept a significant variation in exposure factors or processing without exhibiting a great change in density. On the one hand, wide-latitude film is considered a "forgiving" film. Narrow-latitude or high-contrast film, on the other hand, requires considerably less change in exposure factors or processing to alter the radiographic density.

To maintain simplicity, we will examine film speed in three basic groups:

Fast Film (Ultraspeed):
Has larger silver halide crystals
Requires less exposure by x-rays or fluorescent light from intensifying screens
Produces a grainier image that lacks definition
Has less latitude in exposure factors and processing
Medium Film (Standard or Par Speed):
Is most widely used in veterinary radiography
Represents a compromise between fine grain and speed
Has a medium latitude in exposure factors
Slow Film (High Detail):
Has smaller silver halide crystals
Requires greater exposure by x-rays or fluorescent light from intensifying screens
Produces an image that is less grainy and has greater definition
Has greater latitude in exposure factors

In veterinary radiography, the most common film is medium speed, also known as *standard* or *par speed*. This category is a compromise between fine detail and speed. Medium-speed film is suitable for a wide range of examinations and acts as a standard by which manufacturers rate other films. Medium-speed film is often the only type of film stocked in a veterinary practice.

Film Care

Because of the delicate nature of x-ray film, specifically in terms of the emulsion layer, film handling and storage are of great importance.

Film boxes should be stored on end so that the film is vertical. If the film is stored horizontally for an extended period or if any pressure is placed on the film, the emulsion on each sheet may blend together. The result may be a "block" of x-ray film that is useless. The temperature of storage is also important. The storage area should be cool (10° to 15° C) and have a low relative humidity (40% to 60%). Excessive heat and humidity can result in softening of the film emulsion, causing the film to stick together and, in effect, decrease its shelf life.

Film should not be stored near any source of ionizing radiation or where vapors from formalin, hydrogen peroxide, or ammonia can reach it. These substances can cause fogging.

Close observation of the film expiration date, marked on the end of each box, is also important. If a number of boxes are stored, the film should be used in sequence to avoid expired film.

FILM-SCREEN SYSTEMS

For the technologist to know the speed of the film and screen alone is not enough. Knowledge of the film-screen "combination" is vital. The combined speed or "system speed" is what determines the exposure requirements for any given clinical situation. A wide assortment of film-screen combinations is available. The choice of a system depends on the desired image detail and necessary speed requirements. In some instances the fastest system possible must be used because of the anticipated studies or because of the relatively low-powered equipment.

A numeric value is assigned to each film and screen type. Unfortunately, each film manufacturer has its own manner of speed evaluation, and these may not correlate. In veterinary practice, a medium-speed system (300 to 400) is the most common because of its versatility. See Tables 6-1 through 6-3 for lists of common film-screen system speeds. To acquire specific information concerning the system speed in a given practice, the film manufacturer should be consulted. In general the numeric value for film-screen combination ranges from about 25 to 1200. Although these numbers resemble those of the ASA

TABLE 6-1

KODAK FILM SCREEN SPEED SYSTEMS: GREEN EMITTING

FILM TYPE	Screen			
	LANEX FINE	LANEX MEDIUM	LANEX REGULAR	LANEX FAST
TML	100	300	400	600
PDG	100	300	400	600
TMG	100	300	400	600
OL	100	250	400	600
OG	100	250	400	600
TMH	—	600	800	1200
PDH	—	600	800	1200

TABLE 6-2

AGFA (FORMERLY STERLING/DUPONT) SYSTEM

SCREENS	ORTHOCHROMATIC-G PLUS (GREEN-SENSITIVE FILM)	ORTHOCHROMATIC-GL (GREEN-SENSITIVE FILM)	BLUE-SENSITIVE B FILM	BLUE-SENSITIVE M FILM
GREEN-LIGHT EMITTING				
Ortho 100	100	100		
Ortho 400	400	400		
BLUE-LIGHT EMITTING				
CaWO4			100	—
Blue 800			800	400

TABLE 6-3

3M VETERINARY X-RAY SYSTEM

	Film		
SCREENS	3M ULTRA DETAIL PLUS (GREEN-SENSITIVE FILM)	3M ULTIMATE 2000 (GREEN-SENSITIVE FILM)	3M STANDARD BLUE (BLUE-SENSITIVE FILM)
3M Asymetrix Detail	350	350	
3M Asymetrix Fast Detail	550	550	

(ISO) system for photographic film, the standards are not as rigid.

Key Points

1. Approximately 95% of the exposure recorded on a film is due to the light emitted from the intensifying screens. Only 5% of the exposure of the film results from the ionization of x-rays.
2. A cassette *must* maintain close contact between the intensifying screens and the film.
3. The primary function of the intensifying screen is to reduce the amount of radiation exposure required to produce a diagnostic radiograph.
4. Faster screen speeds require a small exposure and produce less detail; slow screens require a larger exposure and produce greater detail.
5. Screens must be cleaned regularly. Dirt and hair on the screen can cause radiographic artifacts and lead to wrong diagnoses.
6. X-ray film is manufactured with various speeds and latitude.

Review Questions

1. The conversion of x-radiation into visible light occurs via:
   a. double-emulsion x-ray film.
   b. the processor.
   c. intensifying screens.
   d. the cassette.

2. To absorb backscatter, the back of most cassettes is lined with:
   a. lead.
   b. felt.
   c. an intensifying screen.
   d. an x-ray film.

3. Intensifying screens allow:
   a. a higher kVp to be used.
   b. a lower mAs to be used.
   c. a longer exposure time to be used.
   d. a higher mAs to be used.

4. The main advantage of today's rare-earth-coated intensifying screens is:
   a. its emission of light is in the blue region of the UV spectrum.
   b. its ability to convert a latent image into a visible image.
   c. they are easy and inexpensive to separate from the earth.
   d. they have a higher x-ray–to-light conversion efficiency.

5. Which of the following statements is true?
   a. Screen film is more sensitive to ionizing radiation.
   b. Nonscreen film produces poorer detail.
   c. Nonscreen film is highly sensitive to fluorescent light emitted from intensifying screens.
   d. Nonscreen film requires greater exposure.

6. True or false: Both the fluoroscopic image and x-ray image viewed on a view box are considered positive images because the intensity of light emitted by each part of the screen is proportional to the amount of x-rays striking that part of the screen.

7. A processed film that has not been exposed to ionizing radiation or visible light will appear:
   a. black.
   b. green.
   c. clear.
   d. blue.

8. Which of the following are appropriate storage conditions for radiographic film?
   a. 10° to 15° C, 40% to 60% humidity, vertical
   b. 1° to 15° C, 40% to 80% humidity, vertical
   c. 10° to 20° C, 40% to 60% humidity, horizontal
   d. 10° to 15° C, 50% to 60% humidity, horizontal

9. Which of the following film-screen systems is *most commonly* used in veterinary medicine?

   a. High-speed system
   b. Low-speed system
   c. Medium-speed system
   d. The fastest system possible

Suggested Readings

Bushong SC: *Radiologic science for technologists*, ed 7, St Louis, 2001, Mosby.

Eastman Kodak Company: *Kodak: the fundamentals of radiography*, ed 12, Rochester, NY, 1980, Kodak.

Koblik P, Hornof JW, O'Brien TR: Rare-earth intensification screen for veterinary radiography: an evaluation of two systems, *Vet Radiol* 21:224-232, 1980.

Morgan JP, Silverman S: *Techniques in veterinary radiography*, ed 4, Ames, IA, 1987, Iowa State University Press.

Schmidt RA et al: Evaluation of cassette performance: physical factors affecting patient exposure and contrast, *Radiology* 146:801-806, 1983.

chapter 7

Film Processing

CHAPTER OUTLINE

The Darkroom
Film-Processing Solutions
Film-Processing Techniques

Silver Recovery
Film Identification
Film Filing

OBJECTIVES

Upon completion of this chapter, the reader should be able to do the following:

- List and describe the three qualities of a good darkroom
- Describe an organized darkroom
- State the various methods of darkroom lightproofing
- State the correct safelight to be used with blue-light- and green-light-sensitive film
- List the five basic steps of film processing
- Describe the primary function of the developer
- List and describe the six developer components
- State the function of the rinse bath
- State the two basic purposes of the fix bath
- List and describe the six components that make up the fix solution

- Describe the methods of recognizing exhausted chemicals
- Explain how biologic growth can be minimized in processing tanks
- List and describe the nine steps in manual processing
- State the two primary advantages of automatic processing
- Describe how an automatic processor works
- List the basic maintenance procedures recommended for an automatic processor
- List the three methods and reasons for silver recovery
- State the importance of film identification, and list the several methods of film identification available
- State the recommended criteria for filing a radiograph

GLOSSARY

Accelerators: Chemicals that increase the pH of the developer and subsequently increase the rate of developing.

Acidifiers: Compounds that accelerate the fixing process and neutralize the alkaline developer.

Buffers: Compounds in the fixer that maintain proper solution pH.

Clearing agents: Also called fixing agents; a portion of the fixer that dissolves and removes the unexposed silver halide crystals from the film emulsion.

Developer: A chemical solution that converts the latent image on a film to a visible image by converting the exposed silver halide crystals to black metallic silver.

Developing agents: Chemical solutions used to convert a latent image on x-ray film to a visible image.

Fixation: The process by which the unexposed silver halide crystals are removed from the film and the gelatin is hardened.

Fixer: The chemical solution used during fixation.

Hardeners: Chemicals added to the fixing solution or to developers in automatic processors to prevent excessive emulsion swelling.

Latent image: An invisible image on unprocessed x-ray film after it has been exposed to ionizing radiation or light.

Preservatives: Chemicals that prevent rapid decomposition of the developer or fixer.

Restrainers: Often potassium bromide and potassium iodide are used as restrainers or antifoggants. Restrainers limit the action of the developing agent to the exposed silver bromide crystals in the film.

Reticulation: A darkroom artifact produced by variable chemical temperatures that cause irregular expansion and contraction of the film emulsion, resulting in a mottled density appearance.

Rinse bath: A solution (usually water) used to remove excess developer solution before the film is placed in the fix tank.

Solvent: Water; dissolves the ingredients of the developer or fixer and diffuses the chemical into the emulsion of the film.

Stop bath: A solution of acetic acid and water used to "stop" the development of the x-ray film by rapidly neutralizing the alkaline developer solution.

INTRODUCTION

Proper film processing is vital to the production of a quality radiograph. Many believe that the use of appropriate exposure factors is the only component necessary to produce a "good" film. This is far from the truth. The production of a good-quality radiograph depends on many factors, one of which is film processing. When manual processing was the norm in human hospitals, it was said that 90% of all poor-quality radiographs were the result of poor processing. This is still relevant in veterinary radiography. One goal of the radiographer is to eliminate all possible pitfalls that may inhibit quality. A common area for pitfalls is the darkroom. Although quality does not begin in the darkroom, it could possibly end there.

The basic principles of radiographic processing have remained the same over the years, but technology has made remarkable advances toward automation. However, although an increasing number of veterinary practices use automatic film processing, the majority still process radiographs by hand with tanks to hold the processing chemicals. Both methods of processing are discussed in detail in this chapter.

THE DARKROOM

Three qualities constitute a good darkroom. A darkroom must be (1) clean, (2) organized, and (3) lightproof.

Although individual darkrooms may vary in design, all should possess the same qualities. A darkroom should be separate from the radiographic suite and should be used for only one purpose: processing exposed radiographs. Ideally, the room dimensions should be no less than 6 × 8 feet (2.6 × 2 m), and the layout should reduce the possibility of film damage. Most of the work in the darkroom is performed with minimal illumination. Therefore it is important that the darkroom be organized so that all of the equipment can be located quickly and easily. And, of course, cleanliness is crucial. This is the only room where both the intensifying screens and the x-ray film are exposed to the air. If the countertops are dirty and soiled with chemicals, it is easy for both to be sucked into the cassette as it is opened, possibly causing damage to the intensifying screens.

Another factor that is often overlooked in the darkroom is climate control. Because the film emulsion is extremely sensitive to heat and humidity, good ventilation and temperature control are mandatory. A darkroom should be relatively cool and should have low humidity. The specific temperatures and humidity for proper film care are described in Chapter 6.

Organization

There should be essentially two sides to the darkroom: a dry side and a wet side (Fig. 7-1).

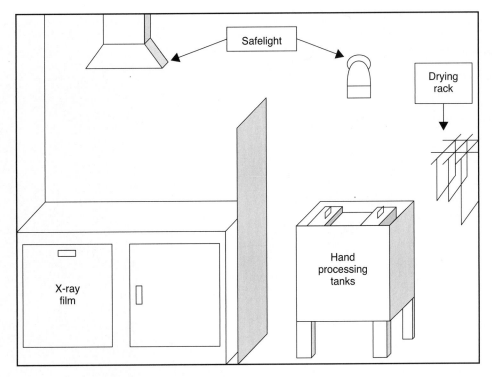

Figure 7-1 *A sample dark room layout showing a wet side and a dry side.*

Dry side. The dry side of the darkroom is where the cassettes are unloaded and reloaded. A countertop or table-top large enough to accommodate the largest cassette in the open position should be available. The tabletop should be constructed of a material that allows frequent cleaning, which is necessary to reduce the source of dark-room artifacts that can potentially get on the film. It must be impossible for chemicals to splash into the dry side. At no time should anything "wet" be brought to the dry side. It is customary to store film under the dry table, either in a cupboard or in a film bin, to allow easy access for reloading cassettes (Fig. 7-2). Film hangers for each size of film should be hung above the table on the dry side on an appropriate bracket. Brackets can be purchased commercially or constructed inexpensively using large hooks found at any hardware store.

Film hangers are available in two designs: channel hangers and clip hangers (Fig. 7-3). Channel hangers tend to retain water and chemicals and need special cleaning and drying to prevent contamination of the dry side. Films must also be removed from the channel hangers to be dried. However, clip hangers are more fragile than the channel type. When the clips are used frequently over a period of time, they become weak and lose the ability to "stretch" the film. The clips also puncture the four corners of the film, which, when filed, can scratch other films in the same envelope. It is important to cut off the corners of films processed with clip hangers before filing to prevent this. When more than one film is processed at the same time in the tanks, the clips on the hangers can scratch neighboring films.

Wet side. The wet side of the darkroom is where the actual chemical processing is performed. A darkroom that hand processes films usually consists of three tanks containing developer, water, and fix solutions. Various tank designs are available. The three tanks can be individually freestanding and warmed as required by an immersion heater (placed in the developer). Alternatively, the developer and fix tanks can be placed in one large tank filled with thermostatically controlled water. The latter system is preferred and can be purchased as a complete package constructed with 3- or 5-gallon (9- or

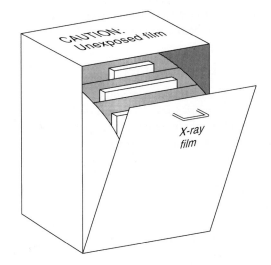

Figure 7-2 *Film storage bin. When closed, the film is stored light-tight in a vertical position.*

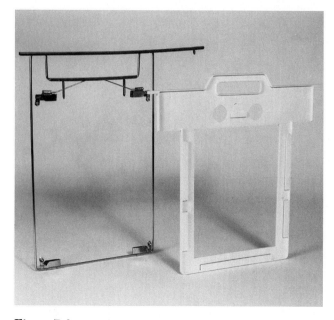

Figure 7-3 *A clip film hanger (left) versus a channel film hanger (right).*

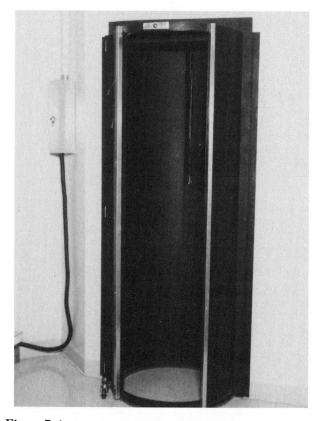

Figure 7-4 *A revolving door for the darkroom. This door is an effective means of entering and exiting the darkroom without risking exposure of the film to light.*

22-L) individual tanks. The water tank is usually four times the size of the smaller developer and fix tanks. The central water tank should have a circulating water system to provide a way to regulate temperature and rinse chemicals off the films during the processing procedure. A thermometer is an essential piece of equipment for the processing tanks because radiographic film is developed for a specified time on the basis of the temperature of the chemicals.

The wet side should also have a film-drying area consisting of either a drying rack or a drying cabinet. The drying rack should be placed in a dust-free area to prevent artifacts from sticking to the wet films. A drying cabinet is a heated forced-air unit that hastens the drying process. A viewing screen is also recommended on the wet side to evaluate radiographs. A "wet" film can be viewed, and, if a second radiograph is required, the radiographer can immediately evaluate the error. This is best achieved in the darkroom before too much time has elapsed.

Darkroom Lightproofing

As mentioned earlier, one criterion of a good darkroom is that it be lightproof. Light leaks in a darkroom can cause significant film fog; therefore taking appropriate measures to lightproof the darkroom is imperative. Lightproofing a room is more difficult than may be expected. The first step is locating the light leaks. Small light leaks may not be perceptible until the eyes have acclimated to the dark, and it may be necessary to spend 5 minutes waiting for the eyes to adapt. To achieve a truly lightproof room, a number of tasks may be necessary.

The entrance to the darkroom is a common site for light leaks. A double-door system or revolving door is preferred but not always practical in a veterinary practice (Fig. 7-4). The first step in lightproofing a standard door is to fit it tightly into its frame against strips of felt or rubber molding. Weather stripping is also useful around doors to prevent the entrance of light. Light entering from underneath the door can be prevented by a vapor seal designed specifically for the bottom of a door. A sliding bolt lock or doorknob lock prevents someone from accidentally entering the darkroom at an inopportune time. A suspended ceiling can be a radiographer's nightmare. It may be necessary to place a large black sheet of plastic above the ceiling tiles to prevent light in adjacent rooms from entering through the seams.

It is a common fallacy that the walls of a darkroom should be "dark." The opposite is true. The walls of the darkroom should be painted white or cream with a good-quality, washable paint. By painting the walls a light color, more reflection of the safelight is produced, providing a more visible work environment. If the quality and intensity of the light are "safe," the illumination reflected from any surface also is "safe," regardless of the color of that surface.

Darkroom safelight. Correct safe lighting in the darkroom is crucial. A "safe" light means that the light produced will not affect the film. Radiographic film is sensitive to ultraviolet light. Safelights use a small-wattage bulb and a special filter to eliminate the light from the blue and

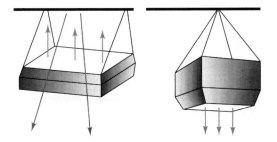

Figure 7-5 *Indirect (left) and direct (right) safe lighting for the darkroom.*

green spectrum. The light bulb should be 15 watts or less. The filter varies by manufacturer. The most common types are a brown filter (Wratten 6B, Kodak) for blue-light-sensitive film and a dark-red filter (Wratten 6BR or GS-1) for green-light-sensitive film. The dark-red filter is recommended because of its versatility: both green-light- and blue-light-sensitive film can be used in this lighting.

Safelights should be positioned so that darkroom work can be performed without fumbling. There are two types of safe lighting: direct and indirect (Fig. 7-5). Direct lighting is a diffused light that shines directly over a work area such as the dry or wet side of the darkroom. Indirect lighting is a filtered light directed toward the ceiling and reflected over the entire room. Indirect lighting is often combined with direct lighting. At no time should the safelight be closer than 4 feet from a work area. A safelight that is too close, has a too-high wattage bulb, or has incorrect filtration may cause film fog.

The efficiency of a safelight can be tested; this is discussed in Chapter 10. Remember, no light is "safe" if the film is exposed to it for a prolonged period. Therefore the film bin should be open only when removing or replacing film. Fogging will result even with a safelight if the bin is left open or if film is left on the counter.

FILM-PROCESSING SOLUTIONS

Film processing, whether it is manual or automatic, comprises five basic steps: (1) developing, (2) rinsing or stop bath, (3) fixing, (4) washing, and (5) drying. The first step in learning how to process a film is a basic understanding of the processing solutions. The chemical solutions can be purchased in a number of forms. Powders and liquid concentrates are those most commonly used in veterinary practice. Water is added to the concentrates according to the manufacturer's instructions to produce the proper amount of solutions for the processing tanks. Preparing the chemicals correctly is important or the resulting solution may adversely affect the radiographic product.

Every effort should be made to keep the chemical solutions at a specified temperature—any variance may adversely affect the radiographic product. At temperatures below those recommended, some of the chemicals may become sluggish in action and may produce an underdeveloped or underfixed radiograph. At temperatures much above those recommended, the chemical activity is too high for manual control.

Keep in mind also that all of the chemical solutions should be the *same* temperature. If the chemicals vary greatly in temperature, film reticulation can result. **Reticulation** appears as a mottled density on a finished radiograph and is caused by irregular expansion and contraction of the film emulsion.

A quality assurance program should be established and maintained in the veterinary practice. This program allows reproducibility, and it gives the radiographer confidence in the exposures used on each radiograph (see Chapter 10).

The Developer

The **developer** is a chemical solution that converts the **latent image** on a film to a visible image. The primary function of the developer is to convert the exposed silver halide crystals to black metallic silver.

The developing time usually is specified by the chemical manufacturer. Keep in mind that the developer temperature affects the developing time. Time-temperature developing is preferred over visual inspection when using the manual processing technique. This manual inspection is called "sight developing," which consists of increasing or decreasing the time according to visual inspection of film density while the film is still in the tank. This technique requires attention and skill and is often subject to error. Sight developing should be avoided if at all possible.

The developer consists of developing agents, accelerators, preservatives, restrainers, hardeners, and a solvent.

1. **Developing agents** are composed of chemical compounds such as hydroquinone or phenidone that can convert exposed grains of silver halide to black metallic silver. The developing agent has little or no effect on the unexposed silver halide crystals.
2. **Accelerators** are chemicals that increase the activity of the developer. Substances such as potassium carbonate or sodium carbonate are used to increase the pH to an alkaline range of 9.8 to 11.4. This increase in pH causes the emulsion to swell and soften, allowing the developing agent to work more effectively.
3. **Preservatives** prevent the rapid oxidation that can occur with alkaline developing agents. They also help maintain a stable development rate and prevent staining of the emulsion layer.
4. **Restrainers** limit the action of the developing agent to the exposed silver bromide crystals in the film.
5. **Hardeners** are often added to developers in automatic processors. They harden the film during processing and prevent excessive swelling of the

emulsion. If the gelatin emulsion were to swell extensively, it could be damaged by the rollers in the automatic processor.

6. The **solvent** consists of water to dissolve the chemicals.

The Rinse Bath

After a film has been in the developer, it retains a substantial amount of developer in the gelatin (approximately 60 mL on a 14- × 17-inch film). If the film were transferred directly into the fixer, the alkaline developer would neutralize the acid of the fixer. The **rinse bath** serves to stop the developing process, rinse the developer from the film, and prevent carryover contamination to the fixer.

Normally, the rinse bath consists of circulating water in which the film is rinsed for 30 seconds. A chemical solution such as acetic acid and water can be used as another method of stopping the development procedure. This chemical solution is called a **stop bath.** In automatic processing, a rinse or stop bath is not necessary because the rollers tend to remove excess developer from the film before it reaches the fix tank.

The Fixer

After a film has been properly developed and the exposed silver halide crystals have been converted to metallic silver, one other step involving the silver crystals remains. The unexposed silver halide crystals remaining on the film are unaffected by the developer solution and must be removed. If these silver crystals were to remain on the film, they would discolor and darken with exposure to light.

The **fixer** serves two basic purposes: (1) it clears the unexposed silver halide crystals from the film, and (2) it hardens the gelatin coating so that it can be dried without damaging the film surface. This process is known as **fixation.** The general guideline is that the film should be fixed for twice the development time to ensure maximum hardening of the emulsion. (Note: A radiograph can be viewed briefly after it has been in the fix for 1 minute and then returned after evaluation.)

The fix solution consists of clearing or fixing agents, preservatives, hardeners, acidifiers, buffers, and a solvent.

1. **Clearing** or fixing **agents** dissolve and remove the unexposed silver halide crystals from the film emulsion. The two most common clearing agents are sodium thiosulfate and ammonium thiosulfate. The agent actually changes the appearance of the film from a milky white to a clear or transparent image. The black metallic silver portion of the film remains the same.

2. **Preservatives** such as sodium sulfite prevent decomposition of the fixing agent.

3. **Hardeners** such as aluminum salt prevent excessive swelling of the gelatinous emulsion during the fixation procedure and softening during the wash procedure. Hardeners shorten the drying time by essentially preventing the film from becoming waterlogged.

4. **Acidifiers** are compounds that accelerate the action of the other chemicals and neutralize any alkaline developer possibly carried over into the acidic fix solution.

5. **Buffers** are chemical compounds added to the solution to maintain the desired pH. Buffers stabilize the acidity against the addition of alkaline developer by carryover. Without the addition of a buffer, the alkaline developer would neutralize the acid of the fix solution, thus shortening the effective life of the fix. Some buffers also prevent sludge formation in the fix bath.

6. The **solvent** consists of water. Its purpose is to dissolve the other ingredients and assist the fixing agent to diffuse into the emulsion layer of the film. Once the fixing agent is in the emulsion layer, it can dissolve the unexposed silver halide crystals. The solvent then helps by carrying the silver halide away from the film.

The Wash Bath

The wash portion of the development procedure is vital to a quality radiograph. Unfortunately, the value of the wash procedure is often underestimated and inadequately performed. The purpose of the wash is to remove the processing chemicals from the film surface. If a film is not washed properly for a long enough period, the image will eventually discolor and fade.

Films should be washed in circulating water so that both surfaces of the film receive fresh water continuously. In manual processing, the average suggested wash time is 20 to 30 minutes with periodic agitation or water circulation. In automatic processing, the water system of the processor keeps a constant flow of temperate water through and around the wash rack and film.

Wetting Agent

A common problem of drip-drying films is the possibility of water spots or other drying streaks. The drying process can be hastened and some artifacts avoided by using a wetting agent bath known as a *surface-tension reducing agent* (a detergent). These agents are commercially available.

Solution Replenisher

In manual processing, chemical depletion is a natural result of chemical carryover into adjacent tanks. As much as 60 mL of developer can be "carried" on a 14 × 17-inch piece of film into the rinse bath. Both the developer and the fixer need frequent replenishment to keep chemicals at a proper level and cover the entire film.

Replenishment solutions are available in powder and liquid concentrate form. The liquids are easier to work with because they eliminate the problem of powder settling on the countertops of the darkroom. Generally, the replenisher has a higher concentration than the original solution to maintain chemical potency.

Solution Replacement

Exhausted processing chemicals (or, more likely, oxidation/ deterioration of chemicals in limited-use situations) are a primary cause of poor-quality radiographs. The developer and fixer solutions are often the last elements checked when a film has poor quality, yet exhausted chemicals are the most common cause. Chemicals that have lost their potency will produce radiographs that have increased film fog and decreased contrast and density.

Determining the need for developer and fixer replacement is based on a couple of clues. In general the developer solution turns from brown to green when it needs to be changed. The developer usually requires less changing than the fixer. Because each film brought into the fix tank brings with it a certain amount of water from the rinse tank, the fix tends to become diluted. The activity of the fix solution, however, cannot be determined by a change in color. The fixer needs to be changed when the "clearing time" is greater than 2 to 3 minutes. Clearing time refers to the amount of time it takes the fixer to clear the unexposed silver halide crystals off the film. If all the silver complexes have not been removed, the film will fog or even turn black when exposed to light. In general chemicals in hand-processing tanks should be changed every 4 to 6 weeks.

Biologic Growth

A common problem encountered in hand-processing tanks is the growth of bacteria and fungi, particularly during the warm seasons of the year. Bacterial and fungal growth can produce slime deposits that can build up in the tanks. The bacteria, fungi, and occasional algae originate from the air, personnel, or incoming water supply. If not controlled, they can cause corrosion of the metal surfaces, as well as artifacts on the films. The growth rate of the organisms is increased in stagnant water.

Biologic growth can be inhibited by good housekeeping. When the chemicals are changed and the processing tanks are drained, they should be scrubbed and quite possibly soaked with 1% chlorine bleach and water. The wash tank of automatic processors should be drained at the end of the day to reduce biologic growth. A simple filtering system can prevent organisms from entering through the water line.

FILM-PROCESSING TECHNIQUES

As mentioned earlier, radiographic film can be processed in one of two ways: manually or with an automatic film processor. The manual process takes approximately 1 hour to produce a finished product. With an automatic processor, a film can be processed and dried in as little as 90 seconds. Both methods produce a quality radiograph, and it is a matter of preference as to which method best suits the clinical situation.

Manual-Processing Procedure

The manual-processing procedure (by hand) should be standardized as much as possible. By establishing a routine and following it, mistakes made in the darkroom are less likely. Normally, the developing tanks are positioned so that the processing procedure starts at the left and ends at the right. In other words, the developing tank is on the left, the wash tank in the center, and the fix tank on the right (Fig. 7-6).

Manual processing is not a difficult procedure, and the technique can be learned in a relatively short period.

Step 1—Preparation. Before the film is processed manually, the chemicals should be at the proper temperature (normally 20° C [68° F]) and should be stirred. Because the chemicals are suspensions, they tend to settle to the bottom of the tanks (Fig. 7-7). The paddles used to stir should not be shared between tanks; the developer paddle should never go into the fix tank and vice versa. (Note: Even slight fixer contamination in the developer can render it useless.) At this point, the white lights should be turned off and the safelight turned on.

Step 2—Unloading the cassette. Care should be taken when removing the film from the cassette. Fingernails should not be used as a tool to remove the film from the

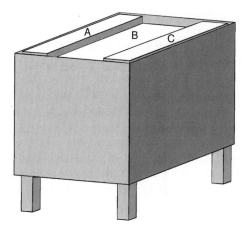

Figure 7-6 *Bird's-eye view of hand-processing tanks. The tank labeled* ***A*** *is the developer,* ***B*** *is the rinse and wash tank, and* ***C*** *is the fix tank.*

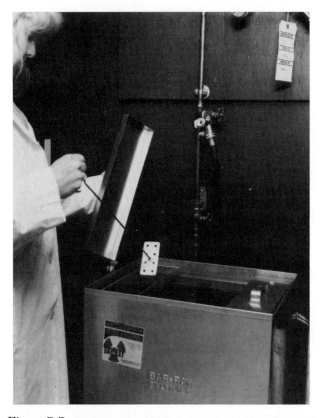

Figure 7-7 *Stirring the chemicals before hand processing is important. The chemicals tend to settle to the bottom of the tanks. Processing without stirring the chemicals could result in unevenly developed film.*

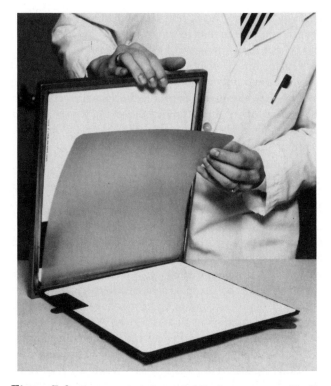

Figure 7-8 *Proper method of removing film from a cassette. The film should be "dumped" out of the cassette rather than "pried" out using fingers.*

cassette corners. This technique can damage the sensitive intensifying screens. The proper method of removing the film is to open the backplate of the cassette and gently shake the top so that the film can be grasped by the corner between the thumb and the forefinger (Fig. 7-8). The x-ray film should be handled by the corners or edges only. The cassette should be closed while it is being labeled and loaded onto the film hanger. Film labeling is discussed at the end of this chapter.

Step 3—Loading the film on a hanger. A tension clip hanger is loaded by inserting the film into the bottom, stationary clips first, then rotating the hanger right side up and inserting the film into the movable spring clips (Fig. 7-9). The film should be stretched so that it is taut enough to "bounce a coin on it." Taut mounting will prevent the film from touching adjacent films or walls in the processing tank.

If a channel hanger is used, it should be held in one hand while sliding the film into the channels with the other. All sides and corners of the film should be checked for correct placement in a channel. Once the film is in position, the top hinge can be closed.

Step 4—Developing the film. The film is immersed in the developing tank, and the hanger is agitated two or

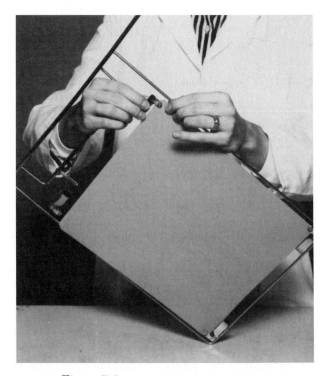

Figure 7-9 *Loading film on a clip film hanger.*

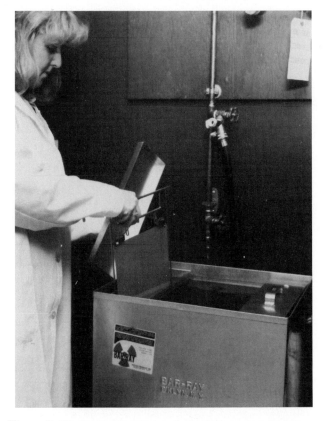

Figure 7-10 *Immerse the film into the developing tank, and agitate two or three times to remove any air bubbles that may be attached to the side of the film. The developer temperature should be 68° F.*

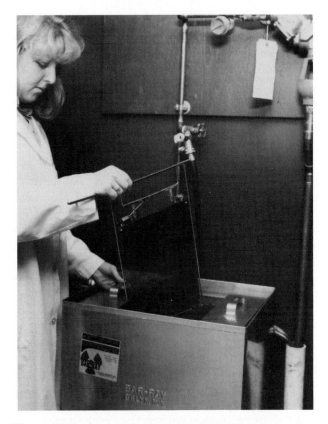

Figure 7-11 *Rinse the film for 30 seconds. Before moving the film to the fix tank, tilt the hanger to allow for faster water drainage.*

three times to remove any air bubbles from the film surface (Fig. 7-10). The lid on the developer tank is replaced, and the timer is set for the appropriate development time. At this juncture, the hands should be dried and the cassette reloaded with film. Care should be taken in the reloading process. The replacement film should meet all four corners of the cassette before closing so that no portion of the film is compressed in the cassette seams.

Step 5—Rinsing the film. When the timer sounds, the film should be removed from the developer rapidly to avoid excessive dripping back into the developer tank (Fig. 7-11). For fast drainage, the hanger should be tilted so that the chemical carryover (spent developer) goes into the rinse or stop bath. Preventing the used developer from adding volume to the developer tank assists accurate tank replenishment. The film is immersed in the rinse bath and agitated for 30 seconds.

Step 6—Fixing the film. After the film has been in the rinse tank for 30 seconds, it should be drained of excess water and immersed in the fix tank (Fig. 7-12). The film is agitated two to three times to remove any air bubbles on the film surface, and the timer is set for the appropriate duration. The duration of the fixation process is usually twice the clearing time and until after the film has

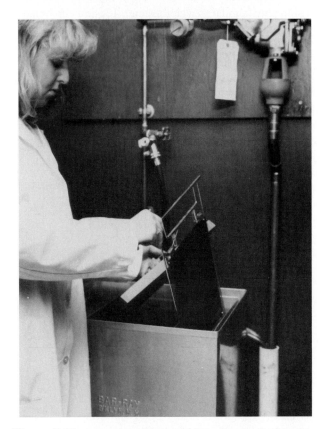

Figure 7-12 *Immerse the film into the fix tank, and agitate the film a few times to remove any air bubbles. The film should be fixed for twice the developing time or a minimum of 10 minutes.*

lost its "milky" appearance. The milky appearance refers to the unexposed silver halide crystals that remain on the film. Once the silver is removed, the image will appear clear or transparent. After the film has been in the fix for 1 minute, it may be viewed briefly to evaluate the quality of exposure and positioning. Putting the film back into the fix tank after evaluation for a total of at least 10 minutes is important to allow maximum hardening of the film surface.

Step 7—Washing the film. The film is removed from the fix quickly so that chemical carryover (spent fixer) enters the wash tank. As with the developer, preventing carryover from entering the fix tank allows for accurate fix replenishment. The film should wash for 20 to 30 minutes (Fig. 7-13). The wash time depends on the water flow and exchange rate of the bath. The flow should have approximately eight complete changes per hour.

Step 8—Optional final rinse. If facilities permit, a wetting agent can speed the drying time and prevent water marks on the film surface. The film is briefly dipped in the wetting agent before drying (Fig. 7-14).

Step 9—Drying the film. The film should be dried in a dust-free area to prevent artifacts from sticking to the wet film surface. If channel hangers are used, the films should be removed from the hangers and hung with clips on a tension wire (similar to a clothesline). Tension clip hangers can be hung on a drying rack (Fig. 7-15).

The films should be well separated and never allowed to touch each other while wet. When the films are dry, the sharp points on the corners of those processed with tension clip hangers must be trimmed before filing. Trimming the sharp points prevents scratching the emulsion of adjacent films. The films can now be inserted into the appropriately labeled envelope.

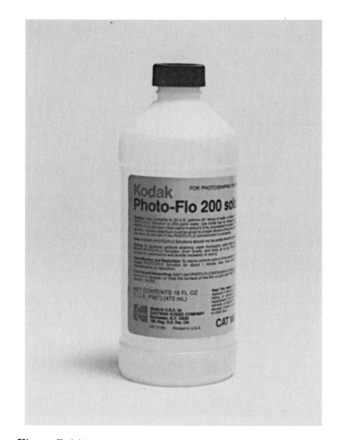

Figure 7-14 *A wetting agent. An optional step in the hand-processing procedure is to immerse the film briefly into a final rinse known as a wetting agent. The wetting agent decreases drying time and the chance of streaking while the film is drying.*

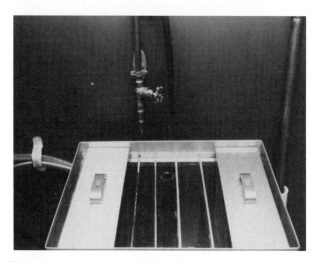

Figure 7-13 *Wash the film for 20 to 30 minutes. If more than one film is being washed at once, provide enough space between each film to allow adequate washing.*

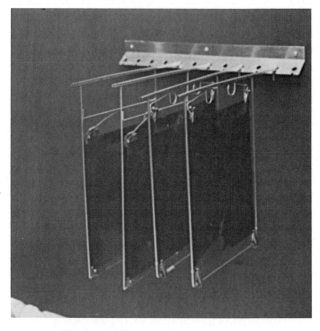

Figure 7-15 *Films drying on a drying rack.*

Automatic Processing

Automatic processing involves the same basic principles as manual processing: the film is developed, fixed, washed, and dried. However, automatic processing has two major advantages over the manual method: (1) It is a highly standardized procedure with consistent quality, and (2) it can produce a dry radiograph in a short time period. In a practice or clinic that has a high radiographic output, the amount of saved labor hours is remarkable. However, the cost of an automatic processor is a primary factor that precludes many veterinary practices from having this convenience. For a low-volume veterinary practice, the expense of an automatic processor may not be justified.

A darkroom is still necessary for automatic processing, except that a much smaller space is required. A counter is necessary on the dry side to unload and load the cassettes, but the wet side consists of the processor only. Because the processor has its own drying mechanism, which uses heated forced air or infrared methods, an exhaust system or extractor fan is necessary to prevent excessive heat and fume accumulation while in operation. Some automatic processors are designed to protrude through the dark-room wall so that a special exhaust system is unnecessary (Fig. 7-16). In this case the film is introduced into the processor in the darkroom, and a finished, dry film exits in the adjacent room.

HOW AUTOMATIC PROCESSORS WORK

Automatic processors involve roughly the same routine as manual processing, except they operate at much higher temperatures and have specially formulated chemicals to speed development. The film is transported through the processor by a series of rollers similar to a conveyer belt in

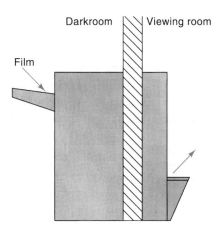

Figure 7-16 *Cross section of an automatic processor that is designed to protrude through the darkroom wall. The film is loaded into the processor in the darkroom, and the finished product is delivered to the adjacent room.*

a factory. The rollers are driven by a motor and move the film at a constant speed (Fig. 7-17). The film must be transported at a controlled speed to ensure that it is developed, fixed, and washed for the proper amount of time.

The exposed film is fed onto the tray of the machine and is then transported through the chemical baths and dryer by the roller assembly. In order to speed development, the rinse between the developer and fix is eliminated. The carryover chemicals are removed by compression as the film passes through squeegee rollers placed between the developer and the fix baths.

PROCESSING CHEMICALS

The solutions are kept in peak condition because fresh chemicals are replenished at a predetermined rate on the

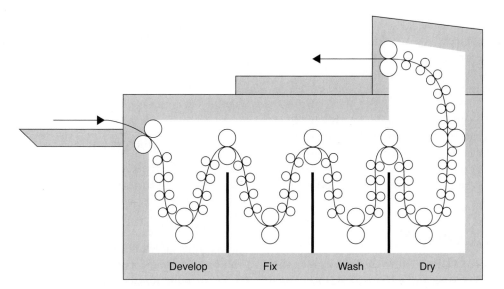

Figure 7-17 *Cross section of an automatic processor showing its series of tanks and rollers. The rollers act as a conveyer belt, carrying the film from the developer, to the fix, to the wash, and finally to the drying racks.*

basis of machine usage. Without replenishment, chemical activity of the processing solutions would decrease with use, as in manual processing. Accurate replenishment is essential to proper processing of film and to long life of the solutions. Generally, when the film is fed into the processor, pumps are activated to infuse replenisher from storage tanks to the baths inside the machine. The added replenisher is blended with the existing processing solutions by the recirculation pumps. Recirculation of the developer and fixer has two functions: to thoroughly mix the solutions and to help maintain the proper temperature and chemical activity. Excess processing solutions flow over the top of the tanks into the drain. Careful observation of the external replenishment tanks is necessary to maintain adequate chemical levels within the machine.

The temperature of the chemicals is constantly monitored and controlled within fine limits by a thermostatically operated water system. As in manual processing, the purpose of the water system is not limited to washing the films. Circulating water controls the temperature of the processing chemicals as well.

The method of water temperature control varies with the design of the processor. Hot and cold water may be blended to a proper temperature by a thermostatic mixing valve before the water enters the machine. Other processors are available with cold incoming water that is electrically heated to the desired temperature.

PROCESSOR MAINTENANCE

As with all mechanical devices, automatic processors can break down and need repair. In order to minimize the need for frequent repairs, proper maintenance is essential (Fig. 7-18). Recommendations for cleaning and maintenance procedures are furnished by the processor manufacturer and may include the following:

> Solution level check
> Replenishment rate check
> Temperature check
> Roller operation check
> Rinsing and wiping of all roller racks
> Regular cleaning of tanks

Although service engineers usually come as quickly as possible in the event of a processor breakdown, a backup processing system is recommended. It is worthwhile to have the necessary chemicals and containers available so that emergency hand processing can be performed if required.

SILVER RECOVERY

In the present age of environmental awareness, recycling has become a national standard. Silver is a valuable natural resource and should be recycled whenever possible. In fact, most states in the United States require silver

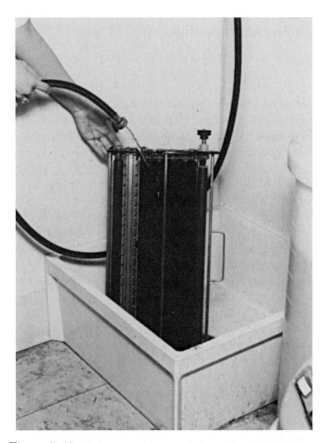

Figure 7-18 *Processor maintenance is imperative to ensure proper film processing. The roller racks should be removed from the processor on a routine basis (at least monthly, depending on its use) and rinsed with warm water to remove any debris.*

recovery as part of pollution control. All heavy metals are considered pollutants and cannot be disposed of in a septic system. Silver recovery is not only environmentally wise but economically prudent.

During the processing procedure, the silver contained in the x-ray film emulsion either is transformed into black metallic silver in the developer solution or is removed by the fix solution. These two byproducts, the fix solution and old radiographs, contain silver that can be recovered.

Three methods of silver recovery from the fix solution exist: (1) metallic replacement, (2) electrolytic recovery, and (3) chemical precipitation.

Metallic Replacement

The metallic replacement method of recovery removes the silver from the exhausted fix by replacing the silver in the solution with another metal. The metal is normally iron in the form of steel wool. The steel wool dissolves in the acid fix solution and physically replaces the suspended silver, thus allowing the silver metal to precipitate to the bottom of the recovery unit.

A metallic replacer unit usually consists of a cartridge loaded with steel wool. The fix is poured into a top receptacle and allowed to "trickle" through the steel wool

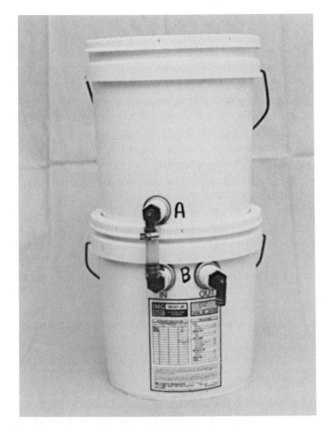

Figure 7-19 *A Vault Junior trickle silver recovery system. The exhausted fix is poured into empty tank A and "trickled" through tank B. The fix containing no silver can then be discarded.*

(Fig. 7-19). The fix containing no silver can then be discarded (according to local pollution control ordinances). Beware, the acid from the fix solution can harm pipes if water flow is low.

Up to 99% of the available silver can be recovered with the metallic replacement method, but the purity of recovered silver is low. This method is relatively inexpensive and is recommended for low-volume hand-processing systems.

Electrolytic Recovery

Electrolytic recovery involves two electrodes (an anode and a cathode) placed either directly into the fix tank or into a separate holding container for the exhausted fix solution. As an electric current passes between the two electrodes, the silver is attracted to the cathode and the silver is plated (collected) on the cathode. The advantage of electrolytic recovery is that the fix solution may be reused; however, this requires much chemical analysis. This method of reclamation recovers high-purity silver but is generally less efficient than metallic replacement.

Chemical Precipitation

The chemical precipitation technique of silver recovery involves addition of more chemical compounds to pre-

cipitate the silver from the fix solution. As the chemicals are added to the fix, the silver floats to the bottom of the receptacle and forms a sludge. The sludge is then filtered, dried, and packed to be sold to a refiner.

Gold and silver refiners and dealers often purchase exhausted fix solution and old radiographs to reclaim the silver that they contain. Companies that purchase fix solutions and discarded radiographs usually are listed in the telephone directory's Yellow Pages.

Before radiographs can be sold for reclamation, however, the veterinary practice is legally required to keep them for a specific length of time. The legal requirement for retaining radiographs is 7 years, but it is advisable to keep them until the patient is deceased.

FILM IDENTIFICATION

Every radiograph should be properly labeled with essential information so that it can be identified at a later date. In many instances, additional radiographs must be taken to evaluate healing or advancement of disease. Without proper labeling, progressive evaluation would be difficult. There is also the legal aspect to consider. If a medicolegal problem were to arise, a radiograph without proper labeling is of little value in a court of law. The only legal labeling of a radiograph is what is in the film emulsion.

Several methods can be used to label a radiograph, and it is a matter of personal preference which method is adopted. All labeling systems should provide the same basic information: (1) name and address of the hospital practice or veterinarian; (2) date the radiograph was taken; and (3) patient identification including name of the owner and patient name, age, sex, and breed.

Lead Markers

One of the simplest methods of film labeling is with lead letters and numbers that are placed directly on the cassette before exposure. The lead digits can be placed in a holder or taped directly to the cassette (Fig. 7-20). The lead absorbs the primary radiation from the x-ray beam so that the film directly under the lead is left unexposed and appears transparent. It is possible to purchase prepared holders that include the name and address of the clinic spelled out permanently in lead letters. With a permanent prepared holder, only the date and identification of the patient must be changed.

The disadvantages of this method of labeling are that it can be time consuming and that the small lead digits are easily lost. In addition, it limits tight collimation because the area outside the patient must be exposed to provide an image of the label.

Lead-Impregnated Tape

Another method of labeling a radiograph during exposure is with disposable lead-impregnated tape. Writing on the

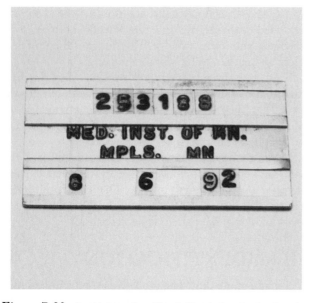

Figure 7-20 *Lead letters placed in a holder designed to be placed on top of a cassette for film identification.*

Photoimprinting Label System

One label system uses a lead blocker placed on the outside of the cassette, an identification card, and a photimprinter. The lead blocker prevents exposure to a 3 × 7 cm area, to which identification can be exposed in the darkroom. Following the removal of the film in the darkroom, but before processing, a typed or written card is placed between the unexposed portion of the film and a light source (photoimprinter). The light is "flashed," and the written information on the card is recorded on the previously unexposed area (Fig. 7-22).

New cassettes can be purchased with the lead blocker already installed, or 3 × 7 cm pieces of lead can be purchased and installed on the cassette face. It is important that the lead blockers be placed in the same corner of all the cassettes. This consistency will prevent "flashing" the wrong corner in the darkroom. Caution should also be taken to ensure that no anatomic area of interest is positioned in the blocker area, where no exposure will be made.

tape with a ballpoint pen or pencil displaces the soft lead, leaving indentations. These indentations create a difference in density that allows x-rays to penetrate to the film. The tape is then placed on a holder that has the name and address of the facility permanently attached (Fig. 7-21). The lead tape can be used to label left or right, time intervals for a series of radiographs, and markers to indicate the direction of the x-ray beam for oblique views.

The lead-impregnated tape is available in 50- or 100-foot rolls or in precut 3-inch strips. The manufacturer of the tape will usually supply the lead-tape holder with the specified facility information.

Miscellaneous Markers

Right (R) and left (L) markers are essential to identify a right or left limb or to identify the right or left side of the thorax or abdomen (Fig. 7-23). Markers may also be necessary at times to identify a unique view, orientation, or beam direction. Labeling the front and rear limbs may be necessary, particularly in equine radiography, because the anatomic structures of the distal limbs of the horse are virtually identical. Time-sequence labels are also available for special procedures to indicate time elapsed after the administration of radiopaque contrast media.

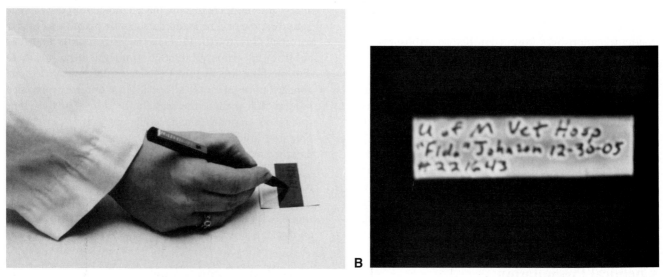

A   **B**

Figure 7-21 *Lead-impregnated tape. **A**, The lead is displaced by means of a pointed writing instrument, leaving indentations. **B**, After the information is written, the tape is adhered to the cassette and exposed during the radiographic procedure.*

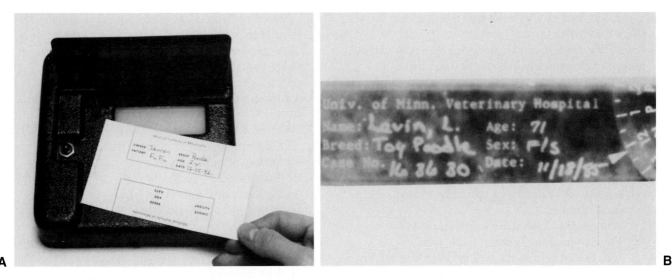

Figure 7-22 *Film identification method known as photoimprinting.* **A,** *The identification card is placed on the photoimprinter with the film placed over the card. The imprinter is then closed, and a light is "flashed" under the card, which exposes the information onto the film.* **B,** *After the film is processed, the identification can be clearly seen in the corner of the film.*

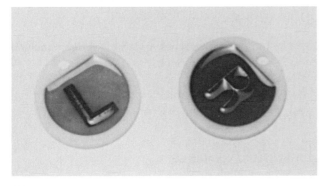

Figure 7-23 *Left (L) and right (R) markers for anatomic orientation.*

Other Identification Methods

If identification was forgotten before exposure, it is possible to write on the film before development with a pencil or other pointed device. The pressure from the pointed device will distort the film emulsion and record the information, which will remain on the film throughout the processing procedure. Scratching the information into the emulsion while it is still wet is also possible. Other methods include a permanent marker or a piece of adhesive tape on the dry film.

All of these identification techniques are considered temporary and are undesirable for routine film identification. They are not considered adequate markings should legal proceedings arise regarding the patient.

FILM FILING

An organized filing system is mandatory in any veterinary practice. It would be pointless to spend time correctly exposing the x-ray film and properly identifying and processing it only to place it indiscriminately in a pile of other radiographs taken in the past. In order to use x-rays for future referral or follow-up examinations, they must be placed in a suitable holder that is labeled appropriately.

Before x-rays are filed, they must be completely dry. When x-ray film is hand processed with tension clip hangers, the corners often remain wet until the film is removed from the hanger and allowed to dry. Cutting the corners of the film where it was attached to the hanger clips may alleviate this problem.

The best method of filing radiographs is in a large, 14 × 17 inch (35 × 43 cm) file envelope, regardless of the film size. Smaller-sized x-ray film could be filed in smaller envelopes, which would be a bit less expensive, but the smaller envelopes tend to get lost among the larger when filed together. Film filing envelopes can be purchased from any radiographic sales service.

Filing the films in a logical manner is crucial. The envelopes should be labeled with a description of the patient, name of owner, date, and type of radiographic examination performed. The type of filing system will vary. Normally, a numeric system is used, employing either a patient case number or a file number. Some clinics have a color-code system for easy retrieval.

*K*EY *P*OINTS

1. The darkroom must be clean, organized, and *completely* lightproof.
2. All chemicals must be kept at the same temperature to prevent reticulation.
3. Bacterial, fungal, and algal growth are a common problem in hand-processing tanks and can be

controlled by cleaning tanks with 1% chlorine bleach when they are drained.

4. Exposed x-ray film can be processed manually in hand tanks or automatically in an automatic processor.

5. The legal requirement for keeping radiographs is 7 years; however, it is advisable to keep them until the patient dies.

REVIEW QUESTIONS

1. The walls of the darkroom should be white or cream colored because:
   a. it is easier to keep these colors clean.
   b. these colors help to detect light leaks.
   c. film can be held to the wall to determine quality.
   d. more reflection of the safelight is produced, providing a more visible working environment.

2. Which of the following is true regarding safelights?
   a. They should be 20 watts or less.
   b. They must be at least 4 feet from the work area.
   c. The brown filter is for blue-light-sensitive film.
   d. Film can be exposed to safelights indefinitely with no ill effects to the film.

3. What is the ideal pH at which to develop radiographs?
   a. 9.8 to 11
   b. 7.2 to 7.4
   c. 2
   d. 7.8 to 9.8

4. Unexposed silver halide crystals remaining on the film are removed at this stage.
   a. Rinsing or stop bath
   b. Washing
   c. Fixing
   d. Developing

5. Advantages of automated film processing include:
   a. consistent quality of processed radiographs.
   b. dry radiographs are produced in a short time.
   c. a much smaller space is necessary.
   d. All of the above.

6. These two byproducts of development contain silver that cannot be disposed of in a septic system:
   a. radiographs and developer.
   b. radiographs and fix solution.
   c. radiographs and rinse.
   d. fix and rinse.

7. Which of the following is not required on the label ID of a radiograph?
   a. Initials of radiographer
   b. Date taken
   c. Patient name and owner name
   d. Name and address of hospital or veterinarian

8. All of the following are legally valid methods of labeling a radiograph except:
   a. lead-impregnated tape.
   b. lead marker.
   c. permanent marker after development.
   d. photoimprinting label system.

9. True or false: The radiographer must recover silver in the veterinary clinic. (explain)

10. The most effective types of darkroom doors include:
    a. doors that do not lock.
    b. revolving door system.
    c. double door system.
    d. Both b and c are correct.

SUGGESTED READINGS

Eastman Kodak Company: *Kodak: the fundamentals of radiography,* ed 12, Rochester, NY, 1980, Kodak.

Gray JE et al: *Quality control in diagnostic imaging,* Rockville, Md, 1983, Aspen.

Morgan JP, Silverman S: *Techniques in veterinary radiography,* ed 4, Ames, Iowa, 1987, Iowa State University Press.

Ticer JW: *Radiographic techniques in small animal practice,* ed 2, Philadelphia, 1984, WB Saunders.

chapter *8*

Radiographic Technique Evaluation

CHAPTER OUTLINE

Physics of Radiography: A Review
Density and Contrast: A Review
Viewing a Radiograph

Evaluation of Radiographic Technique
Practical Applications
Other Error Considerations

OBJECTIVES

Upon completion of this chapter, the reader should be able to do the following:

- Describe briefly how radiography works
- Define density and contrast
- Describe the correct method of viewing a radiograph on a view box
- State the two questions of evaluation for a radiograph
- State the standard change made to kilovoltage to alter the penetration of x-rays
- State the standard change made to milliamperage to alter radiographic density
- List other error considerations that can cause a poor-quality radiograph

• **89** •

Contrast: The measurable difference between two adjacent densities.

Density: The degree of blackness on the radiograph.

Kilovoltage peak (kVp): An exposure factor that is responsible for accelerating the electrons from the cathode to the anode, thereby determining the penetrating power of the x-rays.

Milliamperage-seconds (mAs): An exposure factor that determines the total number of x-rays and the time they can be released from the x-ray tube to expose the film.

INTRODUCTION

The production of a quality radiograph depends on many factors. Chapters 1 through 7 provide a detailed explanation of these factors, yet there is one element that remains to be discussed. This crucial factor involves the evaluation of a finished radiograph.

The ability of the technologist to evaluate a radiograph properly is imperative. Without this ability, the attempt to attain quality is futile. The need for a second radiograph at one time or another is unavoidable, no matter what the skill level of the radiographer. Assessing what is wrong with the radiograph and making the proper corrections are the skills that we seek. Radiographic quality depends on the technologist's understanding of the concepts and variables that produce a good radiograph.

Radiography can be an extremely difficult subject to grasp. The concepts of x-rays and how they are formed is complex. Mastering the physics of radiography is a challenge for all students. Quality radiographs are not attained by "luck" but by a conscious understanding of the variables. This understanding can change a radiographic image into a piece of artwork.

PHYSICS OF RADIOGRAPHY: A REVIEW

X-rays are generated in an x-ray tube, which consists of a cathode side (with a negative electrical charge) and an anode side (with a positive electrical charge). In the tube a stream of fast-moving electrons is attracted and directed from the cathode to the anode. As the electrons collide and interact with the atoms of the target on the anode, a great amount of energy is produced; 1% of this energy is in the form of x-rays.

The cathode consists of a wire filament that emits electrons when it is heated. The temperature of the filament is controlled by the milliamperage (mA) setting on the console of the machine. As the mA is increased, the temperature of the filament increases and the filament produces more electrons. The period during which the electrons (x-rays) are permitted to leave the x-ray tube is in fractions of seconds. The number of electrons and the period set for their release determine how many x-rays are available. Therefore the **milliamperage-seconds (mAs)** controls the total number of x-rays produced.

The anode, which attracts negatively charged electrons, is made of a metal (tungsten) that can withstand high temperatures. This tolerance is necessary because of the great amount of heat produced during the collision of electrons. Ninety-nine percent of the energy produced during the impact of electrons is in the form of heat; only 1% is x-rays. The anode is constructed at an angle so that the electrons are directed downward (toward the cassette) through a window in the metal housing of the x-ray tube.

The electron speed necessary to create a high-energy impact is achieved by applying thousands of volts (kilovolts) across the anode and cathode. The available electrons travel at a tremendous speed toward the positive charge of the anode. High voltage produces x-rays with greater penetrating power and intensity. Therefore the **kilovoltage peak (kVp)** controls the penetrating power of the x-rays.

DENSITY AND CONTRAST: A REVIEW

Chapter 5 gives a detailed explanation of density and contrast. To apply this knowledge in a practical manner, a review of the salient points is necessary.

Radiographic **density** is defined as the degree of blackness on the radiograph. Density is primarily affected by mAs. The higher the mAs, the greater the density and the more blackness on the radiograph. The mAs controls the total number of x-rays available. If x-rays make film black, more x-rays emitted by the machine will cause more blackness on the film. The kVp may also influence density and increase blackness on the radiograph; mAs and kVp can be differentiated because the latter also changes the contrast.

Radiographic **contrast** is defined as the density difference between two areas of a finished radiograph. If the difference between two areas is great, the contrast is described as high. If there is a slight difference in density (an overall gray appearance), the contrast is low.

Radiographic contrast is affected primarily by the kVp. The higher the kVp, the lower the contrast. The kVp governs the penetrating power of the x-ray beam. If a high kVp setting is used, more x-rays reach the film because of the increased penetration (pushing power). The kVp also governs the energy spectrum of the x-ray beam. High-kVp techniques have not only higher peak-energy photons in the beam, which enhance patient penetration, but also have a wider variation of energies among all the photons in the beam, allowing for more variation in the degree of penetration among the photons. This broad photon energy spectrum contributes to the greater gray spectrum (long scale or low contrast), even with high- versus low-kVp techniques. Scatter radiation, which is more prevalent with high-kVp techniques, can influence image contrast as well, but the use of grids and the use of fast screens (i.e., rare-earth screens) minimize this effect.

VIEWING A RADIOGRAPH

To evaluate a film accurately, a radiograph should be viewed on an evenly lit view box in a semidarkened room. The view-box screen should be clean, and all light bulbs should be in working order.

The film position on the view screen is also important. Veterinary radiographers generally follow the medical viewing protocol. Ventrodorsal or dorsoventral anatomy such as an abdomen or a thorax should be placed on the view screen so that the animal's head is at the top (or toward the top of the viewer) and the patient's right is on the viewer's left. In other words, the patient should be in the position to shake the hand of the viewer. All laterally positioned anatomy should face the viewer's left, with the spine at the top.

EVALUATION OF RADIOGRAPHIC TECHNIQUE

In the technical evaluation of a radiograph, two basic questions should be asked:

1. Is the film too light or too dark?
2. Is there proper penetration?

Question 1

The answer to the first question is not always elementary. When examining a radiograph that seems too light, some personnel may conclude that the film is over-exposed. This misunderstanding stems from experience with photography. In taking a picture with a camera, increased exposure time increases the brightness of the picture. Radiography is the opposite of photography in this respect. The x-rays (more exposure) make the film black. If a radiograph is underexposed, it will appear too light. In this case, either kVp or mAs needs to be *increased*.

If the radiograph is too dark, it is overexposed and either the kVp or mAs should be *decreased*. To determine whether the kVp or the mAs should be altered, the second question needs to be asked.

Question 2

When it has been established that the radiograph is either too light or too dark, the next step is to determine why. This leads to the second question, which concerns penetration. This question is the key to finding the solution. If the penetration is inappropriate, then the kVp should be changed (increased for a light film or decreased for a dark film). If the penetration is satisfactory, then the mAs should be changed (increased for a light film or decreased for a dark film). In essence, we need to rule out a problem with kVp. If the kVp is ruled out as the problem, then the solution lies with altering the mAs. The flowchart in Figure 8-1 can be used as a reference for quick evaluation.

Penetration Evaluation of a Radiograph That Is Too Light

When looking at a radiograph that is too light, it is understood that either the kVp or the mAs needs to be increased. The second question, concerning penetration, must be asked: Have the x-rays adequately penetrated the patient and reached the x-ray film? On a film with adequate penetration, the anatomic silhouettes (outlines) are visible. For example, when viewing an abdominal radiograph with adequate penetration, the outlines of the liver, spleen, kidneys, and bowel would be visible. If the penetration is inadequate, the outlines of the abdominal structures would not be visible and the radiograph would look almost completely white in some areas.

Adequate penetration: Increase mAs 30% to 50%
Inadequate penetration: Increase kVp 10% to 15%

Penetration Evaluation of a Radiograph That Is Too Dark

When a radiograph is too dark, either the kVp or the mAs must be decreased. We then need to ask whether the radiograph has appropriate penetration. When a radiograph is overexposed (too dark), the question is not whether there is adequate penetration power, but rather whether there is too much penetration power of the x-ray beam. Overpenetration of a patient is determined by looking at the contrast of the radiographic image, specifically, by looking at the bone tissue compared with the surrounding soft tissues. Remember, as a general rule, high kVp results in low contrast—a gray radiograph. If the bone tissue is gray and not much contrast exists between the bone and adjacent soft tissue, there was too much

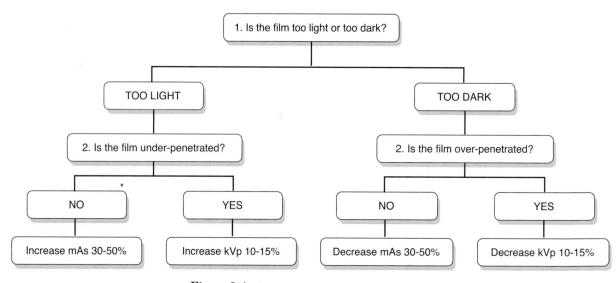

Figure 8-1 *Exposure technique evaluation flow chart.*

penetration of the patient. On the other hand, if the contrast is still acceptable and the bone tissue is relatively white compared with the surrounding soft tissues, it is evident that the kVp is not the problem and that the mAs should be altered.

Not overpenetrated: Decrease mAs 30% to 50%
Overpenetrated: Decrease kVp 10% to 15%

A quality radiograph has adequate penetration, sufficient density, and good contrast. These requirements differ for bone and soft tissue. To be of diagnostic value, a radiograph must have the correct scale of contrast. For soft tissue, low contrast is desirable. An abdominal radiograph, for example, should have many soft grays to assist differentiation of the intraabdominal organs (Fig. 8-2). High contrast is necessary for bone radiography. The image should be well defined, and the bone should be distinct from the surrounding tissue.

PRACTICAL APPLICATIONS

In the four scenarios that follow, evaluate the specified radiographs by answering the two basic questions (Figs. 8-3 to 8-6).

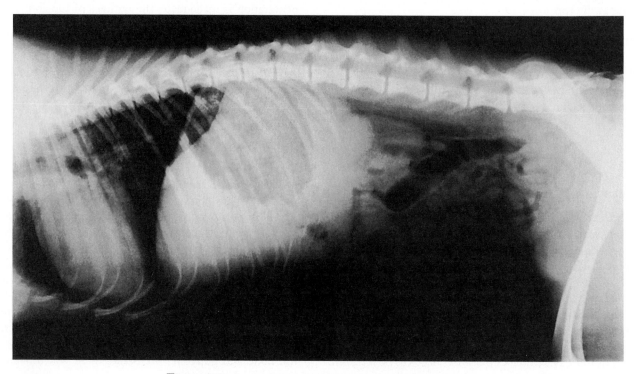

Figure 8-2 *A properly exposed abdominal radiograph (lateral view).*

CASE STUDY 1

EXAMINE THE RADIOGRAPH IN FIG. 8-3

The film is too light. This indicates insufficient kVp or mAs. A close examination shows that the anatomic parts are not clearly visible, especially in the cranial portion behind the diaphragm. This information answers the second question; there is insufficient penetration. The kVp should be increased 10% to 15% to improve the penetration and density and to achieve a suitable scale of contrast for an abdominal radiograph.

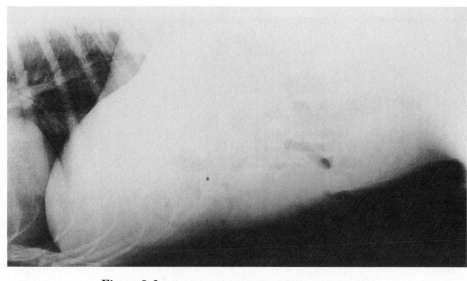

Figure 8-3 *Scenario 1 for evaluating radiographic technique.*

CASE STUDY 2

EXAMINE THE RADIOGRAPH IN FIG. 8-4

Initial examination indicates that the radiograph is too light. On further inspection, the anatomy is visible but lacks density; there is adequate penetration. By increasing the mAs by 50%, the image will be improved by the creation of more blackness on the radiograph. This correction will enhance the overall density and appearance of the film.

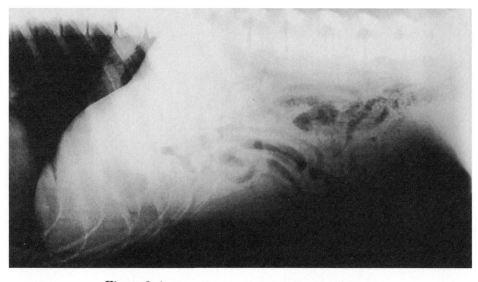

Figure 8-4 *Scenario 2 for evaluating radiographic technique.*

CASE STUDY 3

EXAMINE THE RADIOGRAPH IN FIG. 8-5

The radiograph is too dark. The film has too much density. The problem is difficult to assess until the contrast (which is inappropriate) is examined. Examination of the bone tissue in the radiograph demonstrates that the spine and pelvis are gray, an indication of overpenetration. The radiograph will be of greater diagnostic value if the kVp is decreased by 10% to 15%.

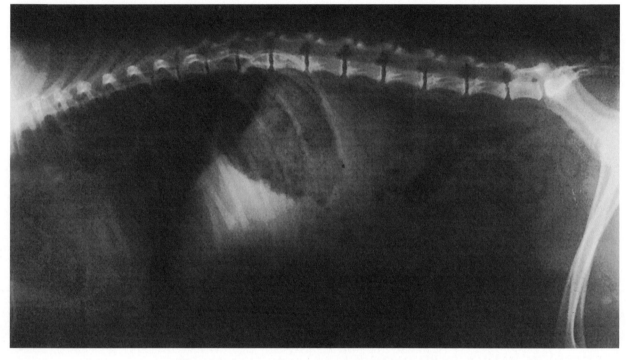

Figure 8-5 *Scenario 3 for evaluating radiographic technique.*

CASE STUDY 4

EXAMINE THE RADIOGRAPH IN FIG. 8-6

This radiograph is also too dark. Close examination of the contrast proves that the radiograph is not overpenetrated. The bone tissue is relatively white compared with surrounding soft tissues, despite the excessive density on the film. On the basis of this observation, it can be concluded that the kVp level is appropriate but that the mAs should be decreased by 30% to 50%.

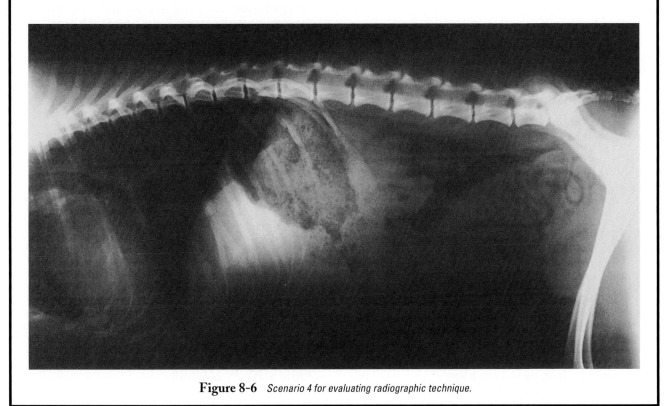

Figure 8-6 *Scenario 4 for evaluating radiographic technique.*

OTHER ERROR CONSIDERATIONS

When evaluating a quality radiograph, the technologist should be aware of other pitfalls that can generate a poor-quality film. Certain standards must be maintained in the darkroom, as well as with the radiographic equipment. A radiograph that has been processed with exhausted chemicals or exposed with a poor film-screen combination, for example, will mimic a film that has been underexposed. In order to eliminate all possible pitfalls, proper quality control should be maintained. Chapter 10 covers this topic in detail.

KEY POINTS

1. When viewing a radiograph of an animal's abdomen in a ventrodorsal or dorsoventral position, the animal's head is at the top of the viewbox and the patient's right is on the viewer's left.

2. A slight difference in density is low contrast (long scale); a high difference in density is high contrast (short scale).

3. The most important question to be able to answer when evaluating the technique of a radiograph is, "Is the film overpenetrated or underpenetrated (an indication of kVp)?" In other words, "Are the outlines of all structures visible?"

4. For soft tissue, low contrast (many shades of gray) is desirable. For bone tissue, high contrast is desirable.

5. The state of chemicals and screen-film combinations can affect the quality of radiographs and mimic inappropriate exposures.

REVIEW QUESTIONS

1. The degree of blackness on the radiograph is:
   a. contrast.
   b. quality.
   c. mAs.
   d. density.

2. Density is determined *primarily* by:
   a. mAs.
   b. kVp.
   c. exposure time.
   d. screen speed.

3. Radiographic contrast is determined *primarily* by:
   a. exposure time.
   b. film speed.
   c. kVp.
   d. mAs.

4. If a radiograph includes many shades of gray, which of the following is also true regarding the image?
   a. High contrast, low kVp
   b. High contrast, high Kvp
   c. Low contrast, high kVp
   d. Low contrast, low kVp

5. When viewing a radiograph of a laterally positioned animal:
   a. the head should be at the top of the viewbox.
   b. the head should face the viewer's left with the spine at the top.
   c. the head should face the viewer's right with the spine at the top.
   d. the head should face the viewer's left with the spine at the bottom.

6. An overexposed film appears _____; to correct this, _____.
   a. too dark; increase mAs or kVp
   b. too light; increase mAs or kVp
   c. too light; decrease mAs or kVp
   d. too dark; decrease mAs or kVp

7. What action should be taken if it is difficult to see anatomic silhouettes on an abdominal film and the film is too light? Why?

   a. Increase kVp by 10% to 15%; shorten wavelength, increase penetrating power
   b. Increase mAs by 10% to 15%; increase the number of x-rays reaching the film
   c. Increase mAs by 30% to 50%; increase density
   d. Decrease mAs by 30% to 50%; lengthen wavelength and decrease penetrating power

8. You have determined that penetration is adequate for a particular abdominal film. All abdominal structures are well outlined. However, the film has an overall appearance of being too light. What should you do next?
   a. Increase mAs by 30% to 50%
   b. Increase kVp by 10% to 15%
   c. Increase mAs by 10% to 15%
   d. Increase kVp by 30% to 50%

9. A thoracic film is too dark. The bone tissue is relatively white. What is the next step?
   a. Increase mAs by 50%
   b. Increase kVp by 15%
   c. Decrease mAs by 15%
   d. Decrease mAs by 50%

10. How does kVp affect scatter radiation?
    a. As kVp increases, scatter radiation decreases.
    b. kVp has no effect on scatter radiation.
    c. As kVp increases, scatter radiation can increase.
    d. As kVp decreases, scatter radiation can increase.

Suggested Readings

Cunliffe-Lavin LM: Radiographic technique: a ray of hope, *Vet Technician J* 12:444-451, 1991.

chapter 9

Developing a Technique Chart

CHAPTER OUTLINE

Suggested Charts
Technique Chart Formulation
Procedure Flowchart: Variable kVp Technique Chart

Other Formulation Methods
Modification Recommendations

OBJECTIVES

Upon completion of this chapter, the reader should be able to do the following:

- State the purpose of a technique chart
- List the factors that influence a technique chart
- List the recommended screen variable kilovoltage peak (kVp) technique charts on the basis of anatomy for a small-animal practice
- Name the equipment necessary for variable kVp technique chart formulation
- Describe how the exposure factors—kVp, milliamperage, and exposure times—are calculated
- List the base milliamperage-seconds (mAs) factors for the three speeds of screens

- Describe the modifications necessary for the exposure technique when using a grid
- State in chronologic order the steps essential for variable kVp technique chart formulation
- Describe how the appropriate mAs setting is chosen for all of the anatomic areas of small animals
- Describe the method of formulating a variable mAs technique chart
- Describe the modifications necessary when a technique chart fails to produce adequate radiographic density because of patient size, condition, or pathology

Santes' rule: Calculation for determining an approximate amount of kilovoltage (kVp) necessary for a given anatomic area on the basis of measurement and the grid being used: (2 × tissue thickness in cm) + source-image distance + grid factor = kVp.

Technique chart: A chart based on tissue thickness and anatomic part that can be consulted for predetermined machine settings.

INTRODUCTION

The **technique chart** is an invaluable resource for a radiographer. Its purpose is to provide a consistent method of choosing the proper exposure factors to create a diagnostic radiograph. On the basis of the thickness of tissue and anatomic area of the body, the radiographer can consult the technique chart for a predetermined machine setting. Without this resource, one would have to calculate a new technique each time a radiograph is taken or use a questionable technique performed previously. A technique chart prevents the need for second radiographs due to inappropriate exposure factors.

Every x-ray machine should have its own formulated technique chart. It is often thought that a successful exposure technique used on x-ray machine A will also work on x-ray machine B. This is not true. Even x-ray machines of the same make and model vary in both quantity and quality of output because of variations in input voltage and calibration. Several other factors influence the chart:

> Speed of screens
> Age of screens
> Speed of film
> Source-image distance (SID)
> Amount of beam filtration
> Temperature and time of film processing
> Type of grid

The factors that affect a technique chart should be standardized as much as possible. The SID, amount of beam filtration, film processing, and type of grid should remain constant. The success of a technique chart depends on the radiographer's willingness to maintain continuity of the variables.

The only variables that should change are the types of film and screens used. The film type and speed should be preselected and limited. The screen speed chosen should fit the needs of the practice and be limited to one or two speeds. A veterinary practice that has a number of screen types must formulate many technique charts. Working with a number of film and screen types that have coinciding technique charts can be confusing and may increase errors.

SUGGESTED CHARTS

Another misconception is that just one technique chart is necessary for an x-ray machine. On the contrary, anatomic and technical differences call for more than one chart. Several charts may be needed and may include the following:

> Screen and nonscreen
> Grid and nongrid
> Various film-screen combinations
> Species specific
> Anatomy specific

In general, five (screen) variable kVp technique charts based on species and anatomy are recommended for a small-animal veterinary practice:

1. Extremity and skull (canine/feline), no grid
2. Abdomen (canine/feline), with grid
3. Thorax (canine/feline), with grid
4. Pelvis and spine (canine/feline), with grid
5. Avian and exotics, no grid

TECHNIQUE CHART FORMULATION

Several methods are used in veterinary practice to formulate a technique chart; they vary slightly, but all are effective. The method presented here is different from others because of a few shortcuts that the technologist may find helpful. The principles of technique chart formulation can be applied to any species and anatomic area. The method presented here applies to x-ray machines that have variable kVp and exposure time settings.

To create a workable technique chart, a series of trial exposures must be made using a cooperative, average-sized patient. Theoretically, by exposing one radiograph, all five suggested technique charts can be formulated.

Equipment needed for this procedure should be gathered before proceeding. A mature dog with average conformation (neither obese nor emaciated) and weighing approximately 50 pounds is an ideal patient for this procedure. With this size dog, a 14- × 17-inch cassette should be used. Use medium-speed x-ray film because of its versatility in veterinary practice.

Exposure Factors

To formulate a variable kVp technique chart, a test radiograph is made of the canine abdomen in lateral recumbency. The measurement is in the range of 11 to 16 cm, and the exposure factors are based on the screen type and grid ratio used. Remember, any measurement exceeding 10 cm necessitates the use of a grid to reduce fog-producing scatter radiation. For an SID of 40 inches, the following information applies:

- *Kilovoltage:* Use **Santes' rule:** (2 × tissue thickness in cm) + 40 inches + grid factor = kVp
- *Milliamperage:* Highest setting possible
- *Exposure time:* Selection based on milliamperage-seconds (mAs) needed for screen type (discussed next)

Base mAs Factors

An mAs chart is shown in Table 9-1. The following base mAs requirements for the intensifying screens are merely starting points for the radiographer. Each radiographic system may require slightly different exposures.

Screen Type	mAs
Fast (high speed)	2.5 to 10
Medium (par speed)	5 to 12.5
Slow (ultradetail)	30 to 40

Exposure Modification for Grid Use

When using a grid, increased exposure is necessary to maintain adequate radiographic density. The addition of a grid usually requires doubling the exposure time. For example, if the exposure technique needed for a tabletop (nongrid) exposure is 2.5 mAs (1/120 second at 300 mA), the new exposure for grid use would be at least 5 mAs (1/60 second at 300 mA).

The kVp will also need to be modified. The amount of modification varies according to the grid ratio being used.

Grid Ratio	Added kVP to Sum of Santes' Rule
5:1	6 to 8
8:1	8 to 10
12:1	10 to 15
16:1	15 to 20

PROCEDURE FLOWCHART: VARIABLE KVP TECHNIQUE CHART

I. Canine abdomen with the use of a grid
   A. Select a dog
      1. Cooperative adult
      2. Moderate muscling
      3. Average weight (≈ 50 lb)
      4. Hair coat clean/medium to short length

TABLE 9-1

MILLIAMPERAGE-SECONDS (MAS) CHART

TIME (SEC)	25 MA	50 MA	100 MA	150 MA	200 MA	300 MA
$1/120$	0.2	0.4	0.8	1.3	1.7	2.5
$1/60$	0.4	0.8	1.7	2.5	3.3	5
$1/40$	0.6	1.3	2.5	3.8	5	7.5
$1/30$	0.8	1.7	3.3	5	6.7	10
$1/24$	1	2.1	4.2	6.2	8.3	12.5
$1/20$	1.25	2.5	5	7.5	10	15
$1/10$	2.5	5	10	15	20	30
$2/10$	5	10	20	30	40	60
$1/4$	6.3	12.5	25	37.5	50	75
$3/10$	7.5	15	30	45	60	90
$4/10$	10	20	40	60	80	120
$1/2$	12.5	25	50	75	100	150
$6/10$	15	30	60	90	120	180
$3/4$	18.8	37.5	75	112.5	150	225
1	25	50	100	150	200	300
$1 1/4$	31.3	62.5	125	187.5	250	375
$1 1/2$	37.5	75	150	225	300	450
2	50	100	200	300	400	600
$2 1/2$	62.5	125	250	375	500	750
3	75	150	300	450	600	900

B. X-ray machine
   1. Evaluate line voltage
   2. Set SID (constant)
C. Exposure technique
   1. Kilovoltage: Use Santes' rule from lateral measurement plus additional kVp for grid use
   2. Milliamperage: Highest setting possible (to achieve shortest exposure time)
   3. Exposure time: Chosen according to required mAs for selected intensifying screen
D. Film-screen system
   1. Select the intensifying screen that best represents an average speed of other screens (fast screens recommended)
   2. Select film that is not expired or damaged (medium-speed film recommended)
   3. A 400- to 600-speed film-screen system is suggested
E. Grid
   1. Ensure grid position
      a. Placed on cassette centered with central x-ray
      b. Under tabletop with Bucky tray centered to central x-ray
F. Test exposure
   1. Use calculated exposure technique
G. Process in standardized darkroom
   1. Solutions adequate strength (hand processing)
   2. Replenisher at recommended rate (automatic processing)
H. Evaluate radiograph
   1. Too dark: Decrease mAs 30% to 50% or kVp 10% to 15%
   2. Too light: Increase mAs 30% to 50% or kVp 10% to 15%
I. Repeat test exposure if initial radiograph was too light or dark
   1. Repeat Step H (evaluation)
J. Formulate and plot technique chart
   1. Increase or decrease kVp by increments of 2 for each centimeter measurement (see examples)

Trial Exposure: Example 1

Known Information
    Lateral abdomen measurement = 13 cm
    Film speed = medium
    Screen speed = medium
    Grid ratio = 8:1
    SID = 40 inches
    Milliamperage capability = 300
    kVp = 120

Calculation for Kilovoltage
    (2 × 13 [cm]) + 40 (SID) + 8 (grid factor) = 74 kVp

Calculations for mAs
    $300 × \frac{1}{120} = 2.5$ mAs
    $300 × \frac{1}{60} = 5$ mAs

    $300 × \frac{1}{40} = 7.5$ mAs
    $300 × \frac{1}{30} = 10$ mAs
    $300 × \frac{1}{24} = 12.5$ mAs

mAs range based on *medium* screen speed

To choose the appropriate mAs for an abdominal radiograph, consider the tissue density being exposed and the grid being used. As stated earlier, the suggested technique charts for the canine are (1) extremity/skull, (2) abdomen, (3) thorax, and (4) pelvis/spine. All of the anatomic areas listed must be assigned a suitable mAs setting. The thorax, for example, possesses fewer x-ray–absorbing tissues than other parts of the anatomy, and therefore fewer x-rays are necessary to produce a proper radiographic density. The thorax requires 50% to 75% less mAs than the abdomen. The pelvis, in comparison, requires 50% to 75% more mAs because of its increased tissue density. The lowest mAs of the base settings is normally sufficient for tabletop extremity/skull use.

The following is a suggested distribution on the basis of the tissue density of each of the anatomic areas and whether or not a grid is necessary.

Based on a machine milliamperage capability of 300, the following calculation can be made to attain the proper time setting:

$$300 \text{ mA} × \underline{\hspace{2cm}} = 7.5 \text{ mAs}$$
$$\text{where}$$
$$\text{time (sec)} = \frac{1}{40}$$

Trial exposure 1: Plotting the chart.
Following is the exposure setting for a 13-cm canine abdomen:

- kVp = 74
- Milliamperage = 300
- Time in seconds = $\frac{1}{40}$

The plotted technique chart is shown in Table 9-2.

Notice that a grid is used for the abdomen even with a measurement thickness of less than 10 cm. It is possible to use a grid with these thicknesses as long as the proper kVp settings are used. Using a grid for *all* measurements of an abdomen, thorax, and pelvis eliminates the confusion created when grid and nongrid techniques are used on the same chart. The use of a grid for measurements less than 10 cm will not decrease radiographic quality. On the contrary, radiographic quality is increased whenever a grid is used. For all technique charts except the extremity/skull chart, a grid can be used for all centimeter thickness increments.

Trial Exposure: Example 2

The x-ray machine used in veterinary radiography often does not have a 300-milliamperage capability. In this

TABLE 9-2

TRIAL EXPOSURE: EXAMPLE 1

AREA: ABDOMEN	Screen/Film: QFD/UVL			
	Grid: 8:1		SID (Inches): 40	
THICKNESS (CM)	KVP	MA	TIME (SEC)	MAS
5	58	300	$1/40$	7.5
6	60	300	$1/40$	7.5
7	62	300	$1/40$	7.5
8	64	300	$1/40$	7.5
9	66	300	$1/40$	7.5
10	68	300	$1/40$	7.5
11	70	300	$1/40$	7.5
12	72	300	$1/40$	7.5
13	74	300	$1/40$	7.5
14	76	300	$1/40$	7.5
15	78	300	$1/40$	7.5
16	80	300	$1/40$	7.5
17	82	300	$1/40$	7.5
18	84	300	$1/40$	7.5
19	86	300	$1/40$	7.5
20	88	300	$1/40$	7.5
21	90	300	$1/40$	7.5
22	92	300	$1/40$	7.5
23	94	300	$1/40$	7.5
24	96	300	$1/40$	7.5
25	98	300	$1/40$	7.5

TABLE 9-3

TRIAL EXPOSURE: EXAMPLE 2

AREA: ABDOMEN	Screen/Film: QFD/UVL			
	Grid: 8:1		SID (Inches): 40	
THICKNESS (CM)	KVP	MA	TIME (SEC)	MAS
5	58	100	$1/12$	8.3
6	60	100	$1/12$	8.3
7	62	100	$1/12$	8.3
8	64	100	$1/12$	8.3
9	66	100	$1/12$	8.3
10	68	100	$1/12$	8.3
11	70	100	$1/12$	8.3
12	72	100	$1/12$	8.3
13	74	100	$1/12$	8.3
14	76	100	$1/12$	8.3
15	78	100	$1/12$	8.3
16	80	100	$1/12$	8.3
17	82	100	$1/12$	8.3
18	84	100	$1/12$	8.3
19	86	100	$1/12$	8.3
20	88	100	$1/12$	8.3
21	90	100	$1/12$	8.3
22	92	100	$1/12$	8.3
23	94	100	$1/12$	8.3

example a 100-milliamperage/100-kVp-capacity machine is used.

Known Information

 Lateral abdomen measurement = 14 cm
 Film speed = medium
 Screen speed = fast
 Grid ratio = 8:1
 SID = 40 inches
 Milliamperage capability = 100
 kVp capability = 100

Calculation for kVp

 $(2 \times 14 \ [\text{cm}]) + 40 \ (\text{SID}) + 8 \ (\text{grid factor}) = 76 \ \text{kVp}$

Calculations for mAs

 $100 \times 1/120 = 0.8 \ \text{mAs}$
 $100 \times 1/60 = 1.6 \ \text{mAs}$
 $100 \times 1/40 = 2.5 \ \text{mAs}$
 $100 \times 1/30 = 3.3 \ \text{mAs}$
 $100 \times 1/24 = 4.2 \ \text{mAs}$
 $100 \times 1/20 = 5.0 \ \text{mAs}$
 $100 \times 1/15 = 6.6 \ \text{mAs}$
 $100 \times 1/12 = 8.3 \ \text{mAs}$

$100 \times 1/10 = 10.0 \ \text{mAs}$
$100 \times 1/8 = 12.5 \ \text{mAs}$

mAs range based on fast screen speed

Trial exposure 2: Plotting the chart.

The following is the exposure setting for a 14-cm canine abdomen:

- kVp = 76
- Milliamperage = 100
- Time in seconds = $1/12$

The plotted technique chart is shown in Table 9-3.

OTHER FORMULATION METHODS

Some x-ray machines limit the alterations made in kilovoltage and milliamperage. Certain older or smaller x-ray machines do not allow for kilovoltage variations in steps as small as 1 or 2 kVp. A compromise between kVp and mAs must be made for this type of machine. For example, if the kVp settings can be altered in 10-kVp intervals only, increased radiographic density may be attained by increasing the mAs. For each centimeter of increased

TABLE 9-4

VARIABLE MILLIAMPERAGE-SECONDS (MAS) TECHNIQUE CHART

THICKNESS (CM)	KVP	MA	TIME (SEC)	MAS	SID	GRID
1	50	100	$1/20$	5	40	No
2	50	100	$1/15$	6.7	40	No
3	50	75	$1/10$	7.5	40	No
4	50	100	$1/12$	8.3	40	No
5	50	100	$1/10$	10	40	No
6	60	100	$1/20$	5	40	No
7	60	100	$1/15$	6.7	40	No
8	60	75	$1/10$	7.5	40	No
9	60	100	$1/12$	8.3	40	No
10	60	100	$1/10$	10	40	No

SUGGESTED DISTRIBUTION

Medium Screens:
5 mAs • Extremity/skull (no grid used)
7.5 mAs • Thorax (grid used)
10 mAs • Abdomen (grid used)
12.5 mAs • Pelvis/spine (grid used)

SUGGESTED DISTRIBUTION

Fast Screens:
2.5 mAs • Extremity/skull (no grid)
5 mAs • Thorax (8:1 grid)
8.3 mAs • Abdomen (8:1 grid)
10 mAs • Pelvis/spine (8:1 grid)

patient thickness, a small amount of mAs is added to the exposure technique. This is called a *variable mAs technique chart.*

Table 9-4 is an example of a variable mAs technique chart. For a tissue thickness of 1 to 5 cm, the same kilovoltage (50) was used. The mAs, on the other hand, was increased approximately 20% to 30% for each centimeter increase. When the chart reaches the centimeter thickness of 6, the kVp is increased to 60, the mAs is decreased to its original value, and the mAs cycle begins again.

MODIFICATION RECOMMENDATIONS

In some instances a technique chart fails to produce a quality radiograph because of excessive patient thickness or pathology. It may be necessary to increase the mAs at a particular centimeter measurement to maintain adequate radiographic density. For example, at the thickness of 15 cm on an abdominal technique chart, the increase in tissue density may demand more milliamperage. The time setting should then be increased for the rest of the centimeter intervals (Table 9-5).

In veterinary radiography, radiographs of patients that are unhealthy are often necessary. Pathologic conditions may require a variation from the standard exposure technique. For patients that are obese or those that have pathologic conditions such as pleural effusion, massive cardiomegaly, or ascites, an increase in exposure factors is necessary to produce adequate radiographic density.

TABLE 9-5

TECHNIQUE CHART EXHIBITING MILLIAMPERAGE-SECONDS (MAS) CHANGE

AREA: ABDOMEN THICKNESS (CM)	Screen/Film: QFD/UVL			
	Grid: 8:1		SID (Inches): 40	
	KVP	MA	TIME (SEC)	MAS
5	58	300	$1/40$	7.5
6	60	300	$1/40$	7.5
7	62	300	$1/40$	7.5
8	64	300	$1/40$	7.5
9	66	300	$1/40$	7.5
10	68	300	$1/40$	7.5
11	70	300	$1/40$	7.5
12	72	300	$1/40$	7.5
13	74	300	$1/40$	7.5
14	76	300	$1/40$	7.5
15	78	300	$1/30$	10
16	80	300	$1/30$	10
17	82	300	$1/30$	10
18	84	300	$1/30$	10
19	86	300	$1/30$	10
20	88	300	$1/30$	10
21	90	300	$1/30$	10
22	92	300	$1/30$	10
23	94	300	$1/30$	10
24	96	300	$1/30$	10
25	98	300	$1/30$	10

Pathologic conditions can decrease radiographic quality by decreasing density and image clarity. Under most circumstances, if an increase in radiographic density is necessary because of fluid-filled lungs or abdomen, the mAs should be increased. Increasing the mAs improves the density without causing excessive scatter radiation, which can fog a radiograph further. If circumstances call for a shorter exposure time, the kilovoltage can be increased 10% to 15% instead of increasing the mAs. The following is a list of suggested modifications:

1. Pleural fluid/massive cardiomegaly: Increase mAs 50%
2. Ascites: Increase mAs 50%
3. Obesity or heavy muscling: Increase mAs 50%
4. Plaster cast: Increase mAs 50%
5. Neonatal dog or cat: Decrease mAs 50%
6. Special procedures using radiographic contrast media: Increase mAs 50%

KEY POINTS

1. Do not assume that two x-ray machines of the same make and model can automatically use the same technique chart.
2. A technique chart usually prevents the need for second radiographs and therefore promotes safety for the patient and personnel.
3. Some pathologic conditions including ascites, pleural effusion, and cardiomegaly require an increase in mAs of up to 50% to increase radiographic density.

REVIEW QUESTIONS

1. Any body part exceeding this measurement requires the use of a grid to reduce fog-producing scatter radiation.
   a. 20 cm
   b. 10 cm
   c. 2.5 cm
   d. 30 cm

2. When taking a test radiograph, the following requirements should be met:
   a. medium-speed film, 75-lb dog in a ventrodorsal position
   b. medium-speed film, 50-lb dog in a dorsoventral position
   c. medium-speed film, 50-lb dog in a lateral position
   d. fast-speed film, 25-lb dog in a lateral position

3. According to the author, when developing a variable kVp technique chart, kilovoltage should be increased or decreased by increments of _____ for each centimeter measurement.

a. 4
b. 2.5
c. 2
d. 10

4. Which of the following variable kVp technique charts is recommended for a small-animal practice?
   a. Canine/feline thorax, with grid
   b. Avian/exotic, no grid
   c. Canine/feline extremity and skull, no grid
   d. Canine/feline abdomen, with grid
   e. All of the above, as well as canine/feline pelvis and spine, with grid

5. Which of the following conditions may require decreasing the mAs to account for increased radiographic density?
   a. Neonatal animals
   b. Ascites
   c. Pleural effusion
   d. Plaster casts

6. If a radiograph is too light after taking a view of the lateral abdomen, what change may be recommended?
   a. Decrease kVp 10% to 15%
   b. Increase mAs 30% to 50%
   c. Increase kVp 30% to 50%
   d. Decrease mAs 30% to 50%

7. Compared with the abdomen, how much mAs does a quality view of the pelvis require?
   a. 50% to 75% less
   b. 30% to 50% less
   c. 30% to 50% more
   d. 50% to 75% more

8. A grid with a ratio of 12:1 will be used with the machine at your clinic. How does this affect the generation of your variable kVp chart?
   a. Need to add 5 to 10 to the sum of Santes' rule
   b. Need to subtract 10 to 15 from the sum of Santes' rule
   c. Need to add 10 to 15 to the sum of Santes' rule
   d. Need to add 8 to 12 to the sum of Santes' rule

9. Your clinic has a 100-milliamperage/100-kVp-capacity machine with an 8:1 grid. You measure a ventrodorsal abdomen on a dog to be 22 inches. Which settings will you set first?
   a. 92 kVp, 100 mA, $^1/_{12}$ sec, 8.3 mA
   b. 90 kvP, 100 mA, $^1/_{12}$ sec, 8.3 mA
   c. 92 kVp, 100 mA, $^1/_4$ sec, 8.3 mA
   d. 92 kVp, 300 mA, $^1/_{12}$ sec, 8.3 mA

10. Using Santes' rule, calculate kVp with the following information:
    Tissue thickness = 11 cm
    Grid factor = 12
    SID = 40 inches
    a. 72
    b. 74
    c. 76
    d. 63

Suggested Readings

Eastman Kodak Company: *Kodak: the fundamentals of radiography,* ed 12, Rochester, NY, 1980, Kodak.

Johns HE, Cunningham JR: *The physics of radiology,* ed 3, Springfield, Ill, 1974, Charles C Thomas.

Morgan JP, Silverman S: *Techniques in veterinary radiography,* ed 4, Ames, Iowa, 1987, Iowa State University Press.

Ticer JW: *Radiographic technique in small animal practice,* ed 2, Philadelphia, 1984, WB Saunders.

Watters JW: Development of a technique chart for the veterinarian, *Compend Cont Educ* 2:568-571, 1980.

QA/QC TESTS FOR THE X-RAY APPARATUS

PERPENDICULARITY

Equipment Needed

Carpenter's level

Objective

To ensure that the x-ray beam is properly centered, we must be sure that the tube stand, collimator, and x-ray tube are perpendicular and properly aligned.

Procedure

1. When the x-ray tube is positioned in the normal position, use the level to confirm that the tube is level and parallel with the table (Fig. 10-3). Stand at the end of the table and look at the tube, collimator, and tube stand. Visually verify that they appear to be perpendicular.
2. Stand alongside the table and verify the same information regarding perpendicularity of the collimator, x-ray tube, and tube stand.
3. If the tube, the collimator, or the tube stand looks crooked or canted, adjust it or have it repaired before attempting any alignment tests or taking any radiographs. This information should be recorded along with whether the test was negative, what was canted, and how it was corrected. If the equipment was serviced, the repair report should be kept for future reference. The information should be recorded for comparison.

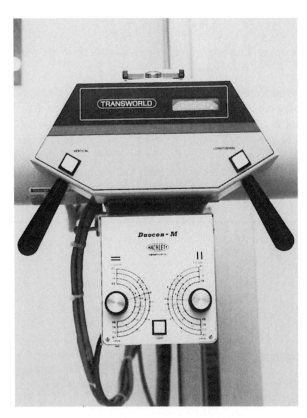

Figure 10-3 *Perpendicularity. A level is used to ensure that the x-ray tube is level and parallel to the tabletop.*

QA/QC TESTS FOR THE X-RAY APPARATUS

TUBE/TABLE/CRANE LOCKS

Equipment Needed
None

Objective
To check the function of the locks to eliminate any unnecessary motion from the x-ray tube, table, or crane.

Procedure
1. Physically place locks on and off to see whether they lock securely and unlock properly.
2. Check to make sure that the lock switch itself is not broken and that it functions properly. This should be recorded for future reference.

QA/QC TESTS FOR THE X-RAY APPARATUS

X-RAY FIELD LIGHT

Equipment Needed
Water and cloth

Objective
To ensure that the field light can be seen properly with the normal lights on in the radiographic room.

Procedure
1. Turn off the power to the machine. Wash the plastic covering of the x-ray collimator with warm water and mild soap. The plastic covering over the tube output area should be clean and free of debris and dirt. If not, artifacts can show up on the radiograph. (Note: On some older equipment, the plastic covering may be part of the filtering of the x-ray beam. If this is the case, do not damage or remove it without having a serviceperson correct the filtration on the equipment.)
2. Turn on the power to the machine. To check the brightness of the light, leave room lights on and turn on the collimator light. If there is no difficulty in seeing the edges of the field, there is no problem.
3. If the dimensions of the light field are difficult to see, there is a problem. A serviceperson should be called to increase the light intensity, and a record should be made for future comparison and reference.

QA/QC TESTS FOR THE X-RAY APPARATUS

LIGHT FIELD SIZE

Equipment Needed
Steel tape measure

Objective
To ensure that the light field determined by the collimator dials is accurate.

Procedure
1. Using the tape measure, verify the SID to the tabletop.
2. Set the collimator size indications at some field size. Remember to use the score for the SID you use routinely. An example of a field size to use is 8 × 10 inches (Fig. 10-4).
3. Turn on the collimator light.
4. Using the tape measure, measure the light field on the tabletop. This measurement should be within 2% of the SID for light field accuracy. This should be recorded for future comparison and reference.

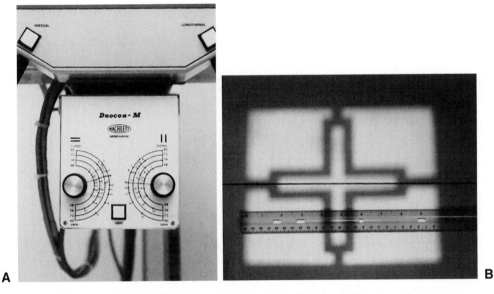

A   B

Figure 10-4 *A, Collimator setting for an 8- × 10-inch field size. B, Field size verification.*

QA/QC TESTS FOR THE X-RAY APPARATUS

COLLIMATOR/CONES/DIAPHRAGMS

If the x-ray equipment does not have a lighted collimator but uses slide-in diaphragms to collimate to the cassette sizes, this test should be conducted.

Equipment Needed

One cassette to match each of the cone/diaphragm sizes or diameters

Objective

To ensure that the cones or diaphragms used are the correct size for the cassettes available for use within the practice.

Procedure

1. Slide the different cones/diaphragms into or onto the x-ray tube, one at a time.
2. Place the appropriate size cassette in the Bucky tray (be sure to recheck the SID).
3. Make an exposure. Use a technique for this exposure that is approximately that for fetlock or carpus.
4. Develop this film. The corners of the developed film will be clear (as if cut off) if the cone/diaphragm used matched the size of the cassette used in the Bucky tray. If there is no Bucky tray and all the radiographs are done tabletop, then do this test tabletop, making sure that the SID is accurate. Record this information in the QA/QC file for future reference.

QA/QC TESTS FOR THE X-RAY APPARATUS

LOCKS/CABLES/OVERHEAD CRANE MOVEMENT

Equipment Needed

None, except the x-ray equipment

Objective

To ensure adequate locking and movement so that the x-ray tube does not drift during the exposure.

Procedure

1. Lock and unlock the locks. When each lock is in the locked position, the item that you are testing should not be able to move. For example, if you are testing the Bucky tray lock, then in the locked position, you should not be able to move it. If you are testing x-ray tube motion, then in the locked position, you should be unable to move the x-ray tube.
2. To assess the overhead crane movement, the x-ray tube must be moved around its known limitations. The tube should move easily and without obstruction. Record this information for future reference.

QA/QC TESTS FOR THE X-RAY APPARATUS

ANGULATION INDICATOR

Equipment Needed
Carpenter's level
Protractor

Objective
To ensure that the angle indicator is correct when using any angulation on the x-ray tube for a radiographic exposure.

Procedure
1. Place the carpenter's level on the tabletop—it should be level.
2. Place the carpenter's level on the bottom of the collimator—this also should be level.
3. Note that at both places the appropriate indicators should be zero.
4. Rotate the x-ray tube to 15 degrees, and using the protractor, measure the degree of angulation. This should also be 15 degrees.
5. Repeat this rotation of the x-ray tube to 30 and to 45 degrees, reading the angle indicator and measuring each degree change with the protractor (Fig. 10-5). Record this information for future reference.

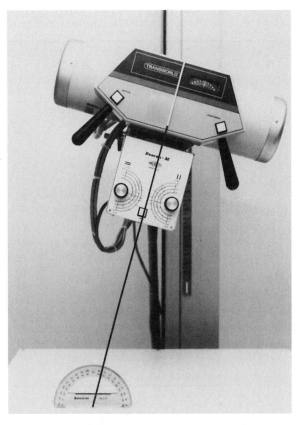

Figure 10-5 *Angulation verification. With the use of a protractor, a rotation of the x-ray tube of 15 degrees is verified.*

QA/QC TESTS FOR THE X-RAY APPARATUS

VIEW-BOX UNIFORMITY

Equipment Needed

Light meter

You can use a photographic light meter if it has a measurement scale. With certain types of photographic light meters, the denominator of the shutter-speed light intensity is in foot-candles.

Objective

To ensure uniform bulb intensity and color for even-light transmittance in radiographic evaluation.

Procedure

1. Unplug the view box from the electrical outlet. Clean the view box inside and out. Use a soft cloth and warm water with mild soap. Do not use nail polish remover or other harsh abrasives because they will scratch the view-box surface.
2. When cleaning inside, ensure that the bulbs are the same brand and the same color (e.g., daylight or soft white).
3. To measure the intensity of the lights, turn on the view box 2 minutes before doing the test. This allows the bulbs to stabilize.
4. Turn off all the room lights.
5. Measure the intensity with the light meter at three different areas on the viewer.
6. Calculate the average of the intensity on the viewer. An average or normal range is 400 to 580 foot-candles. Record this average information to monitor the life of the bulbs and their intensity as they age.

QA/QC TESTS FOR THE X-RAY APPARATUS

LIGHT FIELD/X-RAY FIELD ALIGNMENT

Equipment Needed
Nine pennies
10- × 12-inch cassette loaded with film

Objective
To ensure that the x-ray field is actually going where the light field indicates.

Procedure
1. Center the x-ray tube over the table.
2. Set the SID to 40 inches or your normal SID, and verify that the collimator is level.
3. Put a cassette in the Bucky tray.
4. Center to the tray under the table.
5. Set the collimator field indicators at a field that is approximately 6 × 8 inches.
6. Turn the collimator light on. Place one penny in the middle of each edge of the light field inside the light and one penny in the middle of each edge of the light field outside the light. The edges of the pennies should have the light field running between them, but the pennies should be touching (Fig. 10-6).
7. Make an exposure. The technique should be approximately the same as for a carpus or a stifle.
8. Develop the film. When developed, the radiograph should show the pennies just as they were placed on the table, on either side of the light field. If it does not, the collimator needs adjustment (Fig. 10-7). The width of a penny is 0.75 inch, and 2% of a 40-inch SID is 0.8 inch. Therefore if the x-ray field is off by the width of one penny, it is time to call service personnel.

To ensure that the center of the light and the x-ray field are aligned, draw diagonally from corner to corner on the film itself (all four corners). Make the same drawing from corner to corner on the exposed part. These two pairs of "Xs" also should not be apart by more than 2% of the SID. If they are, realignment by service personnel is necessary. Record this information in the QA/QC file for future reference.

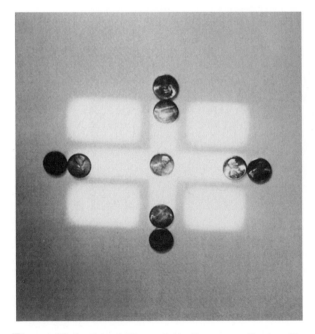

Figure 10-6 *Light field/x-ray field alignment verification. Nine pennies are placed on the edges of the collimator light field, as shown, and an exposure is taken.*

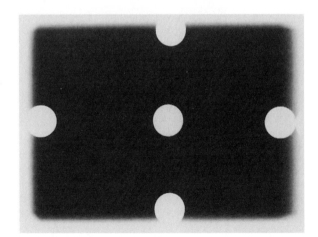

Figure 10-7 *Radiograph of a nine-penny test. This test result is within normal limits.*

QA/QC TESTS FOR THE X-RAY APPARATUS

SCREEN-FILM CONTACT

Equipment Needed
Copper wire mesh contact tool with $\frac{1}{8}$-inch spacing of the wires
Densitometer

Objective
To ensure that the adhesive on the back of the screens within the cassettes is still holding the screen tightly.

Procedure
1. Each cassette to be tested should be allowed to sit for about 10 minutes before this test is performed. This allows any trapped air (from loading the film) to dissipate.
2. Place the cassette on the tabletop.
3. Place the cassette so that the long axis is perpendicular to the anode-cathode axis of the x-ray tube. This is to minimize the anode heel effect.
4. Place the wire mesh over the cassette.
5. Use an SID of at least 40 inches.
6. Cone down to the size of the cassette.
7. Make an exposure using approximately a carpus or a stifle technique for tabletop.
8. Process the film.
9. When viewing the film, place it on a view box in a dimly lit room.
10. Stand approximately 6 to 8 feet back from viewer. You will be looking for areas of darkness or unsharpness on the film. Areas of poor contact appear as dark areas on the film (Fig. 10-8). If this area is in the middle of the cassette or in an area where you are likely to have a patient's area of interest, this screen should be adjusted. This may be as simple as regluing the edges of the screen to the felt. Any household white glue (e.g., Elmer's) can be used, or you can use double-backed tape (e.g., carpet tape). The screens in the cassette may need to be replaced. This test must be done on all cassettes.

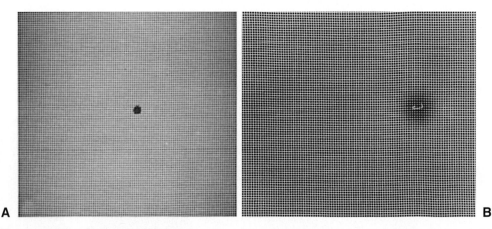

A   B

Figure 10-8 *A, Radiograph of a screen contact test. Note that the grid on the radiograph is well defined. This cassette has good screen-to-film contact. B, Radiograph of a screen-contact test. Note the dark, blurred area. This is an example of poor screen-to-film contact caused by a staple inside the cassette.*

QA/QC TESTS FOR THE X-RAY APPARATUS

UNIFORMITY OF SCREEN SPEED

Equipment Needed
Control cassette for each speed within the practice (usually one that is the newest or most consistent for exposure)
Densitometer
One box of film, to be used with each screen size within the practice

Objective
To determine periodically whether screens have lost speed through wear and tear.

Procedure
Before starting, visually inspect each cassette for properly functioning locks, intact hinges, and screen-felt contact. The screens should be checked for scratches, worn spots, or chips and should be clean.

1. Sort all the cassettes by screen type or speed group (high-speed, par, detail, rare-earth). Test each speed group separately.
2. Select one cassette from a sorted speed group as the control cassette.
3. Record the number of this cassette so that you can repeat this test when needed.
4. Load the cassettes from the film box designated for this procedure. Cutting a 14- × 17-inch film into fourths and placing one fourth into one corner of each cassette helps limit the cost of this procedure. Just remember which corner of the cassette has the film in it.
5. SID should be at least 50 inches if possible. You may have to put the cassettes on the floor to get this distance.
6. Place the corners of the cassettes together.
7. Center the x-ray tube over the area where the cassettes meet.
8. Cone down to approximately 8- × 8-inch field size.
9. Mark the cassette that is the control, and place this cassette into the upper-right-quadrant position of the four cassettes (Fig. 10-9).
10. Make an exposure, using approximately a carpus or a stifle technique. A technique that could be used for a medium-speed system is 10 mAs at 50 to 60 kVp. For a faster speed system, 5 mAs at the same range of kVp would be acceptable.
11. Process these films.
12. Read the density of each film in the center on the densitometer.

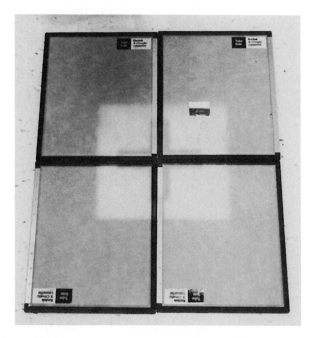

Figure 10-9 *Screen match setup with a marker on the standard cassette.*

Continued

QA/QC TESTS FOR THE X-RAY APPARATUS—cont'd

13. Record the density for each screen.
14. Repeat this procedure until all the screens within the same speed group have been tested.
15. Determine the average density of the films for each speed group. Divide the measured density of each film by the density of the control to determine each screen's ratio.
16. If there is more than one speed in the practice, this procedure must be repeated for the other speed groups, starting from the choice of a control cassette to the recording of the densities. The range of acceptable ratios between screens is between 0.85 and 1.15. Any screen that falls outside the ratio range should be removed from service. Record this information for future reference.

QA/QC TESTS FOR THE X-RAY APPARATUS

MACHINE PARAMETERS FOR CALIBRATION (kVp, mA, TIMER, AND FILTRATION)

Calibration should be conducted at least annually. The rationale for calibrating the x-ray equipment is to ensure that when 80 kVp is chosen, 80 kVp is delivered. Likewise, it is done to ensure that the mA stations and the timer are correct. Calibration involves a series of tests that a serviceperson must perform.

For example, a parameter that can change is kilovoltage. As an x-ray machine ages, kilovoltage can fluctuate. This problem also can be caused by incoming line voltage. Many veterinary clinics do not have a dedicated line for the radiographic equipment, and the voltage can change dramatically with an increase or a decrease in the incoming line voltage. This, of course, affects the penetration on the radiographs. Another possible source of kilovoltage fluctuation is bad internal workings—a computer chip, board, or drive that is not functioning correctly. These problems will be apparent in radiographs that are incorrectly penetrated and need to be repeated.

Darkroom Quality Control

Darkroom cleanliness is so important for good film processing that it is addressed separately. Just wiping up the counter is not enough, but it is a start. There must be no eating and no smoking in the darkroom. Crumbs in the cassettes can cause artifacts that could be interpreted as part of the diagnosis for the patient. Remember that the lit end of a cigarette is not a "safe" light and can fog your radiographs. This type of fog is called darkroom fog. Darkroom fog, no matter what the cause, is unacceptable. Fog can be caused by white-light leaks from around a door, cracked safelights, improper-wattage bulb in the safelight, improper safelight filter, safelight too close to the counter with a too-high wattage bulb, improper chemical temperature, or improper chemical balance.

QA/QC TESTS FOR THE X-RAY APPARATUS

FOG TEST

Equipment Needed
Lightly exposed radiograph
Watch or timer
Densitometer

Objective
To assess any fog in the darkroom that may be adding unwanted density to the radiograph during processing.

Procedure
1. Expose a cassette with a film in it, using a small-extremity technique.
2. Take the cassette into the darkroom.
3. Remove the film from the cassette, place the film on the counter, and cover half of it with the cassette.
4. All the safelights should be on, as in routine processing of a radiograph.
5. Leave the film and cassette in this position for 2 minutes by the watch or timer (Fig. 10-10).
6. Process the film normally.
7. When the film has been processed, notice the difference.
8. Measure each side of the radiograph with the densitometer. The difference should be no greater than 0.08 optical density (OD) for routine film-screen combinations and routine darkroom processing. If the difference is greater than 0.8 OD, the source of the radiographic fog must be located (Fig. 10-11). This test should be done quarterly because it provides a good follow-up on fog. Record this information for future reference.

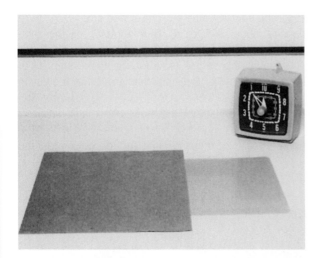

Figure 10-10 *Fog test setup in the darkroom. A piece of unexposed film is placed on the counter in the darkroom, and one half of the film is covered. After 2 minutes, the film is processed and examined.*

Figure 10-11 *Radiograph of a darkroom fog test. Note that the two halves of the film have different densities. This is an example of film fog.*

QA/QC TESTS FOR THE X-RAY APPARATUS

SENSITOMETRY AND DENSITOMETRY

Equipment Needed
Film, one box designated for sensitometry (this should be the same type/speed used every day but of the smallest size [i.e., 8 × 10 inches])
Sensitometer
Densitometer
Sensitometry graph paper
Thermometer

Objective
To ensure that the processing of the radiographs is optimized, thereby providing the best-quality radiograph. This is done by testing the processing procedure using a constant nonradiographic light source.

Procedure
1. In the darkroom, before doing anything else in this procedure, take the temperature of the developer in the processor or hand tank.
2. Using the sensitometer, expose one edge of a piece of radiographic film from the box of film dedicated for sensitometry (Fig. 10-12).
3. Process the film normally.
4. After the film has been processed, read the optical density of the steps with the densitometer and record the result on the graph paper (Fig. 10-13) according to the following procedure.
5. Measure the density in the center area of the film without any exposure.
6. Plot this densitometer reading (number) in the base + fog area on the graph.
7. The base + fog should not increase more than + 0.05 from the original or normal reading.
8. Next, read the steps of the sensitometry exposure and record the numbers on either the film or a piece of scratch paper. These numbers determine which step should be used for the contrast strip and the speed strip.
9. From these numbers, determine which step is within a density range of 1 to 1.3. This is known as the speed step.
10. Plot the density reading for the speed step in the area on the graph. This step is used for the speed step for the entire box of sensitometry film. Variations should not be greater than ± 0.15 of the initial reading. If they are beyond this parameter, corrective action must be taken.
11. Using the numbers for the steps off the scratch paper, determine the density of the steps above and below the speed step.
12. Subtract these two densities for the reading for the contrast strip. These two steps will be used for the contrast strip for the entire box of sensitometry film.

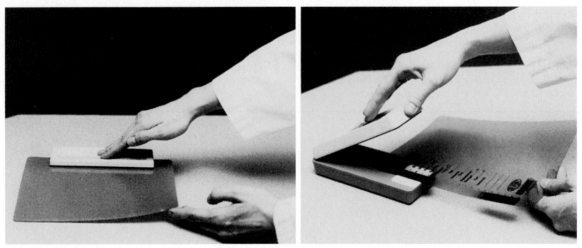

A **B**

Figure 10-12 *A, Exposing a test strip with the sensitometer. B, Reading the test strip with the densitometer.*

Continued

QA/QC TESTS FOR THE X-RAY APPARATUS—cont'd

13. Plot this number on the graph portion for contrast. The variations should not be greater than ± 0.2. If they are beyond this parameter, corrective action must be taken (Fig. 10-14).

14. These densities from the same steps on the sensitometry strip should be read and plotted daily on the graph paper.

It is imperative that this sensitometry and densitometry test be done each day any radiographs are processed. The purpose is to determine the processing environment before films are taken and thereby reduce the need for retaking films. (Note: All sensitometers and densitometers come with detailed instructions on how to do the procedures and the corrective actions to be taken when test results are outside the designated parameters.)

QA/QC TESTS FOR THE X-RAY APPARATUS—cont'd

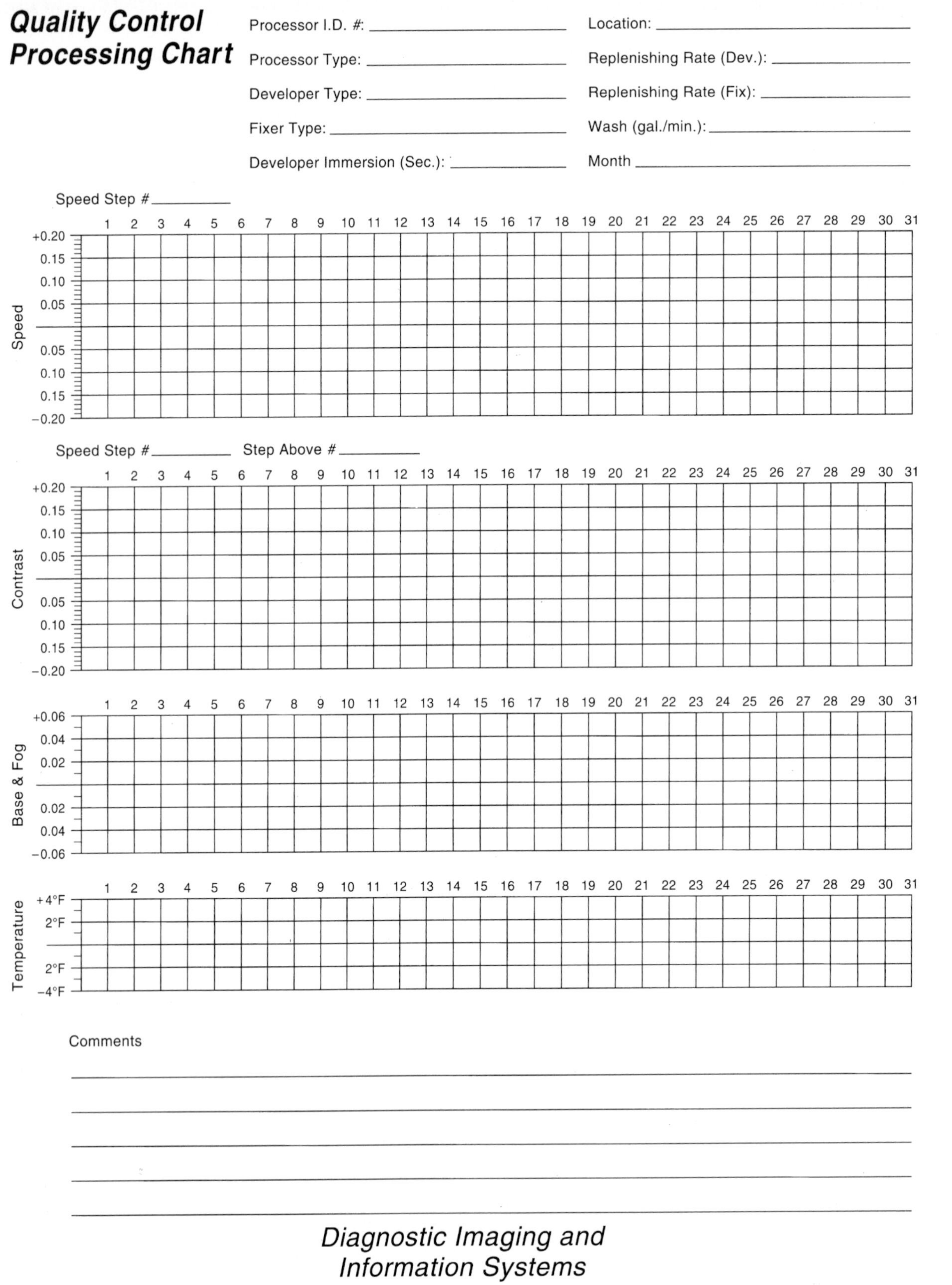

Quality Control Processing Chart

Processor I.D. #: _____

Processor Type: _____

Developer Type: _____

Fixer Type: _____

Developer Immersion (Sec.): _____

Location: _____

Replenishing Rate (Dev.): _____

Replenishing Rate (Fix): _____

Wash (gal./min.): _____

Month _____

Speed Step # _____

Speed

| | 1 | 2 | 3 | 4 | 5 | 6 | 7 | 8 | 9 | 10 | 11 | 12 | 13 | 14 | 15 | 16 | 17 | 18 | 19 | 20 | 21 | 22 | 23 | 24 | 25 | 26 | 27 | 28 | 29 | 30 | 31 |
| +0.20 |
| 0.15 |
| 0.10 |
| 0.05 |
| 0.05 |
| 0.10 |
| 0.15 |
| −0.20 |

Speed Step # _____   Step Above # _____

Contrast

| | 1 | 2 | 3 | 4 | 5 | 6 | 7 | 8 | 9 | 10 | 11 | 12 | 13 | 14 | 15 | 16 | 17 | 18 | 19 | 20 | 21 | 22 | 23 | 24 | 25 | 26 | 27 | 28 | 29 | 30 | 31 |
| +0.20 |
| 0.15 |
| 0.10 |
| 0.05 |
| 0.05 |
| 0.10 |
| 0.15 |
| −0.20 |

Base & Fog

| | 1 | 2 | 3 | 4 | 5 | 6 | 7 | 8 | 9 | 10 | 11 | 12 | 13 | 14 | 15 | 16 | 17 | 18 | 19 | 20 | 21 | 22 | 23 | 24 | 25 | 26 | 27 | 28 | 29 | 30 | 31 |
| +0.06 |
| 0.04 |
| 0.02 |
| 0.02 |
| 0.04 |
| −0.06 |

Temperature

| | 1 | 2 | 3 | 4 | 5 | 6 | 7 | 8 | 9 | 10 | 11 | 12 | 13 | 14 | 15 | 16 | 17 | 18 | 19 | 20 | 21 | 22 | 23 | 24 | 25 | 26 | 27 | 28 | 29 | 30 | 31 |
| +4°F |
| 2°F |
| 2°F |
| −4°F |

Comments

_____

_____

_____

_____

_____

Diagnostic Imaging and Information Systems

Figure 10-13 *Example of a graph used to plot information from the sensitometer/densitometer test strip.*

Continued

QA/QC TESTS FOR THE X-RAY APPARATUS—cont'd

Quality Control Processing Chart

Processor I.D. #: _____ Location: _____

Processor Type: _____ Replenishing Rate (Dev.): _____

Developer Type: _____ Replenishing Rate (Fix): _____

Fixer Type: _____ Wash (gal./min.): _____

Developer Immersion (Sec.): _____ Month _____

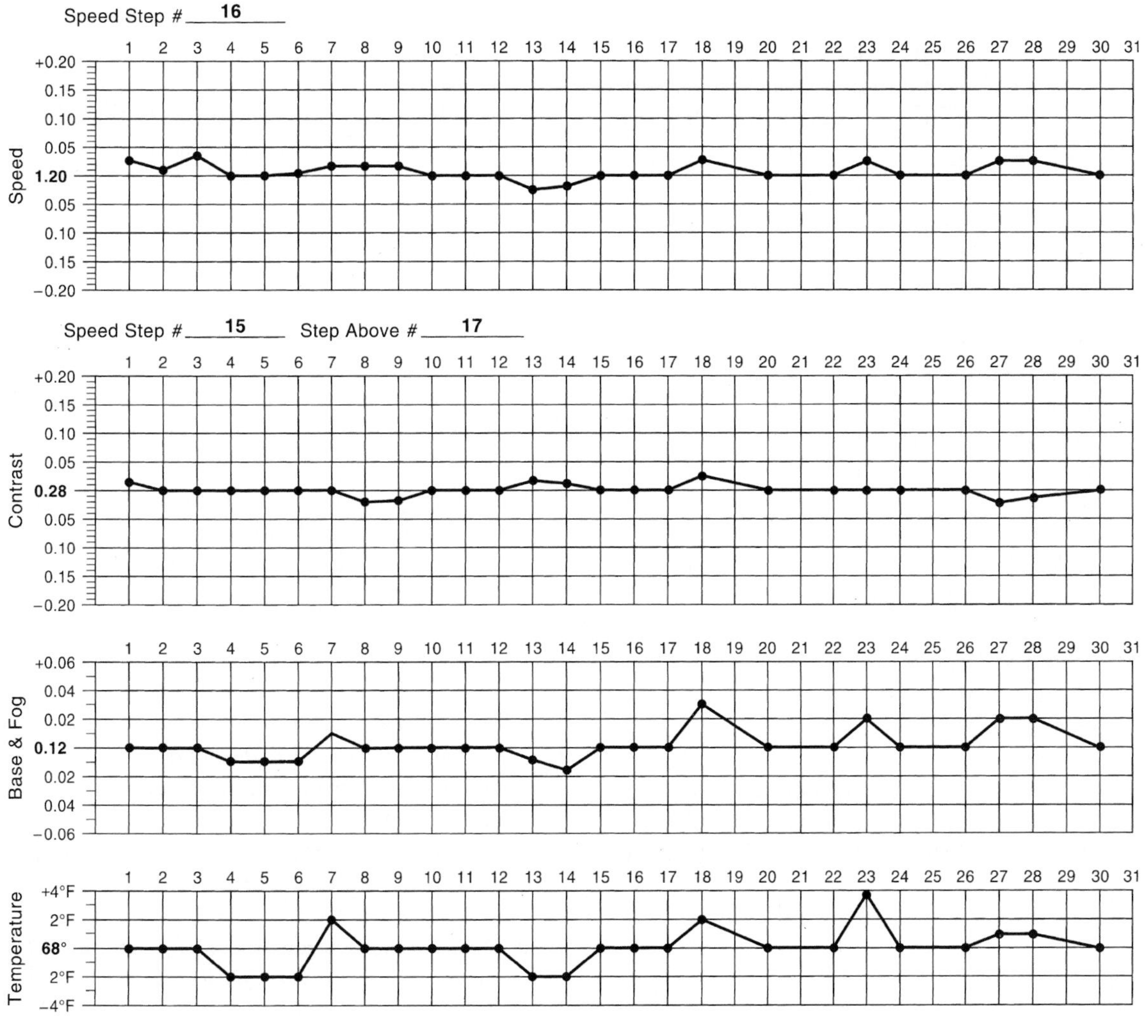

Comments

_____

_____

_____

_____

_____

Diagnostic Imaging and Information Systems

Figure 10-14 *A completed sensitometry/densitometry graph for a month.*

KEY POINTS

1. The purpose of a QA/QC program is to provide a way to minimize the dose of radiation to the patient and personnel, to allow production of quality radiographs to help with an accurate diagnosis, and to decrease the number of repeated films.
2. QA/QC tests are intended to be interpreted objectively. Opinions and personal preferences are inappropriate responses.
3. The majority of QA/QC tests must be performed annually; however, it is important to check the required frequency of each test because some have other than annual schedules.

REVIEW QUESTIONS

1. The source-image distance QA/QC test requires measuring the distance from the bottom one fourth of the end cap of the tube housing to:
   a. the top of the cassette in the Bucky tray.
   b. the bottom of the collimator.
   c. the top of the cassette on the tabletop.
   d. the tabletop.

2. What angles should be measured when performing the angulation indicator QA/QC test?
   a. 10, 20, and 30 degrees
   b. 10, 25, and 40 degrees
   c. 15, 20, and 25 degrees
   d. 15, 30, and 45 degrees

3. When performing the light field/x-ray field alignment QA/QC test with a 40-inch SID, the collimator needs adjustment if the x-ray field differs from the light field by at least:
   a. 3%.
   b. 2%.
   c. 10%.
   d. 5%.

4. When performing the screen-film contact QA/QC test, poor contact between the screen and felt of the cassette is seen as:
   a. whiter/lighter areas on the radiograph.
   b. darker areas on the radiograph.
   c. a completely black film.
   d. a difference of at least 2% between the light field and the x-ray field.

5. When performing the fog test for QA/QC, the optical density between the two sides of the film should be less than:
   a. 0.008.
   b. 0.08.
   c. 0.8.
   d. 8.

6. The sensitivity and densitometry QA/QC test should ideally be performed:
   a. daily.
   b. annually.
   c. weekly.
   d. when the technician suspects that the darkroom environment is not optimal.

7. When performing the uniformity of screen speed QA/QC test, the range of acceptable ratios of the density of each film to the control film within one speed group is:
   a. 1 to 2.
   b. 0.5 to 1.15.
   c. 8.5 to 11.5.
   d. 0.85 to 1.15.

8. The purpose of the quality assurance program is:
   a. equipment calibration.
   b. preventive maintenance.
   c. education of personnel.
   d. None of the above.

9. Darkroom fog:
   a. is tolerable as long as all of the other radiographic parameters are in compliance.
   b. can be caused by an improper wattage bulb in the safelight.
   c. is never acceptable.
   d. Both b and c are correct.

10. The average, acceptable range of intensity for the view-box uniformity QA/QC test is:
    a. 4 to 5 foot-candles.
    b. 40 to 50 foot-candles.
    c. 400 to 500 foot-candles.
    d. 500 to 1000 foot-candles.

READINGS

Gray JE et al: *Quality control in diagnostic imaging*, Rockville, Md, 1983, Aspen.

Thomas W Jr: *SPSE handbook of photographic science and engineering*, New York, 1973, John Wiley.

Technical Artifacts and Errors: Case Studies

Upon completion of this chapter, the reader should be able to do the following:

- State the importance of minimizing radiographic artifacts
- List and describe the common artifacts that occur in veterinary radiography

- State the preventive measures used to eliminate the occurrence of radiographic artifacts
- Identify the artifacts exhibited in each case study and outline their prevention

GLOSSARY

Artifact: Anything that decreases the quality of the radiograph resulting in difficult evaluation and interpretation.

INTRODUCTION

Radiographic **artifacts** are a menace to any radiographer. A radiograph is often marred by artifacts resulting from a number of causes. An artifact not only decreases the quality of the radiograph but may also lead to a misdiagnosis. The radiographer is responsible for recognizing the error and correcting it. This chapter introduces the reader to many possible artifacts and challenges the reader's ability to identify common film faults. Table 11-1 lists common artifacts and their causes. The radiographer should become familiar with this list and understand how to prevent these artifacts from occurring.

If an artifact consistently appears on radiographs, the cassette should be isolated and the screens cleaned and examined for damage. If the fault is persistent, the cassette

TABLE 11-1

COMMON ARTIFACTS AND THEIR CAUSES

ARTIFACT	CAUSE
Film too dark	Overexposure due to too much kVp or mAs Overdevelopment due to too much time in developer or increased developer temperature Overmeasurement of part under examination Machine (meters or timer) out of calibration Source-image distance not correct for grid use
Film too light	Underexposure due to insufficient kVp or mAs Underdevelopment due to decreased temperature or time of development, developer exhausted or diluted X-ray tube failure Incorrect film-screen combination Machine timer out of calibration Drop in incoming line voltage
Film gray/lack of contrast	Too much kVp Radiation fog due to exposure of film to radiation other than desired exposure Light leak in darkroom Storage fog due to conditions that are too hot or too humid Chemical fog due to old chemicals, increased chemical temperature, or increased time of development Film out of date Lack of a grid with use of high kVp Double exposure Incorrect bulb wattage or filter for safelight in darkroom
Lack of detail	Increased object—film distance Blurring due to poor screen-film contact Blurring due to patient motion Blurring due to x-ray tube motion Distorted image due to central x-ray not directed at center of film Double exposure

Continued

TABLE 11-1—cont'd

COMMON ARTIFACTS AND THEIR CAUSES

ARTIFACT	CAUSE
Heavy lines on radiograph (generalized)	Grid lines due to: Grid out of focal range Grid out of alignment to x-ray central beam Grid upside down Damaged grid Roller marks as result of film jammed in automatic processor
Inconsistent film density	Collimation of primary beam Bucky tray not positioned directly under primary x-ray beam Cassette not locked into Bucky tray correctly Light leak into cassette Quantum mottle Target damage (pitted anode) Variable screen-film contact
Black marks (not generalized)	Crimping or folding of film Two films sticking together during development Static electricity Developer on film before processing Fingerprints as a result of developer on hands while loading or unloading cassette
Clear areas on film (white marks; not generalized)	Hair in cassette Scratch in film emulsion Line due to scratch on screen surface Contrast medium on cassette or table Air bubble on film during developing procedure Film touching side of tank during manual processing Fingerprints due to film handling with contaminated hands
Yellow radiograph	Fixer splashes on film before developing Premature age due to improper fixation Film sticking together during fixing process Incomplete washing so that residual fixer oxidizes to yellow powder while destroying the image

should be labeled "faulty screens." However, if the damage could lead to a misdiagnosis, the screens should be discarded and replaced.

After examining the list of artifacts in Table 11-1, read through the following case studies and try to determine the cause and correction of the artifacts before looking at the answers.

CASE STUDY 1

EXAMINE THE RADIOGRAPH IN FIGURE 11-1

This radiograph exhibits a blurred image that lacks detail and definition—a classic example of motion. This artifact can be the result of a number of causes. The most common cause is patient movement during exposure. Patient motion is the most common artifact in veterinary radiography.

To minimize patient motion, a number of preventive measures can be taken. For example, motion can be limited by physical or chemical restraint. Sedation may be necessary for uncooperative patients or for views that are difficult to position without patient compliance. In instances in which the patient is panting, holding the muzzle closed or giving a short, quick blow on the nose while simultaneously making the exposure can effectively stop rapid respiration temporarily. Another method to use is a short exposure time. This can be achieved by using the highest milliamperage possible setting on the x-ray machine and fast intensifying screens.

Another cause of a blurred radiographic image is x-ray tube or cassette motion. This problem occurs primarily in equine radiography, in which a standard x-ray table is not applicable. The cassette must be manually held next to the anatomic area of interest and the x-ray tube positioned on a portable stand. A sturdy tube stand and cassette holder (discussed in Part 2 of this text) can minimize this type of motion.

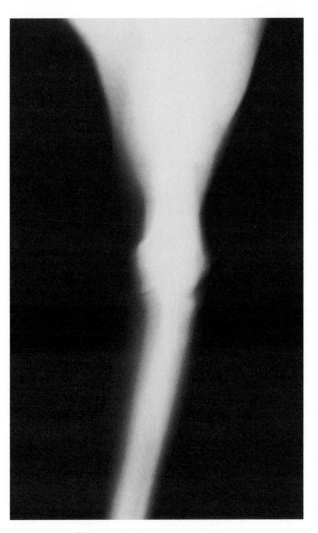

Figure 11-1 *Artifact case study 1.*

CASE STUDY 2

EXAMINE THE RADIOGRAPH IN FIGURE 11-2

This radiograph exhibits a general lack of density. This artifact can be attributed to many causes. On first glance, the radiographer may believe that the radiograph lacks sufficient kilovoltage (kVp) or milliamperage-seconds (mAs). Insufficient exposure factors can certainly cause a radiograph to be too light. However, more than the image is light: the background (area surrounding the patient anatomy) is also light. This type of insufficient film density can be the result of faulty film processing, incorrect film-screen matching, or an x-ray machine out of calibration.

If the processing solutions are expired or are too cold, or if the film is developed for an insufficient length of time, a radiograph such as the one in Figure 11-2 can result. Strict adherence to the standard processing procedure designated for the radiographic film being used and changing the solutions on a regular basis will prevent poor-quality radiographs.

An incorrect film-screen combination can result in a radiograph that is too light or too dark. The intensifying screens must match the film being used. If there is any question, the manufacturer should be consulted.

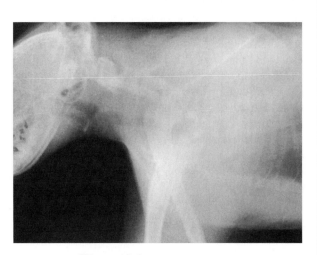

Figure 11-2 *Artifact case study 2.*

CASE STUDY 3

EXAMINE THE RADIOGRAPH IN FIGURE 11-3

Improper film handling is the cause of this radiographic artifact. A black "tree" pattern or a linear dot pattern is caused by a static electrical charge released on the film. Static electricity is most common in dry winter months, when the darkroom has relatively low humidity. To avoid static, eliminate friction by removing the x-ray film from the storage box slowly and placing it in the cassette without dragging across any surface.

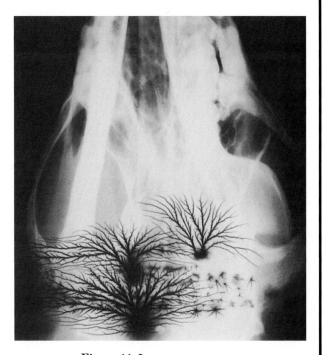

Figure 11-3 *Artifact case study 3.*

CASE STUDY 4

EXAMINE THE RADIOGRAPH IN FIGURE 11-4

This radiograph, similar to the radiograph in Case Study 1, exhibits a blurred image. Under close examination, one can see that two identical images are actually superimposed. This radiograph is an example of a double exposure. Under stressful circumstances, it is possible to inadvertently push the exposure button twice. It is also possible that the audible exposure indicator ("beep" or "ding" during exposure) malfunctioned and a second exposure was then taken. If there is any question of machine function, a service representative should be called.

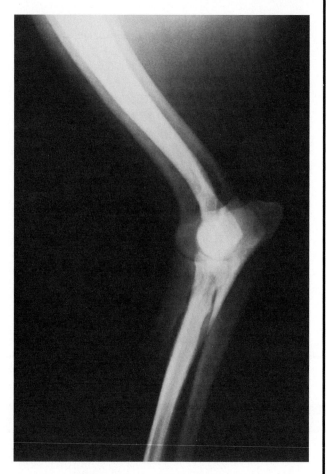

Figure 11-4 *Artifact case study 4.*

CASE STUDY 5

EXAMINE THE RADIOGRAPH IN FIGURE 11-5

The artifact on this radiograph is a classic example of a finger pressure mark caused by incorrect film handling. This artifact is called a finger crescent; it commonly occurs when the radiographer is in a hurry to remove the x-ray film from the cassette. When two fingers are placed on the film a small distance apart and pinched together to remove the film from the cassette, a black crease mark can result from the pressure placed on the film by the fingertips. To avoid this and similar artifacts, x-ray film should be handled by the edges only.

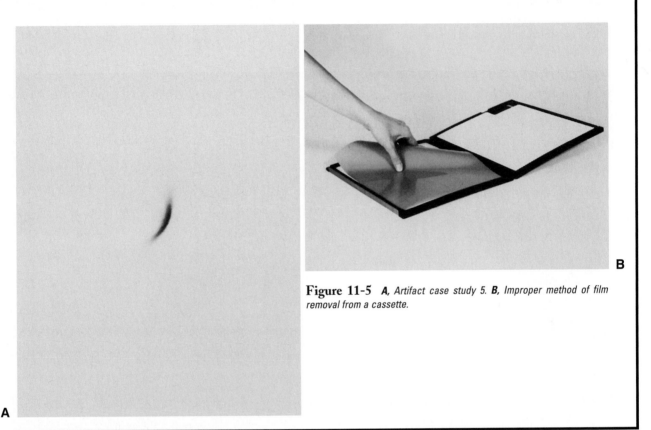

Figure 11-5 *A, Artifact case study 5. B, Improper method of film removal from a cassette.*

CASE STUDY 6

EXAMINE THE RADIOGRAPH IN FIGURE 11-6

The artifact on this radiograph exemplifies the importance of proper animal preparation before radiography. The gray streaks are the result of a wet haircoat. These streaks can potentially inhibit a proper diagnosis or even mimic a pathologic lesion. Radiopaque contrast media, urine, blood, or water can create this artifact.

Before any radiograph is exposed, debris should be removed and the haircoat should be dry. When radiograph-ing a large animal such as a horse, the area of interest should be clean, dry, and free of debris. In equine pedal radiography, the frog of the hoof should be picked and washed, ensuring the removal of dirt, manure, and rocks. Sheep and llama radiography can be a challenge if the wool is long and full of debris. In some instances shearing may be necessary to eliminate excessive artifacts.

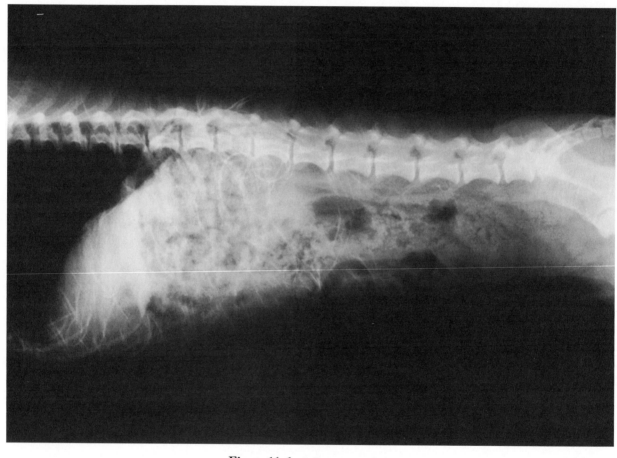

Figure 11-6 *Artifact case study 6.*

CASE STUDY 7

EXAMINE THE RADIOGRAPH IN FIGURE 11-7

This radiographic artifact is one example of what can happen when a technologist is in a hurry to reload a cassette. Care was not taken to ensure that all corners of the film were placed correctly in the corners of the cassette. The film was folded onto itself as the cassette was closed. The fold in the film creates a dark line across the radiograph and a mirror image on either side of the crease. Although this artifact is not common, it is an example of what can occur if the film is not properly loaded into the cassette.

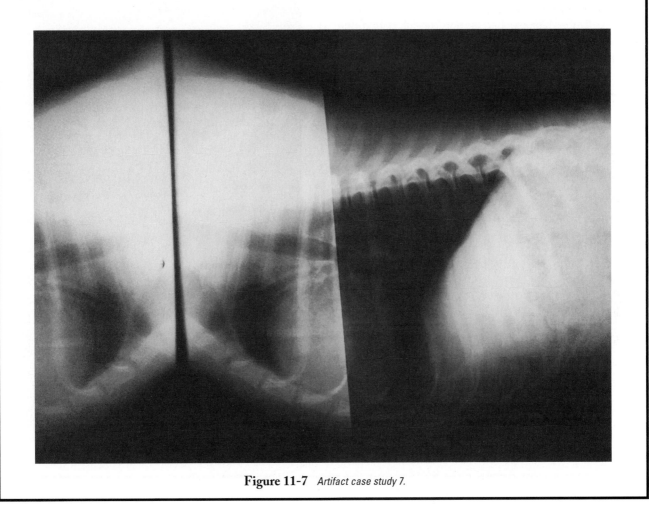

Figure 11-7 *Artifact case study 7.*

CASE STUDY 8

EXAMINE THE RADIOGRAPH IN FIGURE 11-8

The artifact on this radiograph is the result of a foreign object in the cassette, which is a common error. This artifact happens to be a piece of paper that was inadvertently placed in the cassette during the film-loading process. A number of radiographic manufacturers supply x-ray film with a sheet of thin paper between each piece. If the radiographer is not careful during the cassette loading process, it is easy for a sheet of this paper to slip into the cassette with the film.

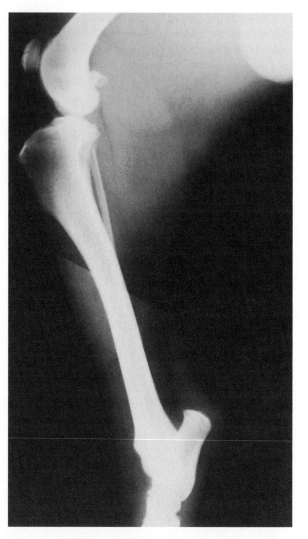

Figure 11-8 *Artifact case study 8.*

CASE STUDY 9

EXAMINE THE RADIOGRAPH IN FIGURE 11-9

The emulsion of the x-ray film is sensitive to damage, especially when wet. This radiograph exhibits a common artifact that occurs during hand processing: a scratch in the emulsion. Unless proper care is taken, the emulsion can become marred through contact with adjacent hangers or other projections. Scratched emulsion is a common occurrence when a number of films are developed at one time. This is especially true with the use of tension clip hangers as opposed to channel hangers. When processing more than one film at a time, be sure there is sufficient space between each film within the tank. Even when a radiograph is completely dry, the emulsion can be damaged. Proper film handling is imperative at all times—before, during, and after processing.

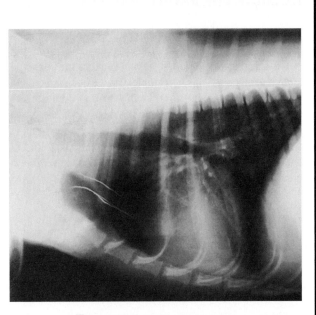

Figure 11-9 *Artifact case study 9.*

CASE STUDY 10

EXAMINE THE RADIOGRAPH IN FIGURE 11-10

The artifact on this radiograph is a classic example of film fog. At some point, either before or after the exposure was made, light exposed a portion of the film. Unwanted light can reach the film in three common ways: (1) the film bin door is ajar, (2) a film box lid is loose or damaged, or (3) the cassette is not closed properly or is damaged.

The film bin in which x-ray film is stored should be light-tight when the door is completely closed. If the technologist is in a hurry and the door is left open or has a faulty seal, light can leak in. In the same respect, if the film boxes are not kept in a film bin and the lid of the box is not secure, film fog is inevitable. In each case more than one film could be fogged. In fact, an entire box of film could be ruined, which would be quite costly to the clinic.

Not latching the cassette completely will allow light to leak in and expose either a portion or all of the film. Improper loading of the cassette can also lead to film fog resulting from a portion of the film's sticking out of the closed cassette. Light can also enter a cassette if it is damaged by being dropped or not handled carefully, preventing a latch from locking. Care when loading and handling a cassette can prevent these problems.

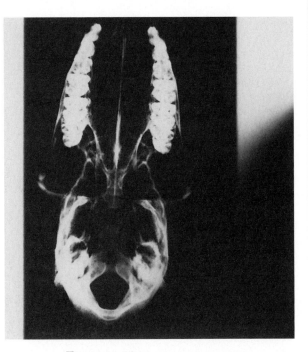

Figure 11-10 *Artifact case study 10.*

CASE STUDY 11

EXAMINE THE RADIOGRAPH IN FIGURE 11-11

This radiographic artifact is uncommon and is a challenging mystery to solve. Notice that the radiograph has a number of superimposed exposures, all of which are too light. The artifact was the result of accidentally leaving an unexposed cassette in the cassette tray while various extremities were exposed with a cassette on the tabletop. Later, when the cassette was found in the tray, it was processed and contained numerous exposures. If a film is suspected of being exposed, it is best to discard or process the film to prevent the need for additional radiographs.

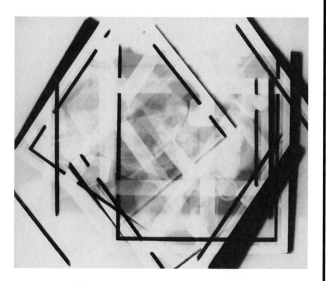

Figure 11-11 *Artifact case study 11.*

EXAMINE THE RADIOGRAPH IN FIGURE 11-12

This radiographic artifact is a common occurrence during or after the use of radiopaque contrast media. Contrast media are used for special radiographic procedures such as an upper gastrointestinal study or cystogram (discussed in Part 2). Whenever radiopaque contrast media are used in veterinary radiography, the possibility of spillage exists. If a contrast medium is present on the cassette or on the x-ray table, it will prevent the x-rays from reaching the film properly. To minimize the occurrence of this artifact, the tabletop and cassettes should be monitored and cleaned frequently if necessary.

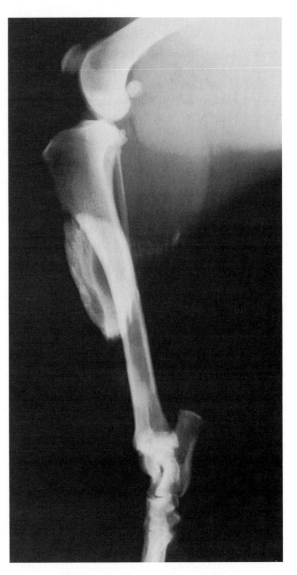

Figure 11-12 *Artifact case study 12.*

CASE STUDY 13

EXAMINE THE RADIOGRAPH IN FIGURE 11-13

The artifact on this radiograph was caused by a portion of the film being unexposed. On one side of the radiograph, there is a definite line where the x-rays are not reaching the film. Collimation can reduce the primary beam field size, but in this case the clear areas on the radiograph would be symmetric (on both sides of the film). Two primary causes for the type of artifact shown here are (1) the central x-ray is not perpendicular to the cassette and (2) the cassette is not directly under the entire primary x-ray beam.

The importance of having the central ray perpendicular (forming a 90-degree angle) to the x-ray film is discussed in Chapter 5. Aiming the central ray at any angle other than 90 degrees not only prevents the entire film from being exposed but causes geometric distortion.

The cause of the artifact in this case study was not the tube angle (no distortion is noted), but the fact that the cassette was not directly under the entire primary x-ray beam. If the cassette is placed into the cassette tray incorrectly, a portion of the primary beam will not reach the film. To ensure proper exposure, the cassette must be locked into the tray with the cassette locks, the tray must be pushed completely under the tabletop, and the center of the cassette tray must be in line with the central x-ray.

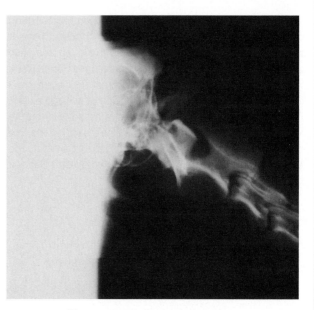

Figure 11-13 *Artifact case study 13.*

CASE STUDY 14

EXAMINE THE RADIOGRAPH IN FIGURE 11-14

The artifact in this radiograph appears as small, clear (white) areas. Close examination reveals that the white blotches are actually fingerprints. This is most likely the result of fix solution on the hands while handling the film before processing. It is imperative that the hands be clean and dry before handling any film. (Remember, fingerprints are a dead giveaway to the culprit of artifactual crime!)

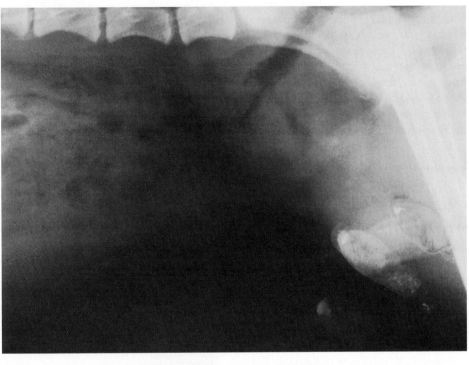

Figure 11-14 *Artifact case study 14.*

CASE STUDY 15

EXAMINE THE RADIOGRAPH IN FIGURE 11-15

This radiograph exhibits numerous white dots. No pattern to the position of the dots exists, but they are located primarily near the caudal portion of the patient. A second view would confirm that this artifact is located inside the body of the patient and is not a problem with the cassette, film, or processing. The white dots are buckshot from a shotgun shell. This patient is most likely a hunting dog that was too close to the hunter's line of fire (or was running away from an unhappy neighbor). This artifact is a common occurrence in field dogs and should not be a cause for alarm. Under most circumstances, the pellets are located in the muscle tissue and remain there or work themselves out of the body with time.

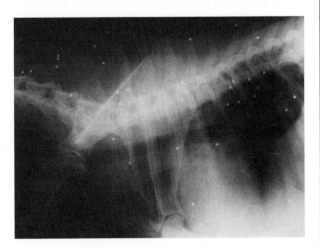

Figure 11-15 *Artifact case study 15.*

CASE STUDY 16

EXAMINE THE RADIOGRAPH IN FIGURE 11-16

The film has been exposed to a low-exposure setting with no animal patient between the x-ray beam and the cassette. This radiograph exhibits a mottled density dispersed over the entire area of the film. No pattern to the mottled density appears to exist. This would indicate the presence of something on the intensifying screens. When the cassette was opened in white light, there was a thin sheet of tissue paper inside. As it turns out, the practice just received new cassettes and neglected to remove the tissue paper that is placed between intensifying screens by the manufacturer for protection.

The lesson: When you purchase new cassettes for your practice, always remember to remove this tissue paper located inside the cassette before loading with film.

Figure 11-16 *Artifact case study 16.*

CASE STUDY 17

EXAMINE THE RADIOGRAPH IN FIGURE 11-17

The film has uneven density where the top of the film is darker than the bottom half of the film. There is also a noticeable wavelike appearance over the entire bottom half of the film. Clearly, this is not an artifact that is on the animal patient because it is dispersed over the entire film. The problem here involves the chemical processing. This film was manually processed using hand tanks. The radiographer failed to stir the chemicals before processing, which resulted in an uneven concentration of developer in the tank. The chemistry subsequently developed the film unevenly. When using hand tank processing, always stir the chemicals before use; otherwise, they tend to settle to the bottom of the tanks. Processing without stirring will result in unevenly developed films.

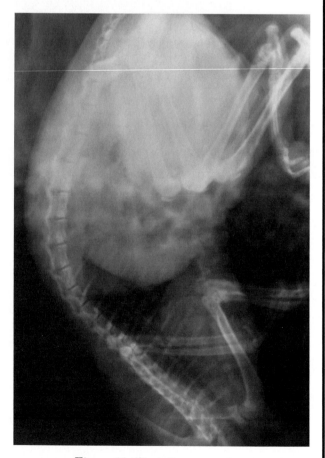

Figure 11-17 *Artifact case study 17.*

KEY POINTS

1. It is essential that the radiographer understand the causes of artifacts and know how to troubleshoot them.
2. Artifacts can mimic pathologic conditions and thus lead to a misdiagnosis.
3. The most common cause of artifacts in veterinary radiology is patient motion.

REVIEW QUESTIONS

1. Which of the following are means of eliminating artifact due to motion?
   a. Short time exposure, highest possible mA
   b. Longer exposure time, highest possible mA
   c. Physical or chemical restraint
   d. Both a and c are correct.

2. A radiograph has appropriate density and contrast. There is a black tree pattern present. What is the most likely cause of this artifact?
   a. Patient motion
   b. Hair in the cassette
   c. Improper film handling
   d. Fixer splashes on film before developer

3. What can the radiographer do to prevent finger crescent artifacts?
   a. Handle the x-ray film by the edges only
   b. Monitor the humidity in the developer room
   c. Do not allow light to leak into the cassette
   d. Do not allow two films to stick together

4. Which of the following can cause light exposure to the film?
   a. A broken cassette that does not close completely
   b. The film bin door is left open to some degree
   c. A film box lid is loose or damaged
   d. All of the above

5. How does spillage of contrast media on the cassette or tabletop cause artifact?
   a. Causes overpenetration of the film in that area
   b. Prevents x-rays from reaching the film properly
   c. Causes linear dot pattern
   d. Causes double exposure

6. If the cassette is not directly under the primary x-ray beam, how will the film look?

7. a. The part of the film not directly under the primary beam is white or unexposed.
   b. The part of the film not under the primary beam is black and unexposed.
   c. The exposed portion will be distorted.
   d. The exposed image will look as if two identical objects are exposed.

7. What should the radiographer do if he or she suspects that the film-screen combination is inappropriate?
   a. Keep a stock of every possible screen speed and try all of them.
   b. Keep a stock of every possible film speed and try all of them.
   c. Consult the manufacturer.
   d. In the future take radiographs without screens.

8. If the radiographer has developer on his or her hands while loading and unloading the cassette, what artifact might be seen?
   a. White marks
   b. Nongeneralized black marks
   c. Generalized image distortion
   d. A yellow radiograph

9. What factor causes film fog?
   a. Light leak in the darkroom.
   b. Incorrect safelight bulb wattage.
   c. Incorrect safelight filter.
   d. All of the above.

10. Which of the following most commonly cause generalized heavy lines on a radiograph?
    a. Grid problems
    b. Roller marks from the processor
    c. Both a and b are correct
    d. None of the above

SUGGESTED READINGS

Douglas SW, Herrtage ME, Williamson HD: *Principles of veterinary radiography*, ed 4, Philadelphia, 1987, Bailliere Tindall.

Eastman Kodak Company: *Kodak: the fundamentals of radiography*, ed 12, Rochester, NY, 1980, Kodak.

Gray J et al: *Quality control in diagnostic imaging*, Rockville, Md, 1983, Aspen.

Morgan JP, Silverman S: *Techniques in veterinary radiography*, ed 4, Ames, Iowa, 1987, Iowa State University Press.

Sweeney RJ: *Radiographic artifacts: their cause and control*, New York, 1983, JB Lippincott.

Ticer JW: *Radiographic techniques in small animal practice*, ed 2, Philadelphia, 1984, WB Saunders.

$\mathcal{R}$adiographic Imaging

General Principles of Positioning

CHAPTER OUTLINE

Positional Terminology
Patient Positioning: Basic Criteria
Film Identification

OBJECTIVES

Upon completion of Chapter 12 of this text, the reader should be able to do the following:

- List and define the proper anatomic positional terminology used in veterinary radiography
- State the four factors that must be considered for accurate reproduction of an anatomic area
- Describe proper patient handling during radiography
- List the basic guidelines for veterinary radiographic positioning
- State the technical preparation necessary before positioning the patient
- Describe how to measure the anatomic area of interest
- List the required views of each anatomic part
- State the advantage of "splitting" a cassette
- Explain the importance of collimation

- List and describe the patient preparation necessary to minimize radiographic inhibitory artifacts
- List and describe the available patient restraint and positioning aids
- State the proper labeling of various anatomic positions
- State the importance of label placement
- Describe the proper radiographic positioning techniques for all anatomic areas of small, large, and exotic animals
- List and describe the common special procedures involving contrast media that are used in small animal radiography

Caudal: Describes parts of the head, neck, and trunk positioned toward the tail from any given point. Caudal also describes those aspects of the limbs above the carpal and tarsal joints that face toward the tail.

Cranial: Describes parts of the neck, trunk, and tail positioned toward the head from any given point. Cranial also describes those aspects of the limb above the carpal and tarsal joints that face toward the head.

Distal: Farther away from the point of origin of a structure.

Dorsal: Upper aspect of the head, neck, trunk, and tail. The term also means toward the upper aspect of the animal. Dorsal also describes the aspects of the legs from the carpus and tarsus joints distally that face toward the head.

Lateral: The x-ray beam enters through either the left or right side of the body and emerges on the opposite side, where the cassette is positioned.

Mediolateral: The x-ray beam enters a limb through the medial side and exits on the lateral side. Most lateral radiographs of the limbs are taken in lateromedial projection in large animal radiography.

Palmar: Used instead of caudal when describing the forelimb from the carpal joint distally.

Plantar: Used instead of caudal when describing the hind limb from the tarsal joint distally.

Proximal: Nearer to the point of origin of a structure.

Recumbent: The animal is lying down when the radiograph is made. Most radiographs of the dog and cat are made with the animal in the recumbent position, and this position should be presumed unless otherwise stated on the radiograph.

Rostral: Parts of the head positioned toward the nares from any given point on the head.

Superior and inferior: Used to describe the upper and lower dental arcades, respectively.

Ventral: Lower aspect of the head, neck, trunk, and tail. The term also means toward the lower aspect of the animal.

POSITIONAL TERMINOLOGY

Understanding the correct terminology for the various anatomic views is essential to a radiographer. The directional terms cited in this text are based on the revised terminology system advocated by the American Committee of Veterinary Radiologists and Anatomists. This relatively new system exactly defines the position and direction of the primary x-ray beam. The correct veterinary anatomic directional terms and abbreviations for radiographic projections follow (Figs. 12-1 and 12-2).

> Left (L) • Dorsal (D)
> Right (R) • Ventral (V)
> Medial (M) • Lateral (L)
> Cranial (Cr) • Rostral (R)
> Caudal (Cd) • Palmar (Pa)
> Oblique (O) • Plantar (Pl)

Beam Direction

The abbreviated term used for the position designates the direction of the x-ray beam. The first letter states where the x-ray beam enters the body, and the second designates where it exits. For example, the abbreviation VD (ventrodorsal) indicates that the x-ray beam enters through the ventral side of the animal and exits on the dorsal side. Directional terms can also be combined for oblique views. For example, DMPaLO of the carpus indicates that the carpus is rotated to a selected-degree angle and the central x-ray enters the dorsal/medial surface and exits the palmar/lateral surface. The radiographer must become familiar with these directional terms to label and expose anatomic areas appropriately.

PATIENT POSITIONING: BASIC CRITERIA

Part 2 of this text instructs the radiographer in correct anatomic positioning. Positioning of small animal patients for radiographic examinations may require sedation or general anesthesia and positional devices. Overt manual restraint should be minimized as much as possible and should be used only when chemical restraint is contraindicated.

Care must be taken to include all essential anatomic regions in the primary beam when positioning patients. The primary goal of positioning for radiography is to find the most suitable posture to produce an accurate reproduction of the anatomic area. Several important factors must be considered if an accurate reproduction is to be made:

1. Welfare of the patient
2. Restraint and immobilization of the patient
3. Minimal trauma to the area of interest
4. The least risk of exposing those assisting with the examination to radiation

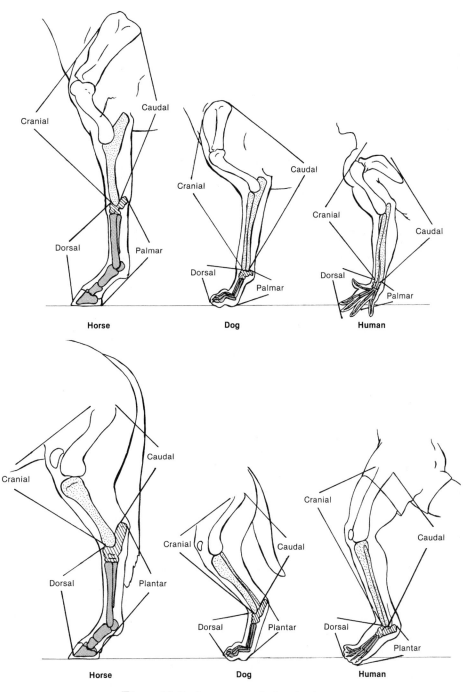

Figure 12-1 *Correct anatomic directional terms.*

The Patient

The comfort and welfare of the patient should be considered at all times. Patience is vital, especially with animals that cannot be sedated. Remember, radiography can be a frightening experience to an animal. The animal is unsure of what is happening and, from its perspective, is certain the procedure will be painful. To minimize anxiety, animals should be handled in a slow, quiet manner. Most animals respond to a calm, soft voice and gentle stroking.

Quick, loud movements and severe restraint usually result in a frightened, tense, and even aggressive patient.

The rotor noise (spinning of the rotating anode) of the x-ray tube often startles animals. Before the actual procedure begins, it is a good idea to start and release the rotor switch when working with patients that exhibit signs of anxiety. The rotor will continue to spin for several minutes, allowing the animal to become accustomed to the noise.

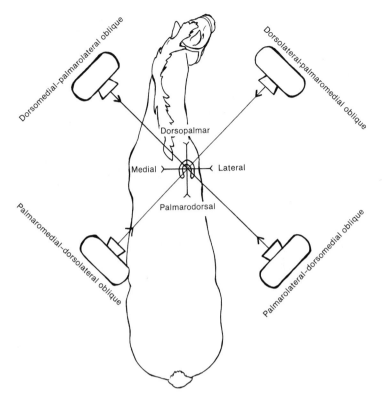

Figure 12-2 *Correct anatomic directional terms for oblique views.*

As much technical preparation for the exposure as possible should be done before the animal is positioned on the table. That is, the patient should be measured, the exposure technique set on the machine console, the cassette placed on the table or Bucky tray, and the label made before positioning the patient. Most animals tolerate being restrained in a particular position for only a short time.

Measurement

A caliper is used to measure the anatomic area of interest. This is an inexpensive device that measures part thickness in centimeter increments (Fig. 12-3). (The site where the measurement should be taken is given for every anatomic area in the positioning series, Chapters 13 to 20.) If the radiographer is unsure where to measure a particular part, the measurement should be made over the part's thickest area. When there is a large difference in thickness in a particular area, it is advisable to make two separate radiographs with different exposures. If only a small difference in tissue density exists, a compromise should be made.

Required Views

Because a radiograph is a two-dimensional picture of a three-dimensional structure, two views of each anatomic area taken at right angles to each other are the minimum recommended. The importance of two views is exemplified

when radiographing a fractured bone. For example, one view of a nondisplaced oblique fracture of a long bone may appear normal. Both a lateral and a craniocaudal view would be necessary to visualize the fracture line.

Another guideline is to position the area of interest closest to the film. This reduces distortion and magnification of the area under examination. In addition, if a limb is being radiographed, it may be helpful to radiograph the opposite corresponding limb. This allows the pathologic structure of one leg to be compared with the normal anatomy of the other.

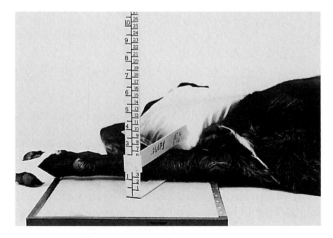

Figure 12-3 *Proper use of a caliper.*

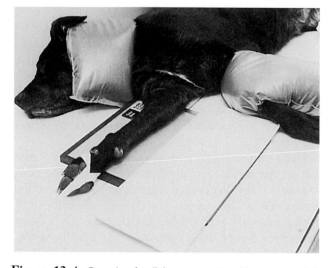

Figure 12-4 *Example of splitting a cassette with a commercially available lead sheet. One view can be exposed on one side of the cassette, and the opposite view can be exposed on the other.*

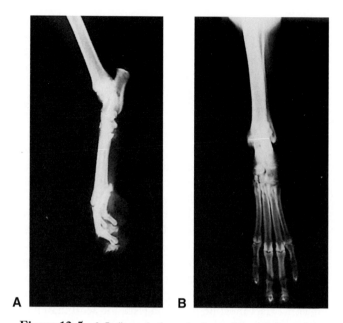

A　　　　　　**B**

Figure 12-5 *A, Radiograph of a canine tarsus, lateral. B, Dorsoplantar views. Note that the toes of the patient are facing the same direction on the film.*

To radiograph more than one view on the same piece of film to minimize the number of films used per patient, the cassette can be "split" by placing a sheet of lead over half to prevent its exposure (Fig. 12-4). Once the first side has been exposed, the lead sheet can be moved to the already exposed area and the other side can be exposed. Lead sheets, which can be purchased from most x-ray supply companies, are usually supplied in preselected sizes, or larger sheets can be purchased and cut to the desired size. The lead should be at least 2 mm thick. If a lead sheet is unavailable, a lead glove can be placed over the area to be shielded.

Splitting a cassette is possible only when the cassette is used on the tabletop, without a film (Bucky) tray or grid, or both. The cassette can be split into any number of areas as long as there is enough space for each anatomic view. When splitting a cassette, it is important to position the animal so that all views of the area are facing the same direction on the film. For example, if a lateral view of the tarsus was exposed with the toes of the patient facing the right side of the cassette, the craniocaudal view should also have the toes facing the right side of the cassette (Fig. 12-5).

Collimation

Collimation of the primary x-ray beam is very important whether or not the technician is splitting a cassette. The smallest field size possible should be used for any given area of the body. For example, when radiographing the carpus of a cat, the collimator light should include the carpus and a small portion of the long bones distal and proximal to the carpus (Fig. 12-6). Exposing a large area surrounding the carpus is not necessary. In fact, such exposure increases the amount of scatter radiation, which decreases radiographic contrast.

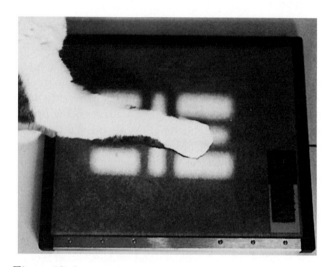

Figure 12-6 *Example of proper collimation ("coning down") for a radiograph of the carpus of a cat.*

Positioning Guidelines

In general, the central x-ray beam should be centered directly over the area of interest. For example, if the x-ray beam is centered over the caudal border of the thirteenth rib for a study of the abdomen, the entire abdomen is included (assuming the proper-size cassette is used).

The measurement for any anatomic region should be taken over the thickest area. This ensures that all regions of the part of interest will be penetrated with sufficient exposure factors.

Specific anatomy must be included for each anatomic area. For example, all radiographs of long bones (humerus and femur) should include the shaft of the bone, as well as the joints both distal and proximal to the bone. For joint radiography, the x-ray beam must be centered over the joint space, and the beam should include a portion of the long bones distal and proximal to the joint.

Patient Preparation

The patient should be clean and free of any debris. If the hair coat of the animal is wet or full of debris, confusing artifacts can appear on the radiograph. Collars, harnesses, and leashes of any sort, especially those made of metal, should be removed. In addition, bandages, splints, and casts should be removed before radiography unless there is a definite medical reason for leaving them in place. Pedal radiography of the horse may require removing the shoes and cleaning the frog of the foot to alleviate any artifacts that may impinge over an area of interest. For radiography of the small animal abdomen, the gastrointestinal tract must be free of ingesta and fecal material. A cathartic such as an enema or a laxative may be indicated to remove the obstructive material. A more detailed discussion of animal preparation for abdominal study is in Chapter 17.

Restraint

As mentioned, chemical restraint is preferred. If manual restraint is required, all personnel in the radiographic suite during exposure must be shielded properly with the appropriate lead apparel. (See Chapter 3 for proper manual restraint and shielding.) With manual restraint, the canine patient usually responds to a calm, authoritative approach, whereas a feline patient will resist too much restraint.

Positioning Aids

To assist in the positioning of the animal patient, devices such as sandbags, foam blocks and wedges, wood blocks, and a radiolucent trough can be used (see Fig. 3-6). Tape, gauze, rope, and compression bands are also useful positioning aids. With these devices, and sedation if necessary, little manual restraint is necessary. Positioning devices are commercially available or can easily be made by hand. Most fabric stores sell foam that can be cut into the desired shape with a scalpel blade or electric knife. Sandbags can easily be sewn and filled with sand for a fraction of the cost of those commercially available. Positioning aids should not be placed under or over the area of interest because none are completely non-radiopaque. Foam tends to produce an air density shadow and absorb and retain liquids that may be radiopaque when dry.

FILM IDENTIFICATION

Proper labeling of a radiograph is mandatory for legal and practical reasons. The film identification should include the appropriate patient information or access number as described in Chapter 7. A marker must also be used to identify the right or left (R or L) side of the patient; the limb being radiographed (front or rear); and the view, if necessary.

Label placement is also important. Anatomic areas that are symmetric (e.g., dorsoventral view of a dog skull) or anatomically identical to another area (e.g., an equine limb distal to the carpus and tarsus) are difficult to distinguish without proper labeling. For example, a lateral view of the front fetlock joint of a horse must be labeled "Left (L) Front."

When a marker is placed on a cassette for craniocaudal or caudocranial views, it should be placed on the lateral aspect of the extremity. In dorsoventral or ventrodorsal views, the marker should be placed on the cassette to identify one side or the other. That is, the lead "R" or "L" should be placed on the appropriate side of the animal. When a lateral projection of the abdomen or thorax is taken, the marker should indicate the side that is down on the table or cassette. For example, if a dog is in left lateral recumbency, the cassette should be labeled "L." When a lateral projection of an extremity is taken, the marker should be placed cranially to (in front of) the leg.

Marking sequential radiographs with appropriate numbers that identify time elapsed or order taken is also important. For example, special procedures such as a gastrointestinal contrast study require sequential radiographs over a period of time. In such an instance each set of radiographs should be labeled with the appropriate time elapsed (hours and minutes).

*K*EY *P*OINTS

1. When radiographing a long bone, the joints immediately distal and proximal to the bone must be included.
2. The smallest field size possible should be used for any given area of the body.
3. Positional terms are named according to where the primary x-ray beam enters and exits the anatomic area of interest.
4. As a general rule of thumb, feline patients tend to resist too much restraint and canine patients respond to a calm, authoritative approach to restraint.
5. The patient's coat should always be checked before taking radiographs to ensure that it is dry and as clean as possible.

REVIEW QUESTIONS

1. Fill in the blanks from the following choices. When radiographing a dorsopalmar view of an animal's limb, the primary x-ray beam enters the _____ of the paw and exits through the _____.
   a. cranial aspect; caudal aspect
   b. dorsal aspect; palmar aspect
   c. medial aspect; lateral aspect
   d. lateral aspect; medial aspect

2. The positional term used to describe the part of the pelvic limb found toward the tail and proximal to the tarsus (hock) is:
   a. Caudal
   b. Plantar
   c. Rostral
   d. Palmar

3. If a body part to be radiographed has a *significant* difference in density between its thickest and thinnest parts, do the following:
   a. Measure and radiograph the thickest part
   b. Measure and radiograph the thinnest part
   c. Use the average measurement to determine the area over which to center the x-ray beam
   d. Take two separate exposures with different measurements

4. True or false (circle one)
   Two views at 180-degree angles from each other are always required for each anatomic part.

5. The anatomic area of interest should be as close to the film as possible in order to do the following:
   a. Reduce distortion
   b. Increase magnification
   c. Enlarge the area of interest as much as possible
   d. Keep the structure as far from the cathode as possible

6. What is the minimum desired thickness of lead sheets used to block films?
   a. 1 mm
   b. 5 mm
   c. 2 mm
   d. 2 cm

7. What can be used in place of a lead sheet to block part of a film?
   a. Another cassette
   b. Collimating as close to the area as possible
   c. Thick books
   d. Lead-lined gloves

8. When radiographing a dog's abdomen, where should the primary x-ray be focused?
   a. Cranial border of eleventh rib
   b. Caudal border of thirteenth rib
   c. Xiphoid
   d. Cranial border of thirteenth rib

9. If an animal's thorax is radiographed while in right lateral recumbency, what marker should be used?
   a. R
   b. L
   c. RF
   d. LF

10. Where should the marker be placed for a limb radiographed in lateral recumbency?
    a. Dorsal to the limb
    b. Caudal to the limb
    c. At the most distal aspect of the limb
    d. Cranial to the limb

SUGGESTED READINGS

Douglas SW, Herrtage ME, Williamson HD: *Principles of veterinary radiography*, ed 4, Philadelphia, 1987, Bailliere Tindall.

Habel RE: *Applied veterinary anatomy*, ed 2, Ithaca, NY, 1978, RE Habel.

Kleine LJ, Warren RG: *Small animal radiography*, St Louis, 1982, Mosby.

Ryan GD: *Radiographic positioning of small animals*, Philadelphia, 1981, Lea & Febiger.

Schebitz H, Wilkins H: *Atlas of radiographic anatomy of the dog and cat*, Philadelphia, 1986, WB Saunders.

Smallwood JE et al: A standardized nomenclature for radiographic projections used in veterinary medicine, *Vet Radiol J* 26:2-9, 1985.

Smallwood JE, Shively MJ: Nomenclature for radiographic views of limbs, *Equine Pract* 1:41-45, 1979.

Ticer JW: *Radiographic technique in small animal practice*, ed 2, Philadelphia, 1984, WB Saunders.

chapter 13

Small Animal Forelimb

CHAPTER OUTLINE

Scapula
Shoulder
Humerus
Elbow

Radius and Ulna
Carpus
Metacarpus-phalanges

SCAPULA

Lateral View

Two methods of radiographing a lateral view of the scapula exist: (1) with the scapula placed dorsal to the vertebral column and (2) with the scapula superimposed over the lung field.

Dorsal to vertebral column.

The best unobstructed view of the scapula is achieved by pushing the leg of interest dorsally so that the scapula is positioned dorsal to the vertebral column (Figs. 13-1 and 13-2).

The patient is placed in lateral recumbency with the affected limb closest to the cassette and held perpendicular to the spine. The limb is then pushed dorsally by grasping it firmly below the elbow and extending the elbow joint. With the elbow in extension, the joint cannot flex, allowing the scapula to be pushed dorsally. As the affected leg is pushed dorsally, the opposite leg is pulled ventrally. By pulling the opposite leg, the thorax becomes slightly rotated, which isolates the scapula dorsal to the body. At this point, the scapula should be seen bulging above the dorsal spinous processes of the thoracic

---

BEAM CENTER: Middle of scapula

MEASUREMENT: Thickest area of scapula

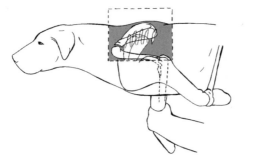

Figure 13-1 *Correct positioning for the lateral view of the scapula positioned dorsal to the vertebral column.*

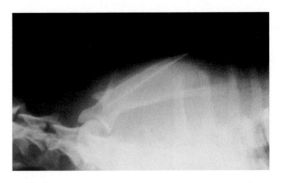

Figure 13-2 *Radiograph of the lateral view of the scapula dorsal to the vertebral column.*

SCAPULA—*cont'd*

vertebrae. Sedation is usually indicated for this view because of the firm manipulation necessary.

Superimposed over cranial thorax.

The view of the scapula superimposed over the cranial thorax is indicated for a patient that is in pain or when excessive manipulation may induce further injury (Figs. 13-3 and 13-4). The body of the scapula is placed over the radiolucent lung fields, allowing visualization of the majority of the bone. Although the entire scapula is not visible, this view is valuable for evaluation of the neck and body.

The patient is placed in lateral recumbency with the affected limb next to the cassette. The affected limb is pulled caudally and ventrally. The upper limb should be extended cranially, out of the area of interest. The sternum can be rotated slightly away from the table to better visualize the dorsal border of the scapula.

Caudocranial View

The patient is placed in dorsal recumbency (on its back) with both forelegs extended cranially (Figs. 13-5 and 13-6). The patient's sternum should be rotated away from the scapula approximately 10 to 12 degrees, which alleviates any superimposition of the ribs of the thoracic cavity over the scapula and gives a clear, unobstructed view of the structure.

BEAM CENTER: Middle of scapula

MEASUREMENT: Cranioventral thorax where scapula is positioned

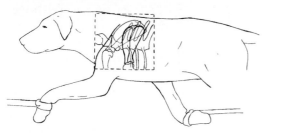

Figure 13-3 *Correct positioning for the lateral view of the scapula superimposed over the cranial thorax.*

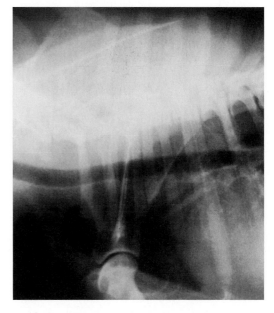

Figure 13-4 *Radiograph of the lateral view of the scapula superimposed over the cranial thorax.*

BEAM CENTER: Middle of scapula

MEASUREMENT: Thickest area (scapulohumeral joint)

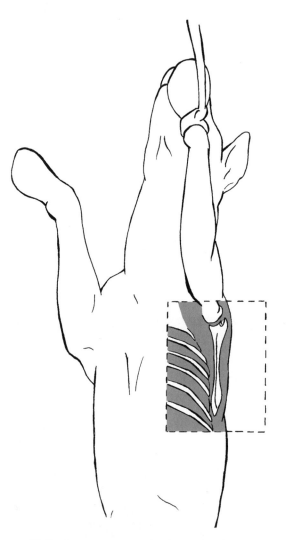

Figure 13-5 *Correct positioning for the caudocranial view of the scapula.*

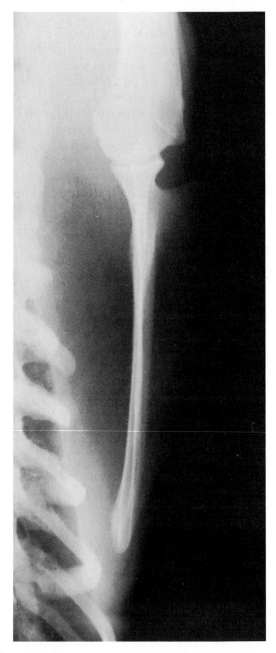

Figure 13-6 *Radiograph of the caudocranial view of the scapula.*

SHOULDER

Lateral View

The patient is placed in lateral recumbency with the shoulder of interest closest to the cassette (Figs. 13-7 and 13-8). To alleviate any superimposition of structures over the shoulder, the leg must be extended cranially and ventrally to the sternum. The opposite limb is pulled in a caudodorsal direction, and the neck is extended dorsally. This gesture rotates the sternum slightly away from the shoulder joint. Care should be taken not to overrotate the thorax because the shoulder may be lifted off the cassette.

BEAM CENTER: To shoulder point

MEASUREMENT: Thickest area over shoulder joint

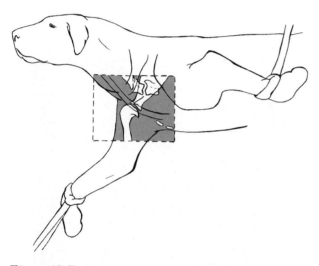

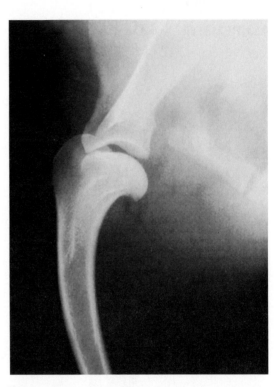

Figure 13-7 *Correct positioning for the lateral view of the shoulder.*

Figure 13-8 *Radiograph of the lateral view of the shoulder.*

SHOULDER—cont'd

Caudocranial View

The position for the caudocranial shoulder is similar to the corresponding view of the scapula. The patient is placed in dorsal recumbency with both forelimbs extended cranially (Figs. 13-9 and 13-10). The limb should be extended so that the humerus is almost parallel to the cassette. Sedation may be necessary to allow such extension. As the forelimb is extended, care must be taken not to rotate the humerus. Any rotation would create an oblique view of the shoulder joint.

In some cases it may be advantageous to expose both shoulders simultaneously. This allows the veterinarian to examine and compare both joints. The only disadvantage to this is that the x-ray beam cannot be centered directly over one joint but is centered in the middle of the two.

BEAM CENTER: To shoulder joint

MEASUREMENT: Over shoulder joint (armpit)

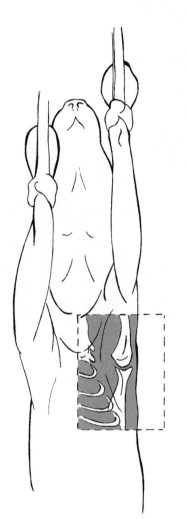

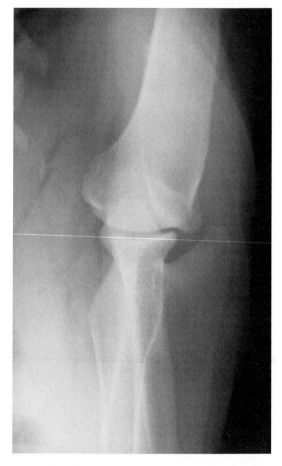

Figure 13-10 *Radiograph of the caudocranial view of the shoulder.*

Figure 13-9 *Correct positioning for the caudocranial view of the shoulder.*

HUMERUS

Lateral View

The patient is in lateral recumbency with the affected limb placed on the cassette. The leg is extended in a cranioventral direction, with the opposite limb drawn in a caudodorsal direction (Figs. 13-11 and 13-12). The head and neck should be extended dorsally. The field of view should include both the shoulder and the elbow joint with the humerus centered to the cassette.

BEAM CENTER: Center of humerus

MEASUREMENT: Thickest area over shoulder joint

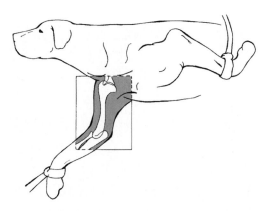

Figure 13-11 *Correct positioning for the lateral view of the humerus.*

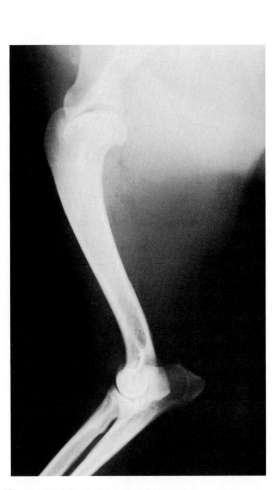

Figure 13-12 *Radiograph of the lateral view of the humerus.*

HUMERUS—*cont'd*

Caudocranial View

The patient is placed in dorsal recumbency with the forelimbs extended cranially (Figs. 13-13 and 13-14). The leg of interest should remain as parallel to the cassette as possible to minimize distortion. The head and neck should remain between the forelimbs to eliminate superimposition and rotation of the body. The humerus should be centered to the cassette, and both the shoulder and the elbow should be included in the field of view.

BEAM CENTER: Middle of humerus

MEASUREMENT: Thickest area over shoulder region

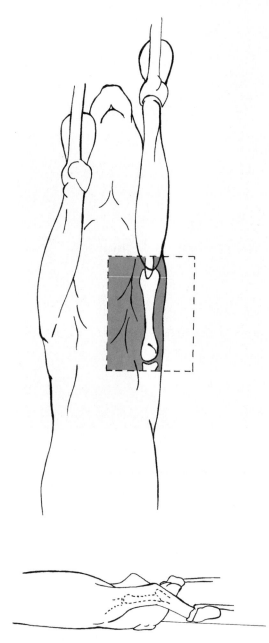

Figure 13-13 *Correct positioning for the caudocranial view of the humerus.*

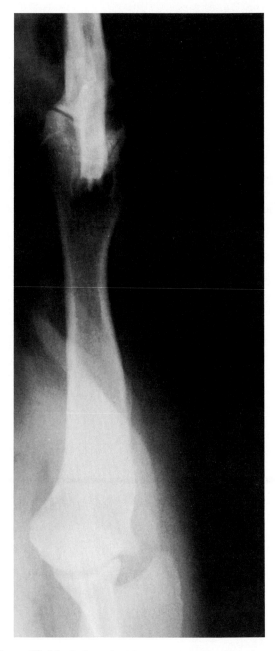

Figure 13-14 *Radiograph of the caudocranial view of the humerus.*

HUMERUS—cont'd

Craniocaudal View

The patient is placed in dorsal recumbency with the affected limb pulled caudally until the line of the humerus is parallel with the cassette (Figs. 13-15 and 13-16). The limb should be abducted slightly from the thorax to alleviate any superimposition of ribs over the area of interest. The field of view should include the shoulder, humerus, and elbow. This view of the humerus has a relatively long object–film distance and usually exhibits some magnification.

BEAM CENTER: Middle of humerus

MEASUREMENT: Thickest area over shoulder region

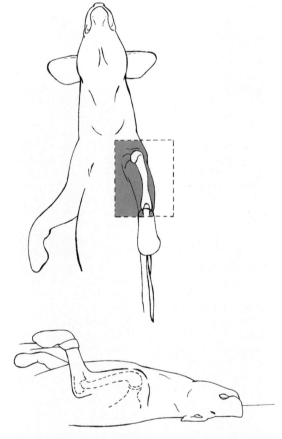

Figure 13-15 *Correct positioning for the craniocaudal view of the humerus.*

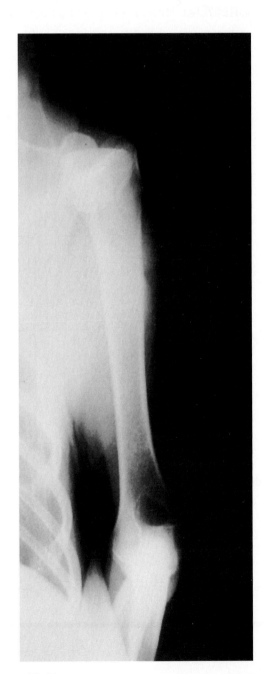

Figure 13-16 *Radiograph of the craniocaudal view of the humerus.*

ELBOW

Craniocaudal View

The patient is placed in sternal recumbency with the affected limb extended cranially (Figs. 13-17 and 13-18). The patient's head should be elevated and positioned away from the affected side. Care should be taken to prevent the elbow from displacing laterally or medially when the head is pulled to one side. To maintain a true craniocaudal position, the olecranon should be placed between the medial and the lateral humeral epicondyles. Placing a foam pad under the point of the elbow may alleviate rolling and prevent rotation.

BEAM CENTER: Over elbow joint

MEASUREMENT: Thickest area (distal humerus)

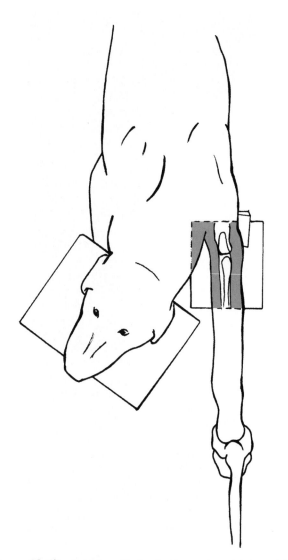

Figure 13-17 *Correct positioning for the craniocaudal view of the elbow.*

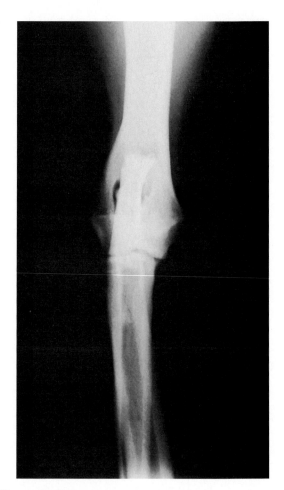

Figure 13-18 *Radiograph of the craniocaudal view of the elbow.*

ELBOW—*cont'd*

Lateral View

The patient is placed in lateral recumbency with the affected limb positioned on the cassette (Figs. 13-19 and 13-20). The head and neck should be extended slightly in a dorsal direction, and the unaffected limb is pulled in a caudodorsal direction. A foam wedge can be placed under the metacarpal region to maintain a true lateral view of the elbow.

BEAM CENTER: Over elbow joint

MEASUREMENT: Distal humerus

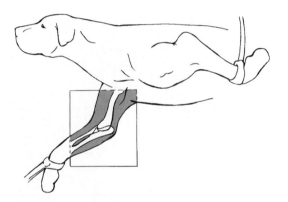

Figure 13-19 *Correct positioning for the lateral view of the elbow.*

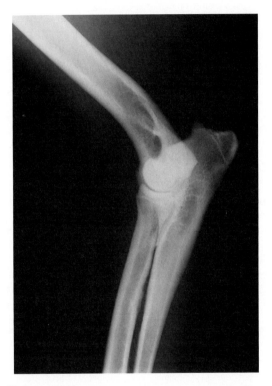

Figure 13-20 *Radiograph of the lateral view of the elbow.*

ELBOW—*cont'd*

Flexed Lateral View

The patient is placed in the same position as for the routine lateral projection. The carpus is pulled toward the neck region, flexing the elbow (Figs. 13-21 and 13-22).

Care should be taken to keep the elbow in a true lateral position during flexion. Keeping the carpus lateral ensures that the elbow remains in a true lateral position.

BEAM CENTER: Middle of elbow

MEASUREMENT: Distal humerus

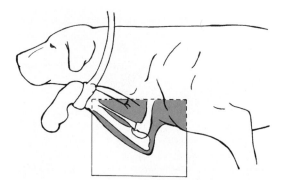

Figure 13-21 *Correct positioning for the flexed lateral view of the elbow.*

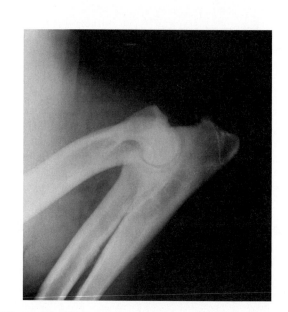

Figure 13-22 *Radiograph of the flexed lateral view of the elbow.*

RADIUS AND ULNA

Lateral View

The patient is placed in lateral recumbency with the affected limb centered on the cassette. The opposite limb is drawn caudally out of the way (Figs. 13-23 and 13-24). The primary x-ray beam should include the elbow and carpal joints.

BEAM CENTER: Middle of radius and ulna

MEASUREMENT: Over elbow

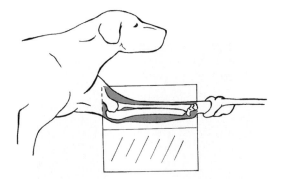

Figure 13-23 *Correct positioning for the lateral view of the radius and ulna.*

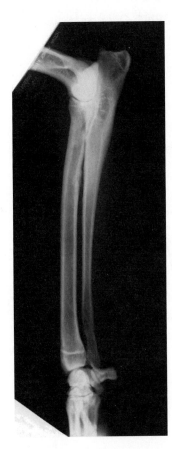

Figure 13-24 *Radiograph of the lateral view of the radius and ulna.*

RADIUS AND ULNA—*cont'd*

Craniocaudal View

The patient is placed in sternal recumbency. The affected limb is extended cranially, with the radius and ulna centered on the cassette. The head should be elevated and positioned away from the affected side (Figs. 13-25 and 13-26). A true craniocaudal position is ensured by confirming the placement of the olecranon between the humeral condyles. The collimated x-ray beam should include the elbow and the carpus.

BEAM CENTER: Middle of radius and ulna

MEASUREMENT: Over distal humerus

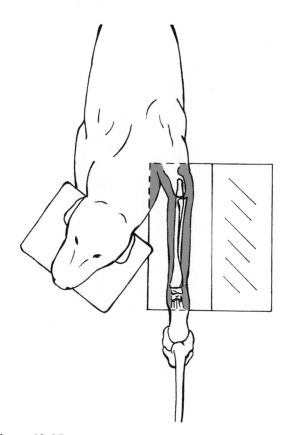

Figure 13-25 *Correct positioning for the craniocaudal view of the radius and ulna.*

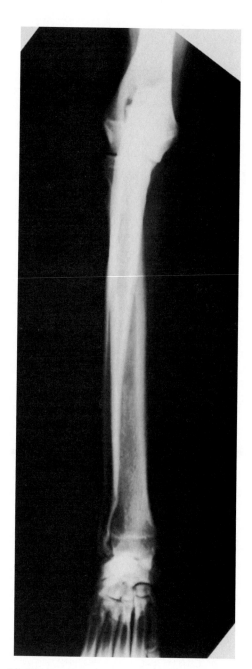

Figure 13-26 *Radiograph of the craniocaudal view of the radius and ulna.*

CARPUS

Lateral View

The patient is placed in lateral recumbency with the affected limb on the center of the cassette (Figs. 13-27 and 13-28). A foam wedge pad can be placed under the elbow to prevent the carpus from moving away from the cassette. The opposite limb is pulled caudally out of the field of view. A flexed lateral view of the carpus can be taken in this position as well, if necessary.

BEAM CENTER: Over distal row of carpal bones

MEASUREMENT: Middle of carpus

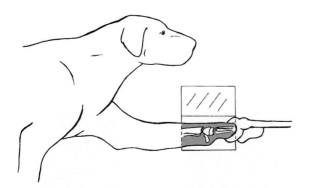

Figure 13-27 *Correct positioning for the lateral view of the carpus.*

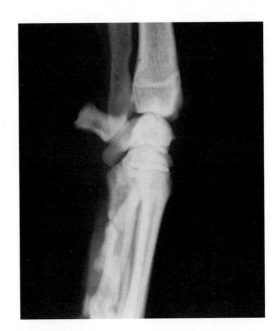

Figure 13-28 *Radiograph of the lateral view of the carpus.*

CARPUS—*cont'd*

Dorsopalmar View

The patient is placed in sternal recumbency with the affected limb extended cranially (Figs. 13-29 and 13-30). The carpus is placed flat on the cassette. A foam pad may be placed under the elbow to prevent rotation.

Because some injuries are difficult to detect radiologically on the standard dorsopalmar and lateral views, oblique views may be helpful. Dorsopalmar-mediolateral and dorsopalmar-lateromedial oblique views are taken at 45 degrees off the dorsopalmar view.

Other views that may be useful to detect joint instability of the carpus are dorsopalmar stressed views. With the affected carpus placed in dorsopalmar position, the radius and ulna are held firmly in place. The paw is pushed medially or laterally with a ruler or wooden paddle. Care should be taken not to apply too much force on the joint to avoid further injury.

BEAM CENTER: Middle of distal row of carpal bones

MEASUREMENT: At beam center site

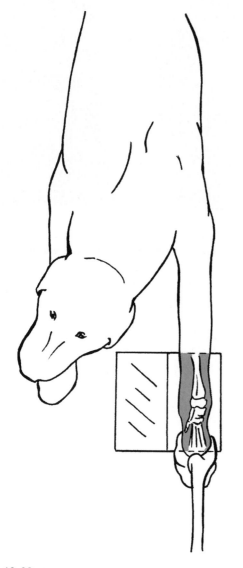

Figure 13-29 *Correct positioning for the dorsopalmar view of the carpus.*

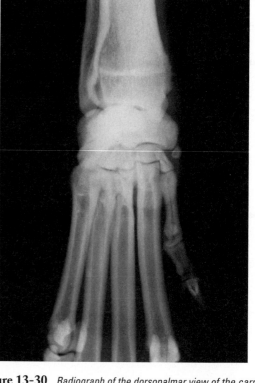

Figure 13-30 *Radiograph of the dorsopalmar view of the carpus.*

METACARPUS-PHALANGES

Dorsopalmar View

The patient is placed in sternal recumbency with the limb of interest extended (Figs. 13-31 and 13-32). The paw is placed flat on the cassette. A piece of adhesive tape can be used to flatten the digits, if necessary. The field size should be large enough to include the carpal joint and the tips of the digits.

BEAM CENTER: Middle of metacarpal bones

MEASUREMENT: Middle of metacarpal bones

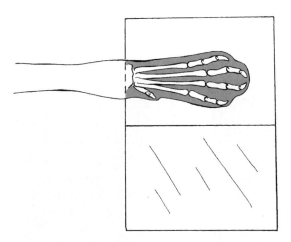

Figure 13-31 *Correct positioning for the dorsopalmar view of the metacarpus-phalanges.*

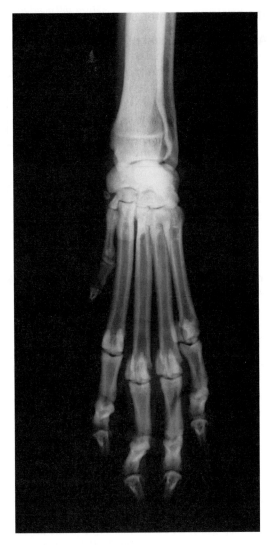

Figure 13-32 *Radiograph of the dorsopalmar view of the metacarpus-phalanges.*

chapter 14

Small Animal Pelvis and Hind Limb

CHAPTER OUTLINE

Pelvis

Femur

Stifle Joint

Tibia and Fibula

Tarsus

Metatarsus-Phalanges

PELVIS

Lateral View

The patient is placed in lateral recumbency with the side of interest closest to the cassette (Figs. 14-1 and 14-2). A foam wedge should be placed between the patient's stifle joints to keep the femurs parallel with the cassette. A foam wedge also alleviates rotation and ensures that the two sides of the pelvis are superimposed. To distinguish the right femur from the left on the finished radiograph, the limb closest to the cassette should be pulled slightly cranial and the top leg slightly caudal. This staggering of the femurs is especially important if the patient has a hip luxation and one femur needs to be differentiated from the other. The field of view should include the entire pelvis and a portion of the lumbar spine and the femurs. The pelvis should be centered in the middle of the cassette.

BEAM CENTER: Over greater femoral trochanter

MEASUREMENT: At level of trochanter

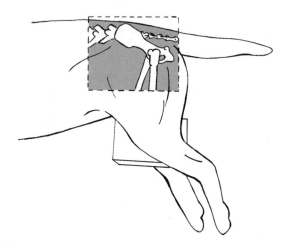

Figure 14-1   *Correct positioning for the lateral view of the pelvis.*

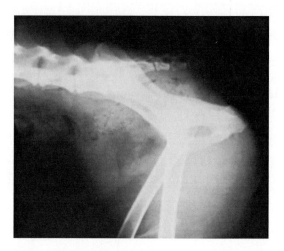

Figure 14-2   *Radiograph of the lateral view of the pelvis.*

PELVIS—*cont'd*

Ventrodorsal View

Frog-leg projection.

The frog-leg view of the pelvis is suitable when pelvic trauma is suspected. Minimal stress and tension are placed on the pelvis and hip joints in this projection.

The patient is placed in dorsal recumbency (Figs. 14-3 and 14-4). A V trough is a useful positioning device to maintain bilateral symmetry. The pelvic limbs can assume a normal, flexed position. The femurs should be at a 45-degree angle to the spine and can be secured in that position by placing sandbags over the tarsal joints. Positioning the limbs identically is important to maintain symmetry.

Extended projection.

The extended view of the pelvis is standard for the evaluation of hip joints for hip dysplasia. Symmetry and precision are vital for this view. Sedation is usually required.

A number of steps are necessary to achieve proper pelvis positioning. The patient is placed in dorsal recumbency with its back in a V trough or maintained with the aid of sandbags. The pelvic limbs are flexed into a frog-leg position, and the tarsal joints are grasped firmly. At this point the stifle joints are rotated medially toward each other. When the stifles are within 1 or 2 inches of each other, the limbs are extended caudally until the femurs are parallel with the cassette or until resistance is encountered. The hind legs can be secured with adhesive tape or handheld with the use of lead gloves (Figs. 14-5 through 14-8).

For correct positioning (Figs. 14-9 and 14-10), the following criteria must be met:

1. Femurs are parallel to each other.
2. Both patellae are centered between the femoral condyles.
3. Pelvis is without rotation; the obturator foramens, hip joints, hemipelvises, and sacroiliac joints appear as a mirror image.
4. The tail is secured with tape (if necessary) between the femurs.
5. Field of view includes the pelvis, femurs, and stifle joints.

BEAM CENTER: Over level of pubis and acetabulum

MEASUREMENT: Over acetabulum (groin)

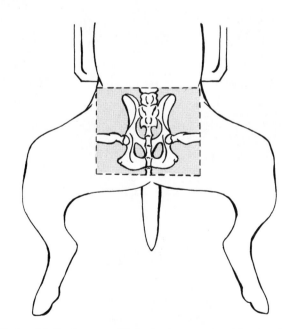

Figure 14-3 *Correct positioning for the ventrodorsal frog-leg view of the pelvis.*

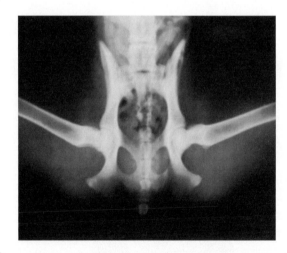

Figure 14-4 *Radiograph of the ventrodorsal frog-leg view of the pelvis.*

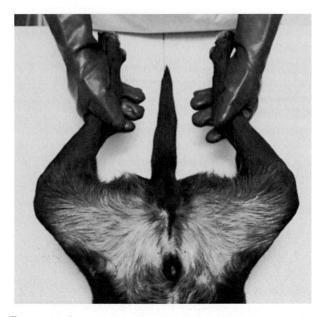

Figure 14-5 *Ventrodorsal extended view of the pelvis: Place the patient in the ventrodorsal frog-leg position.*

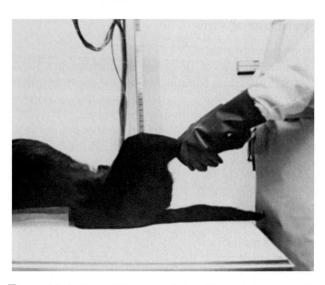

Figure 14-6 *Ventrodorsal extended view of the pelvis: Rotate the stifle joints medially so that they are an inch or two apart.*

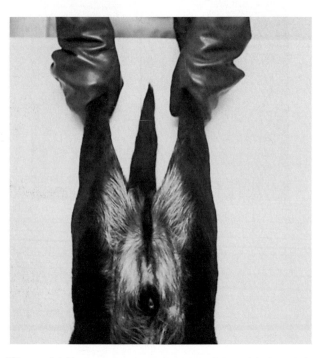

Figure 14-7 *Ventrodorsal extended view of the pelvis: Extend the femurs in a caudal direction while keeping them parallel with the table.*

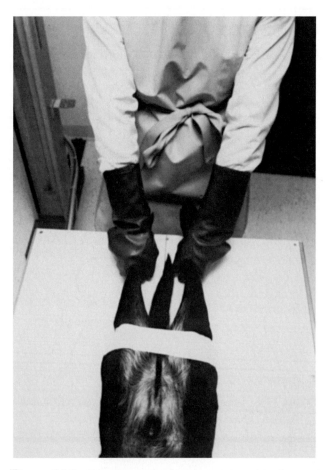

Figure 14-8 *Ventrodorsal extended view of the pelvis: If manual restraint is unwarranted or insufficient, gauze or tape can be used around the distal femurs to secure the pelvis in position.*

BEAM CENTER: Caudal portion of ischium

MEASUREMENT: Over midfemur region

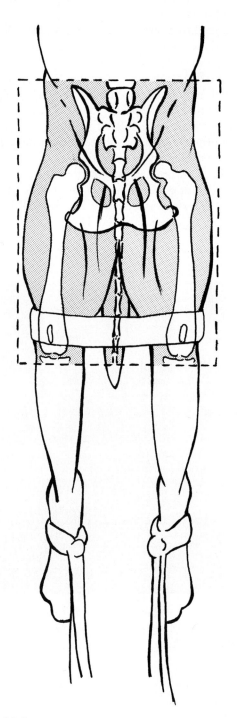

Figure 14-9 *Correct positioning for the ventrodorsal extended view of the pelvis.*

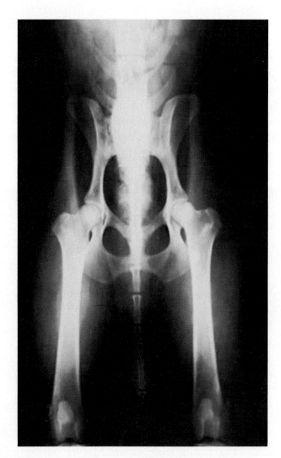

Figure 14-10 *Radiograph of the ventrodorsal extended view of the pelvis.*

The PennHIP method.

In the early 1980s Dr. Gail Smith and a team of researchers at the University of Pennsylvania School of Veterinary Medicine began a scientific investigation to determine a more reliable phenotype to predict canine hip dysplasia. PennHIP, the result of that research effort, refers to a specific diagnostic technique, as well as a provider network and database of hip laxity information. The PennHIP method has been shown to provide a more repeatable and reliable indication of a dog's passive hip laxity than is possible with the hip extended radiograph. The stress radiographic procedure consists of three views: the standard extended view (Fig. 14-11), a compression view with a neutral position, and a distraction view in the same neutral hip position (Figs. 14-12 and 14-13). In the absence of existing degenerative disease, laxity is the single most important component in predicting a dog's susceptibility to canine hip dysplasia.

Individual breed laxity profiles and disease risk curves based on these laxity profiles continue to be developed. Breeding studies have demonstrated high heritability of the PennHIP phenotype, indicating that rapid genetic change will result from selective breeding using hip laxity as a criterion. This PennHIP method has been commercially available since 1994. To perform the PennHIP procedure, the veterinarian or technician must undergo specialized training and certification.

To obtain additional information about PennHIP, contact Synbiotics Corporation at 1-800-248-8099. (PennHIP information courtesy Dr. Steve Peterson of the Synbiotics Corporation, San Diego.)

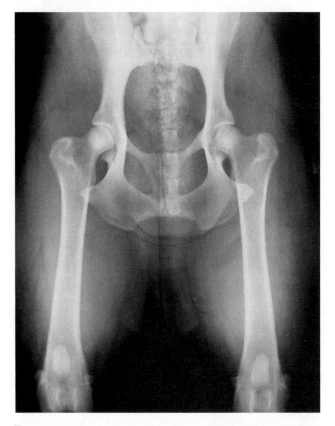

Figure 14-11 *Traditional hip extended view. Orthopedic Foundation for Animals (OFA) rating of "good."*

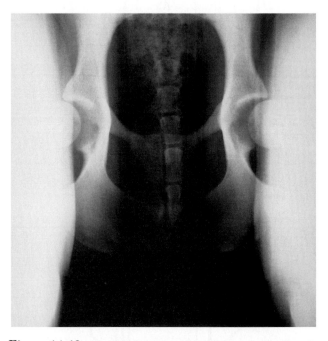

Figure 14-12 *PennHIP distraction view of the same dog. Note the marked laxity present on this view that was not evident from the extended hip view in Figure 14-11.*

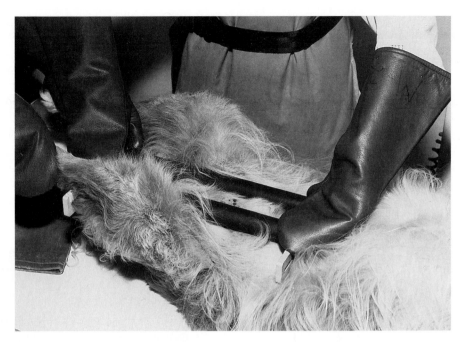

Figure 14-13 *View of the PennHIP procedure showing placement of the distraction device and position of the patient during the PennHIP distraction procedure.*

FEMUR

Lateral View

The patient is placed in lateral recumbency with the affected limb closest to the cassette. The opposite limb is abducted and rotated out of the line of the x-ray beam (Figs. 14-14 and 14-15). A foam pad placed under the proximal tibia can alleviate any rotation of the femur. The field of view should include the hip joint, femur, and stifle joint.

BEAM CENTER: Middle of femur

MEASUREMENT: Middle of femur

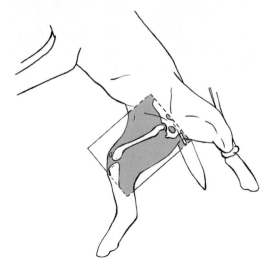

Figure 14-14 *Correct positioning for the lateral view of the femur.*

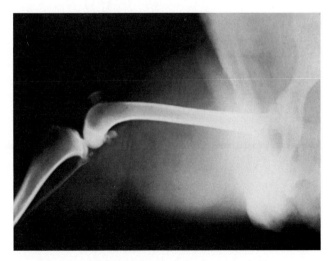

Figure 14-15 *Radiograph of the lateral view of the femur.*

FEMUR—*cont'd*

Craniocaudal View

The patient is placed in dorsal recumbency with the limb of interest extended caudally (Figs. 14-16 and 14-17). Slight abduction of the affected limb eliminates superimposition of the proximal femur over the tuber ischium.

The opposite limb can be flexed and rotated laterally to assist the abduction. Proper alignment is essential so that the femur is in a true craniocaudal position; the patella should be between the two femoral condyles. The field of view should include the hip joint, femur, and stifle joint.

BEAM CENTER: Middle of femur

MEASUREMENT: Middle of femur

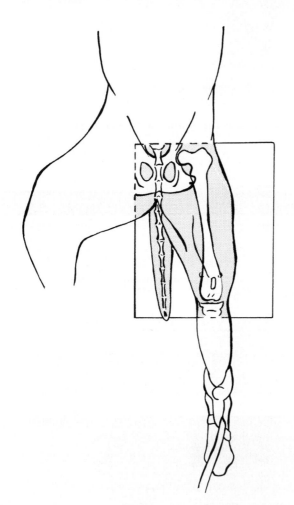

Figure 14-16 *Correct positioning for the craniocaudal view of the femur.*

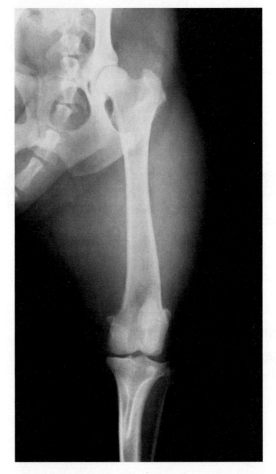

Figure 14-17 *Radiograph of the craniocaudal view of the femur.*

STIFLE JOINT

Caudocranial View

The patient is positioned in sternal recumbency with the affected limb pulled into a position of maximum extension (Figs. 14-18 and 14-19). The opposite limb is flexed and elevated with a sponge or sandbag. Elevation of the opposite limb controls the lateral rotation of the stifle joint under examination. Determining the proper degree of rotation is critical to achieving a true caudocranial view; the patella should be centered between the femoral condyles. Palpation of the femoral condyles and the tibial tuberosity may be helpful to ensure symmetry.

A craniocaudal view of the stifle joint is also possible. The patient is positioned in dorsal recumbency with the limb under investigation extended as for the craniocaudal view of the femur. Although this view may be easier to position, it has the disadvantage of some magnification and distortion of the image due to increased object–film distance.

BEAM CENTER: Over stifle joint

MEASUREMENT: Distal end of femur

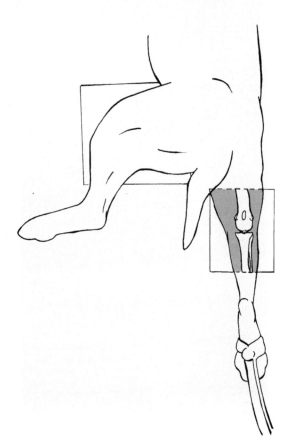

Figure 14-18 *Correct positioning for the caudocranial view of the stifle joint.*

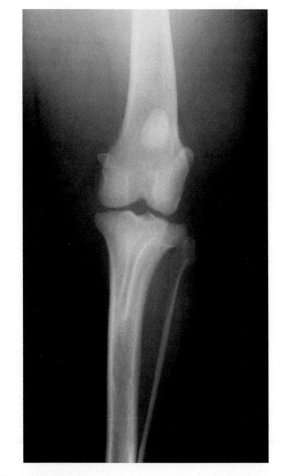

Figure 14-19 *Radiograph of the caudocranial view of the stifle joint.*

STIFLE JOINT—*cont'd*

Lateral View

The patient is placed in lateral recumbency with the affected joint placed and centered on the cassette. The opposite limb is flexed and abducted from the line of the x-ray beam. The stifle joint should be in a natural, slightly flexed position (Figs. 14-20 and 14-21). A sponge pad can be placed under the tarsus so that the tibia is parallel to the cassette surface. Elevation of the tibia ensures superimposition of the two femoral condyles and assists a true lateral projection.

BEAM CENTER: Over stifle joint

MEASUREMENT: Over femoral condyles

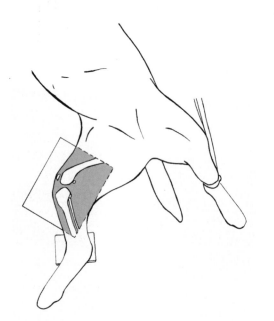

Figure 14-20 *Correct positioning for the lateral view of the stifle joint.*

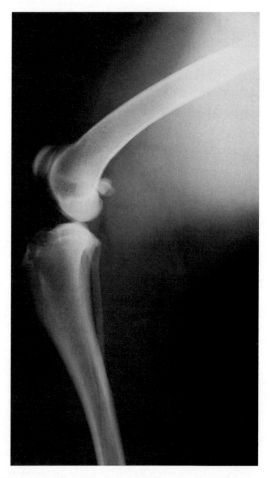

Figure 14-21 *Radiograph of the lateral view of the stifle joint.*

STIFLE JOINT—*cont'd*

Skyline Projection of Patella (Sunrise View)

The skyline projection demonstrates changes that can occur to the patella and the femoral trochlear groove.

The patient is placed in lateral recumbency with the opposite limb down on the table (Figs. 14-22 and 14-23). The affected limb should be in a fully flexed position.

Tape or roll gauze can be placed around the midtibia and femur to hold the stifle joint in this flexed position. The stifle should remain horizontal and can be supported on a foam pad. The cassette is placed behind the stifle joint vertically, and a horizontal x-ray beam is centered to the patella.

BEAM CENTER: Over patella

MEASUREMENT: Site of patellar articulation

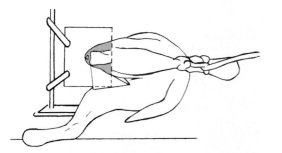

Figure 14-22 *Correct positioning for the skyline view of the patella.*

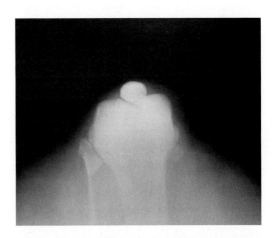

Figure 14-23 *Radiograph of the skyline view of the patella.*

TIBIA AND FIBULA

Lateral View

The patient is placed in lateral recumbency with the affected limb on the cassette. The stifle should be slightly flexed and maintained in a true lateral position (Figs. 14-24 and 14-25). A sponge wedge can be placed under the metatarsus to eliminate any rotation of the tibia. The opposite limb is pulled cranially or caudally so that it is out of the line of the x-ray beam. The field of view should include the stifle joint, tibia and fibula, and tarsal joint.

BEAM CENTER: Middle of tibia and fibula

MEASUREMENT: Over stifle joint

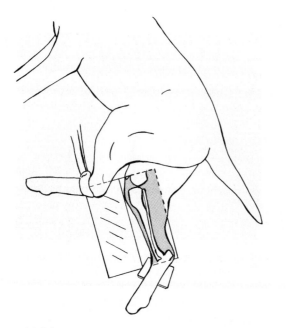

Figure 14-24   *Correct positioning for the lateral view of the tibia and fibula.*

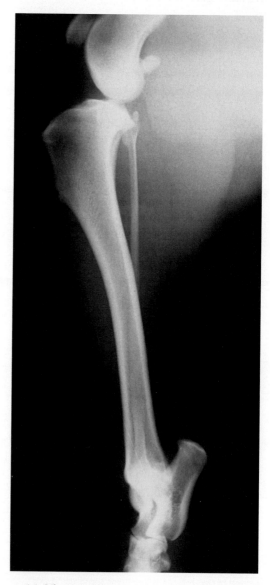

Figure 14-25   *Radiograph of the lateral view of the tibia and fibula.*

TIBIA AND FIBULA—*cont'd*

Caudocranial View

The patient is placed in sternal recumbency with the affected limb extended caudally (Figs. 14-26 and 14-27). The tibia and fibula are centered on the cassette. The body can be supported in position with foam blocks placed beneath the caudal abdomen and pelvic region. Elevation of the hind end minimizes the weight placed on the stifle joint extended caudally and assists positioning. The tibia and fibula should be in a true caudocranial position so that the patella is placed between the two femoral condyles. The opposite limb should be flexed and placed on a sponge pad to control rotation of the limb of interest. If the patient has a long tail, it should be secured with tape out of the field of view. The field of view should include the stifle joint, tibia and fibula, and tarsal joint.

BEAM CENTER: Middle of tibia and fibula

MEASUREMENT: Over level of stifle joint

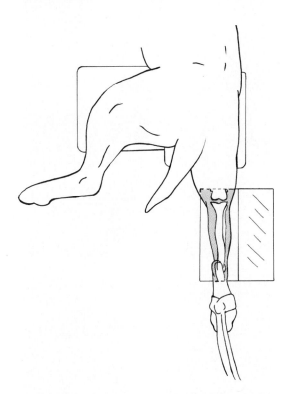

Figure 14-26 *Correct positioning for the caudocranial view of the tibia and fibula.*

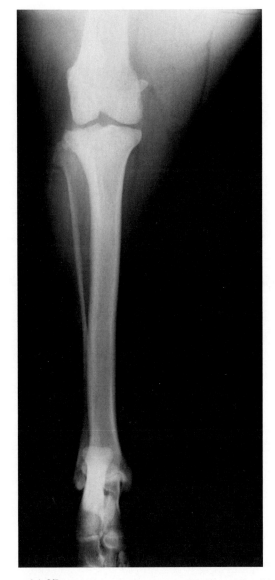

Figure 14-27 *Radiograph of the caudocranial view of the tibia and fibula.*

TARSUS

Lateral View

The patient is placed in lateral recumbency with the affected limb closest to the cassette. The tarsus is placed in a natural, slightly flexed position and centered on the cassette (Figs. 14-28 and 14-29). The tarsus must remain in a true lateral position; a sponge wedge or tape can be used to eliminate any rotation of the limb. The opposite limb should be pulled cranially out of the line of the x-ray beam.

BEAM CENTER: Middle of tarsus

MEASUREMENT: Over thickest area of tarsal joint

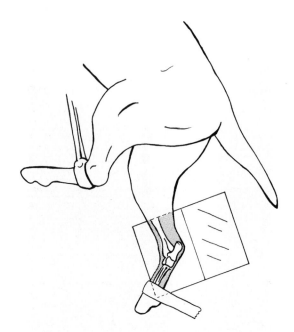

Figure 14-28 *Correct positioning for the lateral view of the tarsus.*

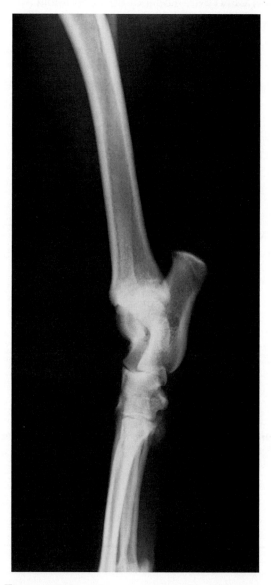

Figure 14-29 *Radiograph of the lateral view of the tarsus.*

TARSUS—cont'd

Plantarodorsal and Dorsoplantar Views

The patient is placed in sternal recumbency with the affected limb extended as for the caudocranial view of the tibia and fibula (Figs. 14-30 through 14-32). The tarsus is centered on the cassette. Foam blocks are placed under the caudal abdomen and pelvic region for patient comfort and to control rotation of the tarsus. A foam wedge should be placed under the stifle joint to achieve maximum extension of the tarsus. If the stifle joint is in a true caudocranial position, the tarsus will naturally follow in a true plantarodorsal position.

The dorsoplantar view of the tarsus may be easier to assist if an animal resists caudal extension of the hind limb. The patient is placed in sternal recumbency with the affected limb extended cranially alongside the body. The limb should be slightly abducted from the body wall to prevent any superimposition over the tarsus. A true dorsoplantar position is ensured by rotating the stifle medially in order to center the patella between the femoral condyles.

BEAM CENTER: Middle of tarsal joint

MEASUREMENT: Thickest area of tarsal joint

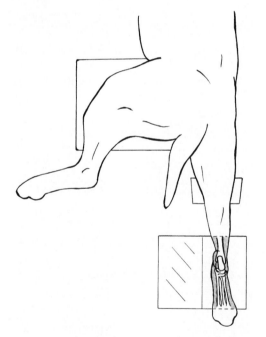

Figure 14-30 *Correct positioning for the plantarodorsal view of the tarsus.*

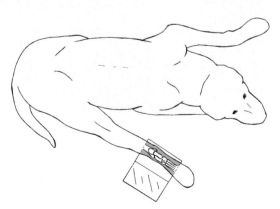

Figure 14-31 *Correct positioning for the dorsoplantar view of the tarsus.*

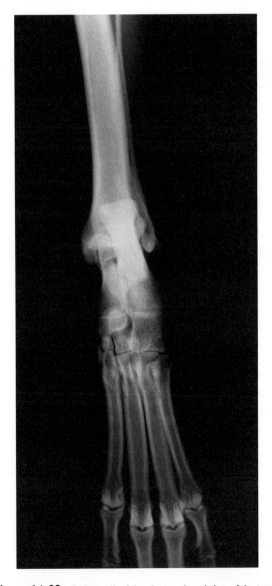

Figure 14-32 *Radiograph of the plantarodorsal view of the tarsus.*

METATARSUS-PHALANGES

Lateral View

The patient is placed in lateral recumbency with the affected metatarsus centered on the cassette (Figs. 14-33 and 14-34). The opposite limb can be pulled caudally or cranially out of view of the x-ray beam. The joint is positioned in a natural flexed position. A sponge pad can be placed under the stifle joint to maintain a true lateral position of the metatarsus. The field of view should include the tarsal joint, metatarsus, and phalanges.

BEAM CENTER: Midmetatarsal region

MEASUREMENT: Distal tarsal joint

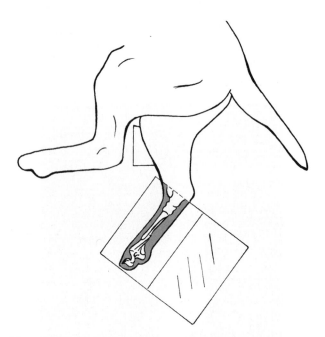

Figure 14-33 *Correct positioning for the lateral view of the metatarsus and phalanges.*

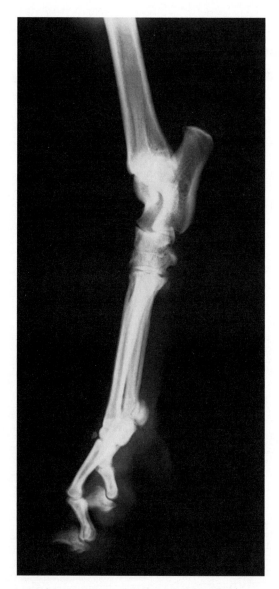

Figure 14-34 *Radiograph of the lateral view of the metatarsus and phalanges.*

METATARSUS-PHALANGES

Dorsoplantar and Plantarodorsal Views

For the dorsoplantar view the patient is placed in sternal recumbency, and the limb of interest is pulled cranially and slightly abducted from the body wall (Figs. 14-35 and 14-36). The metatarsus is centered on the cassette. To achieve a true dorsoplantar view, the stifle joint of the affected limb is rotated laterally and secured with tape. The field of view should include the tarsus, metatarsus, and phalanges.

The plantarodorsal view is positioned the same as the plantarodorsal view of the tarsus.

BEAM CENTER: Midmetatarsal region

MEASUREMENT: Distal tarsal joint

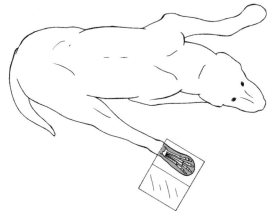

Figure 14-35 *Correct positioning for the dorsoplantar view of the metatarsus and phalanges.*

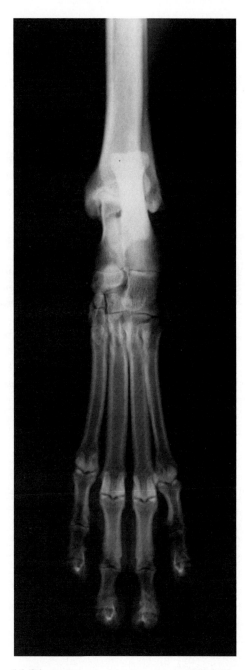

Figure 14-36 *Radiograph of the dorsoplantar view of the metatarsus and phalanges.*

KEY POINTS

1. When radiographing the pelvis in a lateral position, a foam wedge should be placed between the patient's stifles to keep the femurs parallel.
2. Measurement for the lateral pelvic view should be taken over the trochanter, and measurement for the ventrodorsal view should be taken at the acetabulum.
3. To use the PennHIP method of diagnosing canine hip dysplasia, the veterinarian and technician must receive special certification.
4. Sedating the patient is often necessary to take radiographs used to diagnose hip dysplasia.

REVIEW QUESTIONS

1. When radiographing the pelvis in a lateral position, which femur should be slightly more cranial?
   a. The limb farthest from the cassette
   b. The limb closest to the cassette
   c. The limbs must be superimposed
   d. Two lateral views are required—one with the limb closest to the cassette more cranial and the second with the limb farthest from the cassette more cranial.

2. If pelvic trauma is suspected, what view is recommended?
   a. Dorsal recumbency with pelvic limbs extended
   b. Sternal recumbency with pelvic limbs extended
   c. Sternal recumbency with pelvic limbs in a frog-leg position
   d. Dorsal recumbency with pelvic limbs in a frog-leg position

3. To diagnose canine hip dysplasia using the PennHIP method, which positions are required?
   a. Compression view in neutral hip position
   b. Standard extended view
   c. Distracted view in neutral hip position
   d. All of the above

4. Which joints must be included in a radiograph of the femur?
   a. Coxofemoral and stifle
   b. Stifle and sacroiliac
   c. Stifle and tarsus
   d. Coxofemoral and sacroiliac

5. Which view of the stifle is most likely to be magnified?
   a. Lateral
   b. Caudocranial
   c. Extended
   d. Craniocaudal

6. Where is the cassette placed during the skyline projection of the patella?
   a. In the Bucky tray
   b. Horizontally on the tabletop, behind the stifle
   c. Vertically on the tabletop, behind the stifle
   d. Vertically on the tabletop, in front of the stifle

7. Which of the following can assist maintaining a true dorsoplantar view of the metatarsus-phalanges?
   a. Rotate the stifle laterally
   b. Rotate the sternum laterally
   c. Extend the limb as much as possible
   d. Rotate the stifle medially

8. Where should the measurement be taken for a caudocranial view of the tibia and fibula?
   a. Middle of the fibula
   b. Level of stifle joint
   c. Distal fibula
   d. Distal femur

9. Which of the following are aids to securing and maintaining positions of limbs when taking radiographs?
   a. Gloves used as props
   b. Foam wedges
   c. Tape
   d. Both b and c

10. What can the PennHIP method of diagnosing hip dysplasia assess that the extended projection alone cannot assess?
    a. The length of the femurs
    b. The density of the bone
    c. The laxity of the hip joint
    d. Degenerative joint disease

SUGGESTED READINGS

Douglas SW, Herrtage ME, Williamson HD: *Principles of veterinary radiography,* ed 4, Philadelphia, 1987, Bailliere Tindall.

Habel RE: *Applied veterinary anatomy,* ed 2, Ithaca, NY, 1978, RE Habel.

Kleine LJ, Warren RG: *Small animal radiography,* St. Louis, 1982, Mosby.

Morgan JP, Silverman S: *Techniques of veterinary radiography,* ed 4, Ames, Iowa, 1987, Iowa State University Press.

Ryan GD: *Radiographic positioning of small animals,* Philadelphia, 1981, Lea & Febiger.

Schebitz H, Wilkins H: *Atlas of radiographic anatomy of the dog and cat,* Philadelphia, 1986, WB Saunders.

Smallwood JE, Shively MJ: Nomenclature for radiographic views of limbs, *Equine Pract* 1:41-45, 1979.

Ticer JW: *Radiographic technique in small animal practice,* ed 2, Philadelphia, 1984, WB Saunders.

chapter 15

Small Animal Skull

CHAPTER OUTLINE

Skull
Frontal Sinuses
Cranium
Nasal Cavity
Tympanic Bullae

Temporomandibular Joint
Maxilla
Mandible
Teeth

SKULL

Introduction

To obtain a correctly positioned radiograph of the skull, a controlled patient is vital. Anesthesia is usually necessary. If the animal is under general anesthesia, it may be necessary to remove the endotracheal tube in some views to avoid superimposing shadows over the area of interest. The key to a diagnostic radiograph of the skull is precision and symmetry. Any rotation, even slight, may inhibit an accurate diagnosis.

The anatomy of the skull is complicated, and radiography of the area can be just as complex. Familiarity with the anatomy of the small animal skull assists the correct positioning of various views (Figs. 15-1 and 15-2). Furthermore, veterinary radiography deals with many breeds and species and the number of physical variations in skull anatomy adds to the complexity of positioning.

Compare the skull of a collie with that of a Boston terrier—the difference is enormous. However, the principles presented here can be applied to any small animal breed and species.

Lateral View

The patient should be placed in lateral recumbency with the affected side of the skull toward the cassette (Figs. 15-3 and 15-4). To eliminate rotation of the skull, a foam pad of suitable thickness is placed under the ramus of the mandible. The nasal septum should be parallel to the

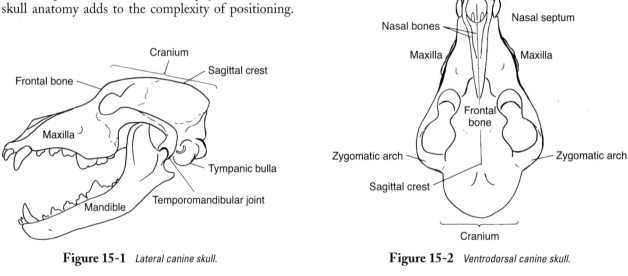

Figure 15-1 *Lateral canine skull.*

Figure 15-2 *Ventrodorsal canine skull.*

BEAM CENTER: Lateral canthus of eye

MEASUREMENT: Over high point of zygomatic arch (for demonstration of nares, measurement should be taken at nasal notch)

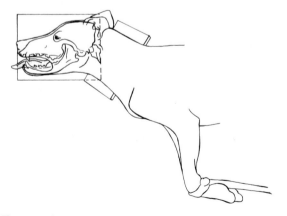

Figure 15-3 *Correct positioning for the lateral view of the skull.*

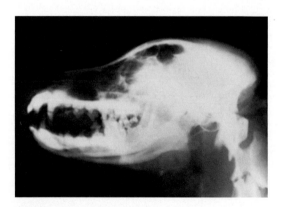

Figure 15-4 *Radiograph of the lateral view of the skull.*

surface of the cassette. From the view of the x-ray tube (bird's-eye view), the mandibular rami should be super-imposed. Placing a pad under the cranioventral cervical region and pulling the front limbs caudally may help maintain the skull in a true lateral position. The field of view should include the entire head from the tip of the nose to the base of the skull.

Dorsoventral View

The patient is placed in sternal recumbency with the head resting on the cassette (Figs. 15-5 and 15-6). Gentle

pressure can be placed over the cervical region with a sandbag to keep the skull next to the cassette in a dorso-ventral position. The front limbs can remain in a natural position alongside the head but out of view of the x-ray beam. Check the final positioning by looking in a rostro-caudal direction. The sagittal plane of the head should be perpendicular to the cassette. If the head consistently rotates to one side or the other, a strip of adhesive tape can be placed over the cranium in the desired position. The field of view should include the entire head from the tip of the nose to the base of the skull.

BEAM CENTER: Lateral canthus of eye

MEASUREMENT: Over high point of cranium

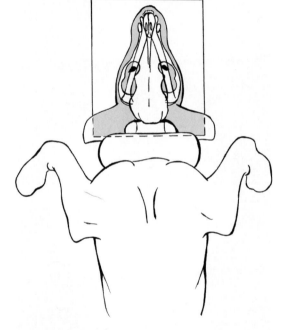

Figure 15-5 *Correct positioning for the dorsoventral view of the skull.*

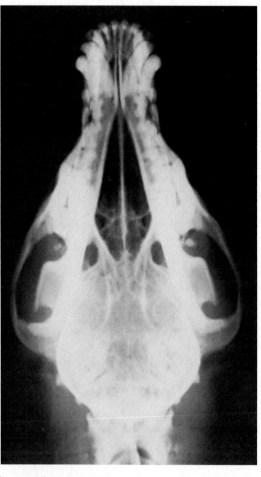

Figure 15-6 *Radiograph of the dorsoventral view of the skull.*

SKULL—*cont'd*

Ventrodorsal View

The patient is placed in dorsal recumbency (Figs. 15-7 and 15-8). A V trough or sandbags may be used to keep the animal in position. The front limbs are extended caudally and secured. A foam pad should be placed under the midcervical region to properly position the skull on the cassette. The nose must remain parallel to the cassette, and the skull must be balanced in a true ventrodorsal position. Rotation of the skull is a problem with animals that have a prominent external occipital protuberance. A thin sponge pad placed under the cranium helps prevent this type of rotation. The field of view should include the entire head from the tip of the nose to the base of the skull.

BEAM CENTER: Lateral canthus of eye

MEASUREMENT: Lateral canthus of eye

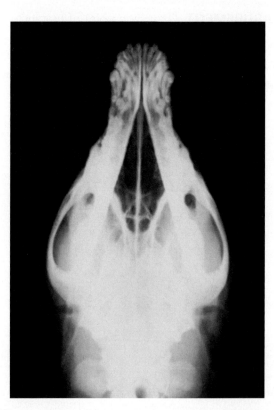

Figure 15-8 *Radiograph of the ventrodorsal view of the skull.*

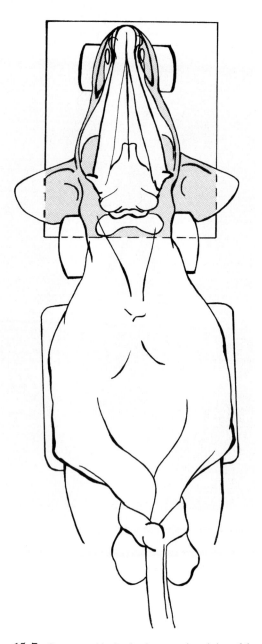

Figure 15-7 *Correct positioning for the ventrodorsal view of the skull.*

FRONTAL SINUSES

Rostrocaudal View

The patient is placed in dorsal recumbency with the nose pointing upward (Figs. 15-9 and 15-10). The front legs should be pulled caudally alongside the body. The nose is positioned perpendicular to the cassette. A length of roll gauze or tape can be tied around the nose to stabilize the patient in this position. The frontal sinuses should be centered on the cassette, and the field of view should include the entire forehead of the patient. The collimator central beam should be aimed perpendicularly to the cassette and centered between the eyes.

BEAM CENTER: Through center of frontal sinuses, between eyes

MEASUREMENT: Over site of nasal sinuses ("nose stop")

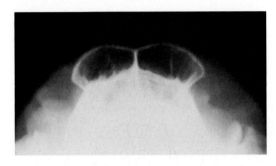

Figure 15-10 *Radiograph of the rostrocaudal view of the front sinuses.*

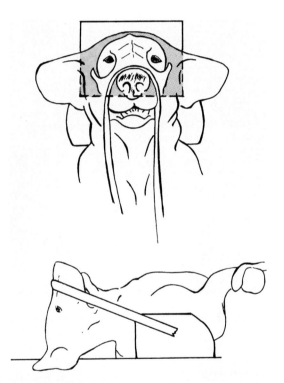

Figure 15-9 *Correct positioning for the rostrocaudal view of the frontal sinuses.*

CRANIUM

Rostrocaudal View

The patient is placed in dorsal recumbency with the nose pointing upward and the front limbs pulled caudally alongside the body (Figs. 15-11 and 15-12). This view is similar to the frontal sinus projection, except that the angle of the nose is directed slightly in a caudal direction.

With a length of roll gauze or tape, the nose is pulled caudally approximately 10 to 15 degrees. If an endotracheal tube is in place, care must be taken not to crimp the tube while flexing the animal's neck. The cranium should be centered to the cassette, and the field of view should include the entire cranium.

BEAM CENTER: Midpoint between eyes

MEASUREMENT: Site of frontal sinuses

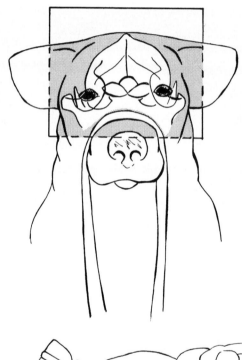

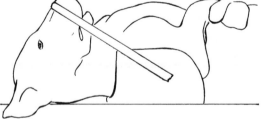

Figure 15-11 *Correct positioning for the rostrocaudal view of the cranium.*

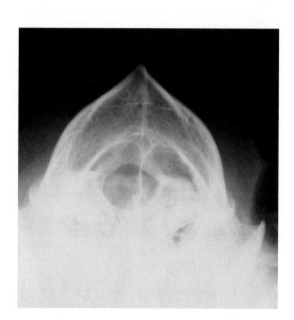

Figure 15-12 *Radiograph of the rostrocaudal view of the cranium.*

NASAL CAVITY

Ventrodorsal Open-Mouth View

The patient is placed in dorsal recumbency with the front legs extended caudally alongside the body. The maxilla remains parallel with the cassette and is secured with a strip of tape placed inside the mouth, with the ends of the tape adhered to the table on either side of the patient's head. A length of roll gauze or tape is tied around the mandible and pulled in a caudal direction so that the mouth is wide open (Figs. 15-13 and 15-14). The mouth may also be propped open with a tongue depressor placed between the canine teeth of the upper and lower arcades.

Keep in mind that the tongue depressor may cast a slightly superimposing shadow over the nasal cavity. If an endotracheal tube is in place, it should be tied to the mandible or removed before exposure to prevent superimposition of this structure over the area of interest.

The x-ray tube should be angled 10 to 15 degrees so that the x-ray beam is directed inside the mouth. The nasal cavity should be centered to the cassette, and the field of view should include the entire maxilla from the tip of the nose to the pharyngeal region.

BEAM CENTER: Through level of third upper premolar

MEASUREMENT: Over level of third upper premolar

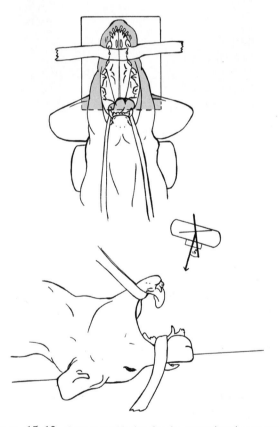

Figure 15-13 *Correct positioning for the ventrodorsal open-mouth view of the nasal cavity.*

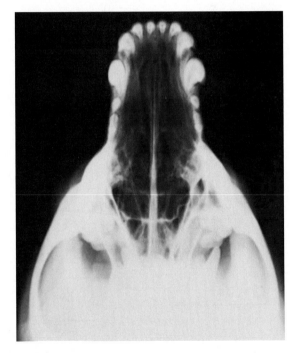

Figure 15-14 *Radiograph of the ventrodorsal open-mouth view of the nasal cavity.*

TYMPANIC BULLAE

Rostrocaudal Open-Mouth View

The patient is placed in dorsal recumbency with the nose pointing upward and the front legs pulled in a caudal direction alongside the body. The mouth is held open with gauze or another suitable mouth speculum (Figs. 15-15 and 15-16). The nose is pulled approximately 5 to 10 degrees in a cranial direction, and the mandible is pulled caudally. The amount of cranial pull on the maxilla varies with the shape of the skull of the breed. The bullae should be projected free from the mandible and the hard palate of the maxilla. The field of view should include the entire nasopharyngeal region of the skull.

BEAM CENTER: At level of commissure of lips

MEASUREMENT: At level of commissure of lips

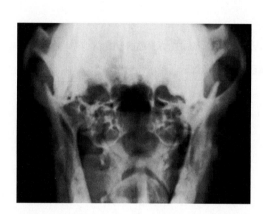

Figure 15-16 *Radiograph of the rostrocaudal open-mouth view of the tympanic bullae.*

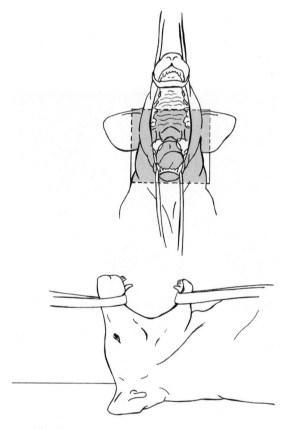

Figure 15-15 *Correct positioning of the rostrocaudal open-mouth view of the tympanic bullae.*

TYMPANIC BULLAE—*cont'd*

Lateral Oblique View

The patient is placed in lateral recumbency with the unaffected tympanic bulla toward the cassette (Figs. 15-17 and 15-18). The front legs should be extended caudally slightly to assist the skull lying in a natural oblique position. In most instances, the skull has a natural lie of 8 to 12 degrees of rotation from true lateral. This degree of rotation allows the tympanic bullae to offset one another and provides adequate isolation of the structures. This view of the bullae can also be used to examine an oblique projection of the temporomandibular joints.

BEAM CENTER: Over center of tympanic bullae

MEASUREMENT: At level of tympanic bullae

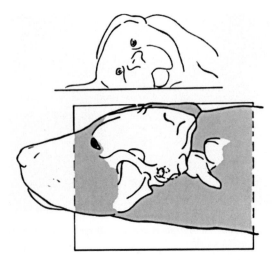

Figure 15-17 *Correct positioning for the lateral oblique view of the tympanic bullae.*

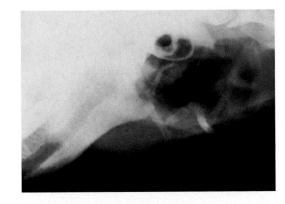

Figure 15-18 *Radiograph of the lateral oblique view of the tympanic bullae.*

TEMPOROMANDIBULAR JOINT

Ventrodorsal Oblique View

The patient is placed in lateral recumbency with the affected side toward the cassette. The skull is initially placed in a true lateral position. The cranium is then rotated approximately 20 degrees toward the cassette (Figs. 15-19 and 15-20). A sponge wedge under the mandible secures the skull in this position. This rotation prevents superimposition by the opposite temporomandibular joint and other surrounding structures. The ventrodorsal oblique projection can be taken with the mouth either open or closed.

BEAM CENTER: Over center of temporomandibular joint

MEASUREMENT: Over lateral canthus of eye

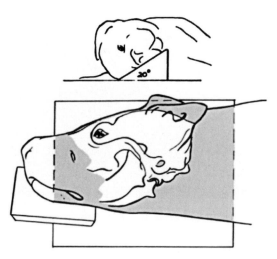

Figure 15-19 *Correct positioning for the ventrodorsal oblique view of the temporomandibular joint.*

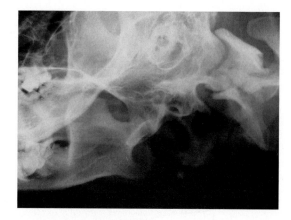

Figure 15-20 *Radiograph of the ventrodorsal oblique view of the temporomandibular joint.*

MAXILLA

Dorsoventral Intraoral View

The patient is placed in sternal recumbency with the head in straight alignment with the spine (Figs. 15-21 and 15-22). A nonscreen packaged film is placed in the mouth to the level of the commissure of the lips. A cassette can be placed in the mouth, but it is difficult to insert because of its size. The corner edge of the film is introduced into the mouth first to allow more of the maxilla to be radiographed. Because the source–image distance (SID) is reduced as a result of the film being elevated off the table, the x-ray tube should be raised accordingly to compensate.

BEAM CENTER: Over site of interest

MEASUREMENT: At level of commissure of lips

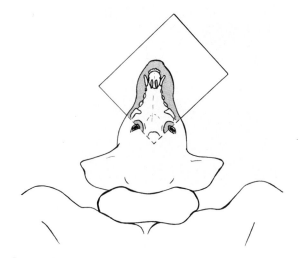

Figure 15-21 *Correct positioning for the dorsoventral intraoral maxilla.*

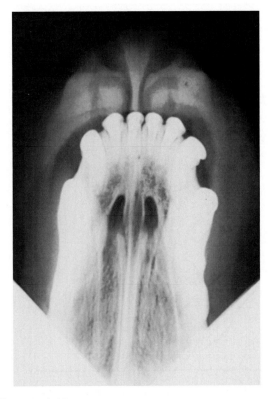

Figure 15-22 *Radiograph of the dorsoventral intraoral maxilla.*

MAXILLA—*cont'd*

Upper Dental Arcade

Open-mouth ventrodorsal oblique view.
The patient is placed halfway on its back with the maxillary arcade of interest closest to the cassette. The head is rotated approximately 45 degrees to the cassette and stabilized with a sponge wedge pad or cotton (Figs. 15-23 and 15-24). The rotation of the head eliminates superimposition of the contralateral arcade. The mouth should be maintained in an open position with a tongue depressor or other suitable radiolucent mouth gag.

BEAM CENTER: Over third premolar

MEASUREMENT: At proximal hard palate

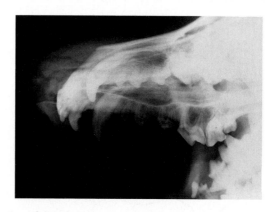

Figure 15-24 *Radiograph of the ventrodorsal open-mouth oblique view of the maxilla (upper dental arcade).*

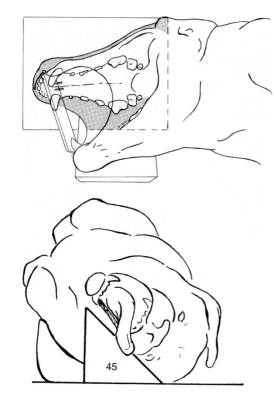

Figure 15-23 *Correct positioning for the ventrodorsal open-mouth oblique view of the maxilla (upper dental arcade).*

MANDIBLE

Ventrodorsal Intraoral View

The patient is placed in dorsal recumbency with the head extended in a cranial direction (Figs. 15-25 and 15-26). A nonscreen packaged film is placed in the mouth with the corner edge of the film introduced first. The film is inserted until the edges of the film reach the commissure of the lips. The tongue should be pulled cranially to eliminate unequal density over the mandibular area. Because the SID is reduced as a result of the film being elevated off the table, the x-ray tube should be raised accordingly to compensate.

BEAM CENTER: Over site of interest

MEASUREMENT: At commissure of lips

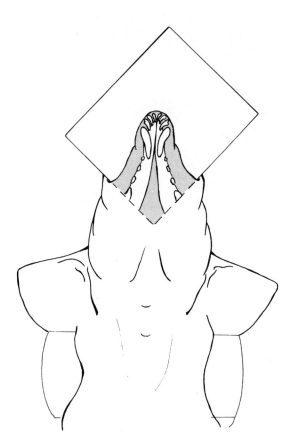

Figure 15-25 *Correct positioning of the ventrodorsal intraoral view of the mandible.*

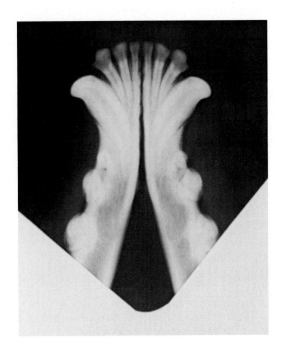

Figure 15-26 *Radiograph of the ventrodorsal intraoral view of the mandible.*

MANDIBLE—*cont'd*

Lower Dental Arcade

Open-mouth dorsoventral oblique view.

The patient is placed in lateral recumbency with the affected mandible closest to the cassette (Figs. 15-27 and 15-28). A radiolucent mouth gag is placed to separate the upper and lower arcades. The cranium should be rotated approximately 20 degrees away from the tabletop and maintained in this position with a sponge wedge pad or cotton.

BEAM CENTER: Over site of interest

MEASUREMENT: At level of first molar

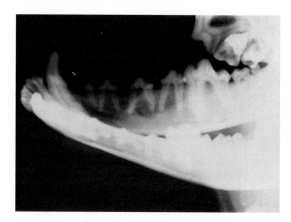

Figure 15-28 *Radiograph of the dorsoventral oblique open-mouth view of the mandible (lower dental arcade).*

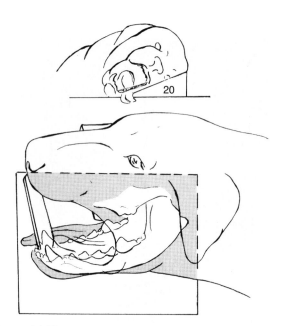

Figure 15-27 *Correct positioning for the dorsoventral oblique open-mouth view of the mandible (lower dental arcade).*

TEETH

Lateral Intraoral View

The most accurate method of visualizing a tooth and tooth root is with intraoral, nonscreen dental film.

The patient is placed in lateral recumbency with the unaffected side on the table and the area of interest uppermost (Figs. 15-29 and 15-30). The film is inserted into the mouth and placed against the medial border of the maxilla or mandible behind the affected tooth. It may be difficult to insert the film against the medial border of the maxilla and mandible because of the normal anatomy of the canine and feline mouths. That is, the hard palate of the dog and cat is relatively flat, which makes film positioning difficult. The film is maintained in position with a pair of forceps. If necessary, the angle of the x-ray tube or skull of the patient should be altered to keep the film perpendicular to the x-ray beam.

BEAM CENTER: Over site of interest

MEASUREMENT: At site of interest (exposure factors are usually approximated and depend on patient's size—consult film manufacturer)

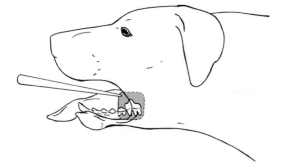

Figure 15-29 *Correct positioning for a lateral intraoral view of the teeth using nonscreen dental film.*

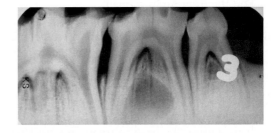

Figure 15-30 *Radiograph of a lateral intraoral view of the teeth using nonscreen dental film.*

KEY POINTS

1. If an endotracheal tube is in place while radiographing a rostrocaudal view of the skull, special care must be taken not to crimp it.
2. The lateral oblique view of the tympanic bullae requires placing the *unaffected* side of the skull closest to the cassette.
3. The nasal septum must be parallel with the cassette on a lateral view of the skull.

REVIEW QUESTIONS

1. Which of the following may be helpful for proper positioning of the skull in a lateral view?
   a. Place a foam pad under the ramus of the mandible.
   b. Pull the front limbs cranially.
   c. Place a pad under the caudodorsal cervical region.
   d. The mandibular ramus closest to the cassette should be slightly ventral to the ramus farthest from the cassette.

2. What is the disadvantage of a more prominent external occipital protuberance?
   a. It may cause the head to rotate in a ventrodorsal view.
   b. It may cause the head to rotate in a lateral view.
   c. It may cause the head to rotate in a dorsoventral view.
   d. It requires kVp to be increased.

3. Where should the beam be centered for a rostrocaudal view of the frontal sinuses?
   a. Through the center of the frontal sinuses
   b. Over the point of the nose
   c. At the symphysis of the rami
   d. At the top of the head

4. What is the appropriate angle and direction of the x-ray tube in a ventrodorsal open-mouth view of the nasal cavity?
   a. 15 to 20 degrees directed inside the mouth
   b. 10 to 15 degrees directed at the top of the frontal sinuses
   c. 10 to 15 degrees directed inside the mouth
   d. 20 to 25 degrees directed inside the mouth

5. What views are most helpful to view the tympanic bullae?
   a. Rostrocaudal open-mouth, lateral
   b. Rostrocaudal open-mouth, lateral oblique
   c. Lateral oblique, ventrodorsal open-mouth
   d. Ventrodorsal open-mouth, rostrocaudal open-mouth

6. What is the appropriate degree of rotation of the head for a ventrodorsal oblique view of the temporomandibular joint?
   a. Approximately 20 degrees
   b. Approximately 15 degrees
   c. Approximately 25 degrees
   d. Approximately 10 degrees

7. Why is the source–image distance decreased in a dorsoventral view of the maxilla?
   a. The film is in the Bucky tray.
   b. The head is elevated off the table.
   c. The film is on the tabletop.
   d. The film is in the mouth off the tabletop.

8. Where is the beam centered for the open-mouth ventrodorsal view of the upper dental arcade?
   a. Over the third premolar
   b. At the commissure of the lips
   c. Over the canine tooth
   d. Over the first premolar

9. Because even the slightest rotation of the skull can lead to a wrong diagnosis:
   a. it is often necessary to use tape to secure the skull.
   b. general anesthesia helps to maintain symmetry.
   c. it is best if several radiographers assist with manual restraint.
   d. Both a and b are correct.

10. Where is the film placed for a lateral intraoral view of the teeth?
    a. Against the lateral border of the maxilla or mandible behind the affected tooth with the unaffected side on the table
    b. Against the medial border of the maxilla or mandible behind the affected tooth with the unaffected side on the table
    c. Against the medial border of the maxilla or mandible behind the affected tooth with the affected side on the table
    d. None of the above

SUGGESTED READINGS

Douglas SW, Herrtage ME, Williamson HD: *Principles of veterinary radiography,* ed 4, Philadelphia, 1987, Bailliere Tindall.

Habel RE: *Applied veterinary anatomy,* ed 2, Ithaca, NY, 1978, RE Habel.

Kleine LJ, Warren RG: *Small animal radiography,* St Louis, 1982, Mosby.

Ryan GD: *Radiographic positioning of small animals,* Philadelphia, 1981, Lea & Febiger.

Schebitz H, Wilkins H: *Atlas of radiographic anatomy of the dog and cat,* Philadelphia, 1986, WB Saunders.

Smallwood JE, Shively MJ: Nomenclature for radiographic views of limbs, *Equine Pract* 1:41-45, 1979.

Ticer JW: *Radiographic technique in small animal practice,* ed 2, Philadelphia, 1984, WB Saunders.

chapter 16

Small Animal Spine

CHAPTER OUTLINE

Cervical Spine
Thoracic Spine
Thoracolumbar Spine

Lumbar Spine
Sacrum
Caudal Spine

To obtain a diagnostic radiograph of the vertebral column, two factors must be considered. First, the vertebral column must always be as parallel to the tabletop as possible. Second, the disk spaces of the spine must be nearly perpendicular to the tabletop and in parallel alignment with the central axis of the primary x-ray beam. These criteria can be met through a number of means.

On rare occasions no manual assistance may be necessary to achieve correct positioning of animal patients placed in recumbency. However, it is usually necessary to alter the lateral recumbent position of the animal and positioning devices such as foam sponges, sandbags, or

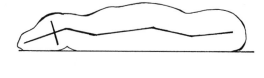

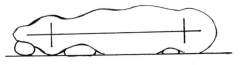

Figure 16-1 *Positioning alterations necessary for a lateral spine study. Sponges are used to support the midcervical, midlumbar, and skull regions to keep the spine parallel to the table.*

cotton may be helpful. Usually, efforts to improve the patient's positioning focus on elevating the sternum and hind legs and providing support for the skull and midcervical and midlumbar regions (Figs. 16-1 and 16-2). Remember, any positioning device superimposed on an area of interest must be radiolucent.

Another method that can be used to achieve correct positioning is manual traction. By pulling the front and rear legs in opposite directions for views of the thoracolumbar spine, the vertebral column naturally extends to a near-parallel position, and the intervertebral disk spaces are opened. This positioning method is contraindicated for patients that have spinal column injuries such as fractures or luxations.

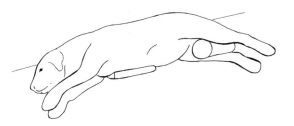

Figure 16-2 *Positioning alterations necessary for a lateral spine study. Sponges are used to support the sternum and between the hind legs to prevent rotation of the spine.*

CERVICAL SPINE

Ventrodorsal View

The patient is placed in dorsal recumbency with the head extended cranially and the front limbs pulled caudally alongside the body (Figs. 16-3 and 16-4). The patient must be restrained in a true ventrodorsal posture, and the cervical spine must be parallel with the cassette. A sponge pad or cotton can be placed under the midcervical region to eliminate any distortion in this area. The field of view should include the base of the skull, the entire cervical spine, and the first few thoracic vertebrae.

For large patients that weigh more than 50 lb, it may be necessary to radiograph the cervical spine in two separate areas. Two radiographs are required because of the extreme difference in thickness between the caudal and the cranial cervical spine. For example, the first area should include the base of the skull and C-1 to C-4, centering the x-ray beam at C-2 to C-3. The second area should include C-4 to T-1, centering the x-ray beam at C-5 to C-6.

Extended Lateral View

The patient is placed in lateral recumbency with the head and neck extended and the front limbs pulled in a caudal direction. Gentle traction should be placed on the cervical region by pulling the head of the patient in a cranial direction. This traction can be accomplished manually by stretching the cervical spine, or a length of roll gauze can be tied around the nose behind the canine teeth and pulled cranially (Figs. 16-5 and 16-6). A foam wedge pad is placed under the mandible to eliminate skull obliquity. To position the cervical spine parallel with the cassette, it may be necessary to place a sponge wedge pad or cotton under the midcervical region. The field of view should include the base of the skull, the entire cervical spine, and a few thoracic vertebrae.

For large patients that weigh more than 50 lb, it may be necessary to radiograph the cervical spine in two sections, making sure to overlap the two views. For example, the first section of the spine should include the base of the skull to C-4, centering the x-ray beam at the C-2 to C-3 interspace. The second section then includes C-4 to T-1, with the x-ray beam centered at the C-5 to C-6 interspace.

BEAM CENTER: Over C4-5 intervertebral space

MEASUREMENT: C5-6 intervertebral space

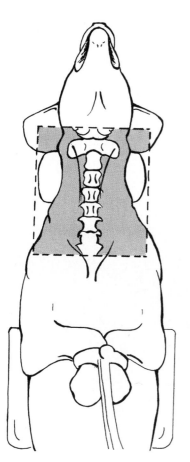

Figure 16-3 *Correct positioning for the ventrodorsal view of the cervical spine.*

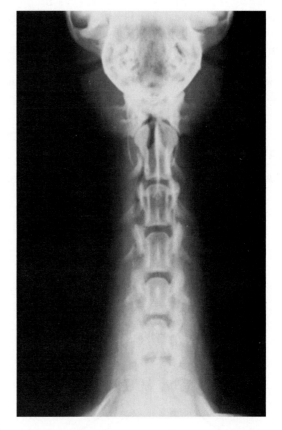

Figure 16-4 *Radiograph of the ventrodorsal view of the cervical spine.*

BEAM CENTER: Intervertebral space of C-4 and C-5

MEASUREMENT: Over level of C-7 (thoracic inlet)

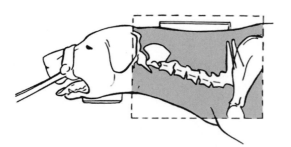

Figure 16-5 *Correct positioning for the lateral view of the cervical spine.*

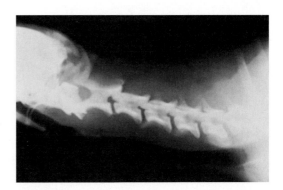

Figure 16-6 *Radiograph of the lateral view of the cervical spine.*

CERVICAL SPINE—*cont'd*

Flexed Lateral View

The patient is placed in lateral recumbency with the front limbs pulled in a caudal direction. A length of roll gauze or rope is tied around the mandible behind the canine teeth, and the free end of the line is placed between the forelimbs. Gentle traction is placed on the free end of the gauze, and the head is pulled caudally toward the humeri (Figs. 16-7 and 16-8). Care must be taken not to hyper-flex the neck, which may cause tracheal trauma or collapse of an endotracheal tube. It may be necessary to elevate the vertebrae to the level of the thoracic spine with a sponge wedge pad or cotton. An appropriately sized cassette should be used so that the field of view includes the area from the base of the skull to the first few thoracic vertebrae.

BEAM CENTER: C3-4 intervertebral space

MEASUREMENT: Over level of C-7 (thoracic inlet)

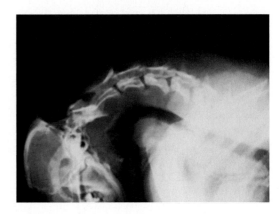

Figure 16-8 *Radiograph of the flexed lateral view of the cervical spine.*

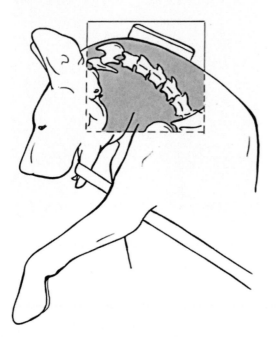

Figure 16-7 *Correct positioning for the flexed lateral view of the cervical spine.*

CERVICAL SPINE—*cont'd*

Hyperextended Lateral View

The patient is placed in lateral recumbency with the front limbs extended caudally. The head and neck region is extended in a dorsal direction until resistance is met (Figs. 16-9 and 16-10). A foam wedge pad or cotton is placed under the mandible to alleviate skull obliquity and under the midcervical region to align the vertebrae. The field of view should include the area from the base of the skull to the first few thoracic vertebrae.

BEAM CENTER: C3-4 intervertebral space

MEASUREMENT: Over level of T-1 (thoracic inlet)

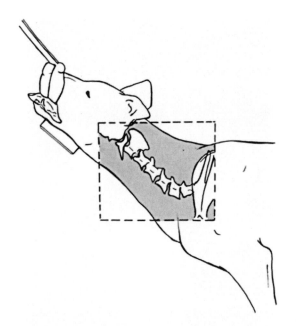

Figure 16-9 *Correct positioning of the hyperextended lateral view of the cervical spine.*

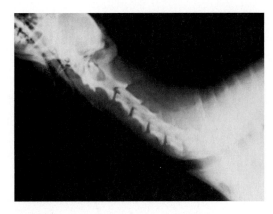

Figure 16-10 *Radiograph of the hyperextended lateral view of the cervical spine.*

THORACIC SPINE

Ventrodorsal View

The patient is placed in dorsal recumbency with the front limbs extended cranially (Figs. 16-11 and 16-12). The rear limbs can assume a normal position. The animal must be maintained in a true ventrodorsal position so that the sternum is superimposed on the thoracic spine. A V trough placed under the lumbar region can assist in maintaining this position. The field of view should include all of the thoracic vertebrae from C-7 to L-1.

BEAM CENTER: Over level of caudal border of scapula (T-6)

MEASUREMENT: At highest point of sternum

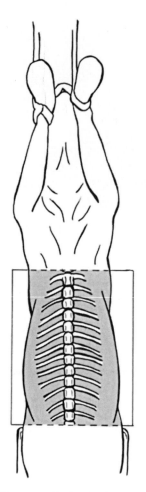

Figure 16-11 *Correct positioning for the ventrodorsal view of the thoracic spine.*

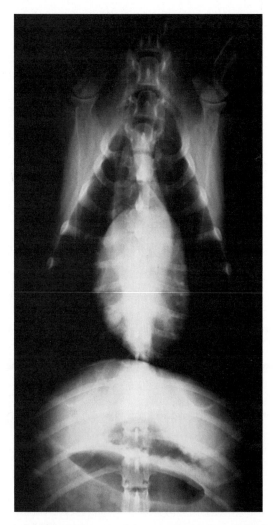

Figure 16-12 *Radiograph of the ventrodorsal view of the thoracic spine.*

THORACIC SPINE—*cont'd*

Lateral View

The patient is placed in lateral recumbency with the front and rear limbs moderately extended in opposite directions away from the body (Figs. 16-13 and 16-14). The sternum is elevated with a sponge wedge pad to eliminate any rotation of the thoracic vertebrae. To ensure proper positioning, the sternum should be at the same distance from the tabletop as the thoracic spine. The thoracic spine is centered to the cassette, and the field of view should include the area from the seventh cervical vertebral body to the first lumbar vertebral body.

BEAM CENTER: Over seventh thoracic vertebral body

MEASUREMENT: At level of seventh rib

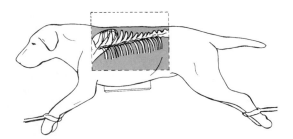

Figure 16-13 *Correct positioning for the lateral view of the thoracic spine.*

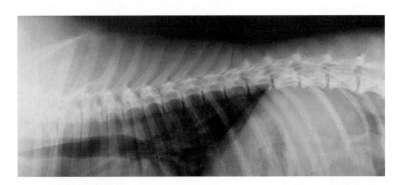

Figure 16-14 *Radiograph of the lateral view of the thoracic spine.*

THORACOLUMBAR SPINE

Ventrodorsal View

The patient is placed in dorsal recumbency with the front limbs extended cranially (Figs. 16-15 and 16-16). The hind limbs can assume a normal position. The patient must be maintained in a true ventrodorsal position, with the sternum superimposed over the thoracic spinal column. A V trough may be helpful in stabilizing the animal. The spine is centered to the cassette, and the field of view should include all of the thoracic and lumbar vertebrae.

BEAM CENTER: Over thoracolumbar junction

MEASUREMENT: At thoracolumbar junction

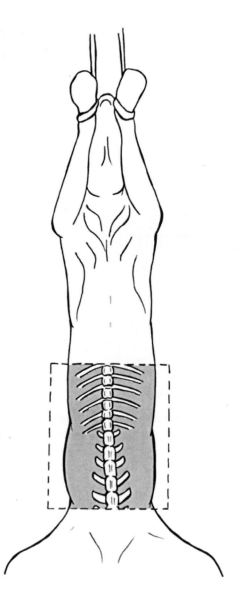

Figure 16-15 *Correct positioning for the ventrodorsal view of the thoracolumbar spine.*

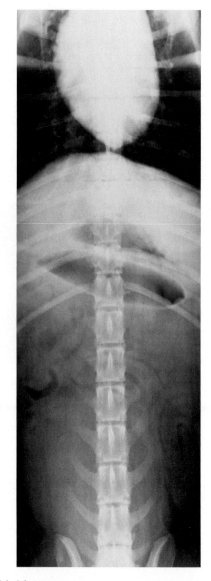

Figure 16-16 *Radiograph of the ventrodorsal view of the thoracolumbar spine.*

THORACOLUMBAR SPINE—*cont'd*

Lateral View

The patient is placed in lateral recumbency with the front and rear limbs pulled in opposite directions away from the body (Figs. 16-17 and 16-18). A sponge wedge pad is placed under the sternum so that it is elevated to the same horizontal plane as the thoracic vertebrae. The spine should be centered to the cassette, and the field of view should include the entire thoracolumbar spine.

BEAM CENTER: Over thoracolumbar junction

MEASUREMENT: At thoracolumbar junction

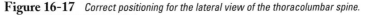

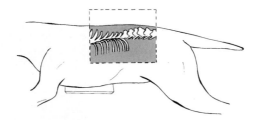

Figure 16-17 *Correct positioning for the lateral view of the thoracolumbar spine.*

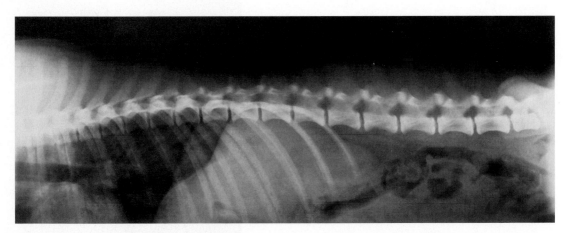

Figure 16-18 *Radiograph of the lateral view of the thoracolumbar spine.*

LUMBAR SPINE

Ventrodorsal View

The patient is placed in dorsal recumbency with the front limbs extended cranially and the rear limbs in a normal position (Figs. 16-19 and 16-20). To maintain a true ventrodorsal position, a V trough can be placed under the thoracic region. The spine should be centered to the cassette, and the field of view should include the entire lumbar spine from the thirteenth thoracic vertebral body to the first sacral vertebral body.

BEAM CENTER: Over fourth lumbar vertebral body

MEASUREMENT: At level of first lumbar vertebral body

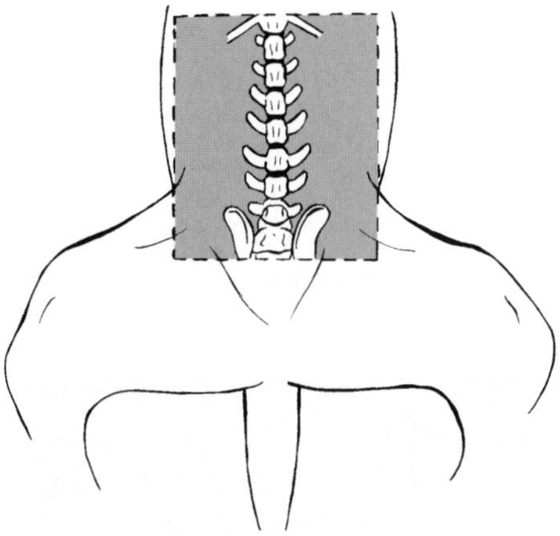

Figure 16-19 *Correct positioning for the ventrodorsal view of the lumbar spine.*

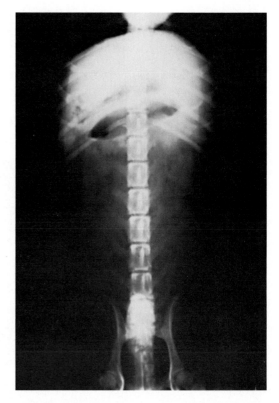

Figure 16-20 *Radiograph of the ventrodorsal view of the lumbar spine.*

LUMBAR SPINE—*cont'd*

Lateral View

The patient is placed in lateral recumbency with the front and rear limbs in moderate extension (Figs. 16-21 and 16-22). A sponge wedge pad should be placed under the sternum to eliminate any rotation of the lumbar spine. Placing a sponge pad or cotton under the midlumbar region may be necessary to achieve proper alignment. The lumbar spine is centered to the cassette, and the field of view should include the entire lumbar vertebrae from the thirteenth thoracic vertebral body to the first sacral vertebral body.

BEAM CENTER: Over level of fourth lumbar vertebral body

MEASUREMENT: At level of first lumbar vertebral body

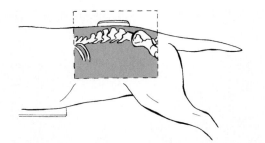

Figure 16-21 *Correct positioning for the lateral view of the lumbar spine.*

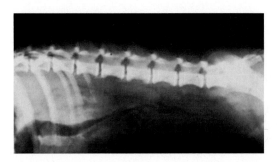

Figure 16-22 *Radiograph of the lateral view of the lumbar spine.*

SACRUM

Ventrodorsal View

The patient is placed in dorsal recumbency with the rear limbs in a normal position (Figs. 16-23 and 16-24). A V trough can be placed under the thoracic region to maintain a true ventrodorsal position. The sacrum is centered to the cassette. The x-ray tube is directed at a 30-degree angle toward the head and centered over the sacrum. The field of view should include the area from the sixth lumbar vertebral body to the iliac crests.

Positioning for the lateral sacrum is the same as for the lateral pelvis.

BEAM CENTER: Over level of sacrum

MEASUREMENT: At level of sacrum

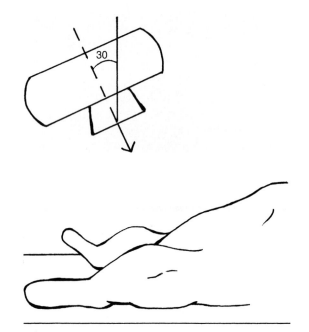

Figure 16-23 *Correct positioning for the ventrodorsal view of the sacrum.*

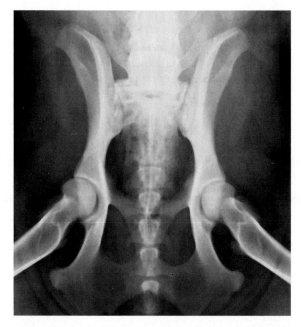

Figure 16-24 *Radiograph of the ventrodorsal view of the sacrum.*

CAUDAL SPINE

Ventrodorsal View

The patient is placed in dorsal recumbency with the rear limbs in a normal position (Figs. 16-25 and 16-26). The body can be maintained in a true ventrodorsal position with the aid of a V trough placed under the thoracic region. The tail is extended in a caudal direction and centered in the middle of the cassette. For animals that have a natural curl to the tail, it may be necessary to tape the tail to the cassette.

BEAM CENTER: Over area of interest

MEASUREMENT: At proximal tail

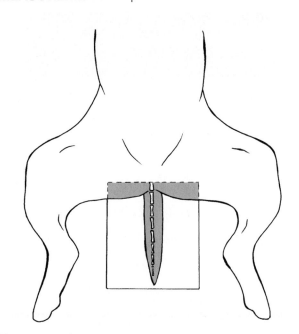

Figure 16-25 *Correct positioning for the ventrodorsal view of the caudal spine.*

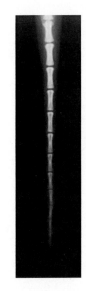

Figure 16-26 *Radiograph of the ventrodorsal view of the caudal spine.*

CAUDAL SPINE—*cont'd*

Lateral View

The patient is placed in lateral recumbency with the tail extended in a caudal direction (Figs. 16-27 and 16-28). Raising the cassette and maintaining it on a foam block of appropriate thickness may be necessary. Elevation of the cassette allows the tail to remain parallel to the tabletop and in alignment with the rest of the spine. The tail is centered on the cassette.

BEAM CENTER: Over area of interest

MEASUREMENT: At proximal tail

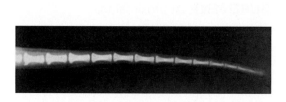

Figure 16-28 *Radiograph of the lateral view of the caudal spine.*

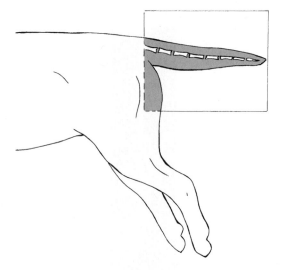

Figure 16-27 *Correct positioning for the lateral view of the caudal spine.*

Key Points

1. A foam wedge should be placed under the sternum to elevate it to the same horizontal level as the spine for a lateral thoracic and thoracolumbar view.
2. To obtain optimal radiographs of the spine, the disk spaces must be nearly perpendicular to the tabletop and in parallel alignment with each other.
3. Manually extending a patient's front and rear limbs for a spinal view is contraindicated if the patient has a spinal column injury.

Review Questions

1. Which of the following is true?
   a. Any positioning device(s) superimposed on an area of interest must be radiodense.
   b. Any positioning device(s) superimposed on an area of interest must be radiolucent.
   c. Disk spaces must be near parallel to the tabletop for a diagnostic radiograph of the vertebral column.
   d. Using positioning devices under the thoracolumbar area is usually necessary for a lateral view of the spine.

2. What is the field of view for the cervical spine?
   a. Base of the skull, entire cervical spine, and first few thoracic vertebrae
   b. Base of the skull and first few thoracic vertebrae
   c. Base of the skull and cervical vertebrae
   d. Skull, cervical vertebrae, and first few thoracic vertebrae

3. Where is the measurement taken for a hyperextended lateral view of the cervical spine?
   a. C5-6
   b. C6-7
   c. T2-3
   d. T-1 (thoracic inlet)

4. What indicates that a thoracic radiograph is in a true ventrodorsal position?
   a. Humeri are parallel.
   b. The heart is parallel on either side of the thoracic spine.
   c. The sternum is superimposed over the thoracic spine.
   d. The sixth rib is superimposed over the scapulohumeral joint.

5. Which of the following is true?
   a. For a flexed lateral view of the cervical spine, the head should be pulled cranially.
   b. For an extended lateral view of the cervical spine, the head should be pulled caudally.
   c. For a flexed lateral view of the cervical spine, the head is pulled caudally.
   d. For an extended lateral view of the cervical spine, the head is extended rostrally.

6. Where should the measurement be taken for a lateral view of the thoracic spine?
   a. Seventh thoracic vertebra
   b. Sixth thoracic vertebra
   c. Eighth thoracic vertebra
   d. Thickest area of the thorax

7. Which vertebrae must be included in a ventrodorsal view of the thoracolumbar spine?
   a. T11-L3
   b. T11-L2
   c. T12-L2
   d. All of the thoracic and lumbar vertebrae

8. How should the rear limbs be positioned during a lateral lumbar view?
   a. Pulled cranially
   b. Pulled caudally
   c. Frog-leg
   d. The limb closest to the cassette is pulled slightly cranially

9. At what angle should the x-ray tube be positioned for a ventrodorsal view of the sacrum?
   a. 30 degrees toward the tail
   b. 20 degrees toward the head
   c. 30 degrees toward the head
   d. 40 degrees toward the tail

10. Where should the cassette be placed for a ventrodorsal view of the caudal spinal?
    a. Under the sacrum
    b. In the Bucky tray
    c. On the tabletop
    d. Perpendicular to the tabletop

Suggested Readings

Douglas SW, Herrtage ME, Williamson HD: *Principles of veterinary radiography,* ed 4, Philadelphia, 1987, Bailliere Tindall.

Habel RE: *Applied veterinary anatomy,* ed 2, Ithaca, NY, 1978, RE Habel.

Kleine LJ, Warren RG: *Small animal radiography,* St Louis, 1982, Mosby.

Ryan GD: *Radiographic positioning of small animals,* Philadelphia, 1981, Lea & Febiger.

Schebitz H, Wilkins H: *Atlas of radiographic anatomy of the dog and cat,* Philadelphia, 1986, WB Saunders.

Smallwood JE, Shively MJ: Nomenclature for radiographic views of limbs, *Equine Pract* 1:41-45, 1979.

Ticer JW: *Radiographic technique in small animal practice,* ed 2, Philadelphia, 1984, WB Saunders.

chapter 17

Small Animal Soft Tissue

CHAPTER OUTLINE

Pharynx
Thorax
Abdomen

INTRODUCTION

The term *soft tissue* describes the areas of the body that surround the skeletal structures. Unlike radiography of bone tissue, visualization of soft tissue can be difficult because it involves only slight differences in radiographic density. Production of a soft tissue radiograph that has high contrast between the various adjacent soft structures is almost impossible without the use of contrast media. To achieve the correct contrast, density, and visualization, a number of factors must be considered:

1. To attain a long scale of contrast with good visualization of the internal soft tissue structures, a relatively high kilovoltage and low milliamperage-seconds are used.
2. A grid is necessary for areas of dense tissue to maintain image clarity and radiographic detail.
3. An exposure time of $^1/_{30}$ second or less is necessary for thorax radiography to minimize motion caused by cardiac and respiratory movement.
4. Proper preparation is necessary for abdominal radiography. The patient should be fasted for 12 to 24 hours and given a cleansing enema at least 1 hour before radiography.
5. Exposure of the thorax and abdomen must be taken during the correct phase of respiration: inspiration for the thorax and expiration for the abdomen.

PHARYNX

Lateral View

The patient is placed in lateral recumbency with the forelimbs pulled in a caudal direction. The head and neck are extended cranially and placed in a true lateral position (Figs. 17-1 and 17-2). A sponge wedge pad placed under the mandible helps eliminate obliquity of the skull and frees the larynx from the mandible to allow better visualization of the laryngeal region. The air passages of the upper respiratory tract act as a negative contrast agent and permit the soft tissue structures of the pharyngeal region to be differentiated. The field of view should include the entire area of the neck between the lateral canthus of the eye and the third cervical vertebral body.

BEAM CENTER: Over pharynx

MEASUREMENT: At level of base of skull

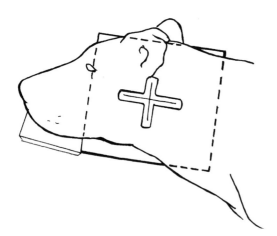

Figure 17-1 *Correct positioning for the lateral view of the pharynx.*

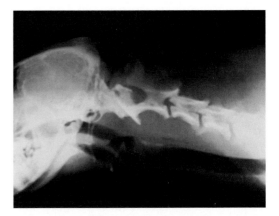

Figure 17-2 *Radiograph of the lateral view of the pharynx.*

THORAX

Dorsoventral View

The dorsoventral view of the thorax is preferred for the evaluation of the heart because the heart is closer to the sternum and is in near-normal suspended position within the thorax. Unfortunately, it may be difficult to position larger dogs for the dorsoventral projection because of their deep chests. The dorsoventral view requires great care to ensure that the sternum is superimposed over the vertebral column. If this position is impossible to execute, it may be necessary to attempt a ventrodorsal projection.

The patient is placed in sternal recumbency with the thoracic vertebrae superimposed over the sternum (Figs. 17-3 and 17-4). The forelegs are pulled slightly forward to prevent the elbows from tucking under the thorax. The rear legs are allowed to flex in a natural crouching position. This crouched position may be difficult for the canine patient with hip dysplasia, and it may be necessary to consider the ventrodorsal view. The head is lower and is placed between the two forelimbs. The field of view should include the entire thorax. The rule is "the thorax is inside the rib cage"; if you include all of the ribs, you will radiograph the entire thorax.

The exposure must be taken at the peak of inspiration to allow complete radiographic visualization of the lung tissue. The patient's breathing should be observed several times before making the exposure. This allows the radiographer ample time to make the exposure at the proper phase of respiration.

BEAM CENTER: Over caudal border of scapula

MEASUREMENT: At level of caudal border of scapula

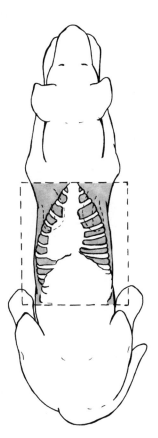

Figure 17-3 *Correct positioning for the dorsoventral view of the thorax.*

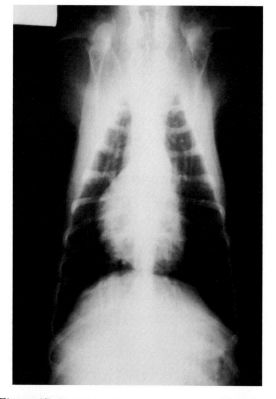

Figure 17-4 *Radiograph of the dorsoventral view of the thorax.*

THORAX—*cont'd*

Ventrodorsal View

The ventrodorsal view of the thorax is advocated when a full view of the lung fields is necessary. This projection provides a better view of the accessory lung lobes and caudal mediastinum. Although it is easier to control a patient in ventrodorsal position, this view is contra-indicated for patients in obvious respiratory distress. Placing such an animal on its back would be dangerous and could possibly cause further respiratory problems.

The patient is placed in dorsal recumbency with the forelimbs extended cranially (Figs. 17-5 and 17-6). The hind limbs can assume a normal position. Great care must be taken to ensure that the patient is in a true ventrodorsal posture. The sternum must be superimposed over the spine. If rotation is encountered, a V trough or sandbags placed under the pelvic region may be helpful. The field of view should include the entire thorax. The rule is "the thorax is inside the rib cage"; if you include all of the ribs, you will radiograph the entire thorax.

The exposure is taken at the peak of inspiration. The patient's breathing should be observed several times before making an exposure. This allows the radiographer ample time to make the exposure at the proper phase of respiration.

BEAM CENTER: Over caudal border of scapula

MEASUREMENT: At level of caudal border of scapula

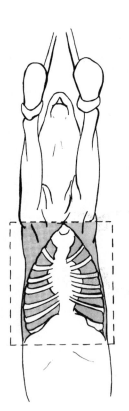

Figure 17-5   *Correct positioning for the ventrodorsal view of the thorax.*

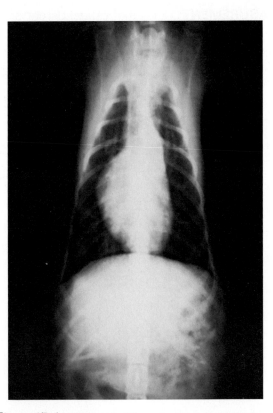

Figure 17-6   *Radiograph of the ventrodorsal view of the thorax.*

THORAX—*cont'd*

Lateral View

A right lateral study of the thorax has been recommended for a more accurate view of the cardiac silhouette. Not all veterinary radiologists agree with this recommendation, and some prefer a left lateral thorax. We will not argue either point here. In some instances it is necessary to expose both right and left lateral projections when subtle lung metastasis is suspected.

The patient is placed in lateral recumbency, left or right side down, with the front limbs extended cranially (Figs. 17-7 and 17-8). Extension of the forelimbs helps eliminate superimposition of the triceps and humeri over the cranial aspect of the thorax. The hind limbs should be pulled in a slightly caudal direction to maintain a proper degree of symmetry of the thoracic cage. The head is extended slightly to avoid displacement of the trachea. The sternum is elevated with the use of a foam wedge pad to a level above the x-ray table equal to that of the thoracic vertebrae. Elevation of the sternum prevents rotation of the thorax. The field of view should include the entire thoracic cavity from the line of the manubrium sterni caudally to the first lumbar vertebral body. The rule is "the thorax is inside the rib cage"; if you include all of the ribs, you will raddiograph the entire thorax.

The exposure should be taken at the peak of inspiration.

BEAM CENTER: Over caudal border of scapula

MEASUREMENT: At level of caudal border of scapula

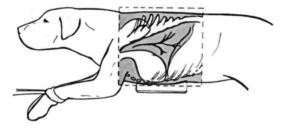

Figure 17-7 *Correct positioning for the lateral view of the thorax.*

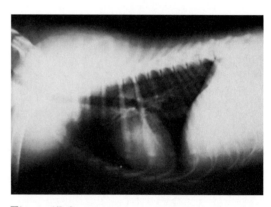

Figure 17-8 *Radiograph of the lateral view of the thorax.*

THORAX—*cont'd*

Lateral View with Horizontal Beam

The lateral view with a horizontal beam is used to confirm the presence of fluid or free air in the thoracic cavity and to assist its quantification. Two positions can be used: (1) the standing lateral (Fig. 17-9) and (2) the sternally recumbent lateral (Fig. 17-10). The standing lateral view is not as desirable because of superimposition of the humeral soft tissues over the cranial thorax in a natural standing posture.

For the sternally recumbent lateral view, the patient is placed in sternal recumbency on top of a foam pad that is approximately 5 to 10 cm thick. The height of elevation is determined by the size of the animal and the cassette used. The forelimbs and head are gently extended in a cranial direction. The hind limbs are allowed to assume a natural crouched position. The cassette is placed in a vertical position against the lateral side of the patient. A commercially available cassette holder or positioning device helps support the cassette in place. The thorax should be centered to the cassette, and the field of view should include from the manubrium sterni caudally to the first lumbar vertebral body. The field of view should include the entire thorax. The rule is "the thorax is inside the rib cage"; if you include all of the ribs, you will radiograph the entire thorax. (Note: The same projection can be performed for the abdomen.)

BEAM CENTER: Over caudal border of scapula

MEASUREMENT: At level of caudal border of scapula

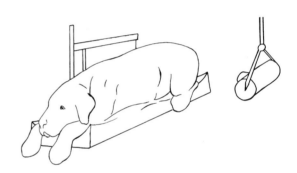

Figure 17-10 *Correct positioning for the recumbent lateral view of the thorax using a horizontal x-ray beam.*

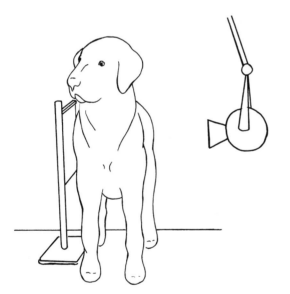

Figure 17-9 *Correct positioning for the standing lateral view of the thorax using a horizontal x-ray beam.*

THORAX—*cont'd*

Lateral Decubitus View (Ventrodorsal View with Horizontal Beam)

The lateral decubitus projection, like the standing lateral view, is used to confirm quantitative thoracic fluid or air. This study is made with the animal in lateral recumbency and with a horizontal x-ray beam directed ventrodorsally. The position is further specified according to the side that is down (e.g., left decubitus).

The patient is placed in lateral recumbency on top of a 5- to 10-cm thick foam pad (Figs. 17-11 and 17-12).

The foam pad is necessary to elevate the patient off the tabletop and to allow visualization of both sides of the thorax. The forelimbs and the head are extended cranially. The hind limbs are pulled slightly in a caudal direction to keep the spine of the patient close to the cassette. The thorax is centered to the cassette, which is placed behind the patient in a vertical posture. The field of view should include the entire thorax. (Note: The same projection can be performed for the abdomen.)

BEAM CENTER: Over caudal border of scapula

MEASUREMENT: At level of caudal border of scapula

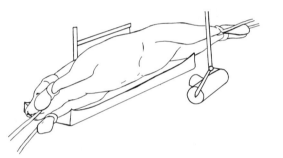

Figure 17-11 *Correct positioning for the ventrodorsal decubitus view of the thorax using a horizontal x-ray beam.*

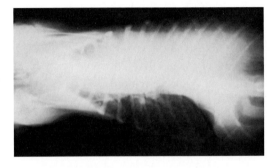

Figure 17-12 *Radiograph of the ventrodorsal decubitus view of the thorax (exhibiting fluid) using a horizontal x-ray beam.*

ABDOMEN

Ventrodorsal View

The patient is placed in dorsal recumbency with the hind limbs positioned in normal flexion (Figs. 17-13 and 17-14). A V trough or sandbags placed under the thoracic region may help maintain a true ventrodorsal posture. The field of view should include the entire abdomen from the diaphragm to the level of the femoral head. With larger patients, it may not be possible to include the entire abdomen on one cassette. In this case two radiographs should be taken: one of the cranial abdomen and the other including the caudal abdomen.

The exposure for an abdominal radiograph is taken during the expiratory pause so that the diaphragm is in a cranial position and not placing any compression on the abdominal contents.

BEAM CENTER: Over caudal aspect of thirteenth rib (for feline patients, center two to three fingerbreadths caudal to the thirteenth rib)

MEASUREMENT: At level of caudal aspect of thirteenth rib

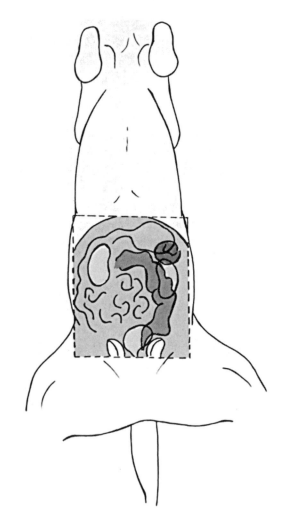

Figure 17-13 *Correct positioning for the ventrodorsal view of the abdomen.*

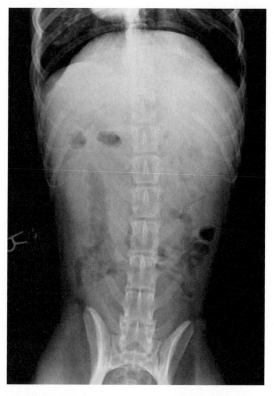

Figure 17-14 *Radiograph of the ventrodorsal view of the abdomen.*

ABDOMEN—*cont'd*

Lateral View

The patient is placed in right lateral recumbency with the hind limbs extended in a caudal direction (Figs. 17-15 and 17-16). The right lateral view is chosen to assist longitudinal separation of the kidneys. Pulling the hind limbs caudally helps eliminate superimposition of the femoral muscles over the caudal portion of the abdomen. A foam pad of suitable thickness is placed between the femurs to eliminate rotation of the pelvis and caudal abdomen. Another foam pad should be placed under the sternum to elevate it to the same level as the thoracic spine. The abdomen should be centered to the cassette, and the field of view should include the diaphragm caudally to the femoral head.

The exposure is made during the expiratory pause so that the diaphragm is displaced cranially.

BEAM CENTER: Over caudal aspect of thirteenth rib (for feline patients, center two to three fingerbreadths caudal to thirteenth rib)

MEASUREMENT: At level of caudal aspect of thirteenth rib

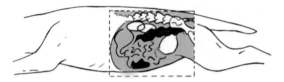

Figure 17-15 *Correct positioning for the lateral view of the abdomen.*

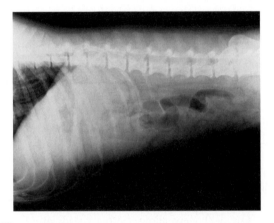

Figure 17-16 *Radiograph of the lateral view of the abdomen.*

KEY POINTS

1. A ventrodorsal thoracic view is contraindicated in a patient in respiratory distress.
2. When subtle lung metastasis is suspected, both right and left lateral views of the thorax are recommended.
3. The thorax should be radiographed during peak inspiration, and the abdomen should be radiographed during peak expiration.

REVIEW QUESTIONS

1. What must the field of view include for the pharynx?
   a. Third premolar, third cervical vertebra
   b. Base of skull, third cervical vertebra
   c. Zygomatic arch, third cervical vertebra
   d. Lateral canthus of eye, third cervical vertebra

2. When should a dorsoventral view of the thorax be taken?
   a. One at the peak of expiration and one at the peak of inspiration
   b. One at the peak of inspiration
   c. One at the peak of expiration
   d. One at the peak of inspiration and one any time during expiration

3. What is one advantage of taking a ventrodorsal view of the thorax as opposed to a dorsoventral view?
   a. The VD view allows better visualization of the caudal mediastinum and accessory lung lobe.
   b. The VD view allows better visualization of the heart.
   c. The VD view is more comfortable for the patient in respiratory distress.
   d. All of the above

4. Where is the measurement taken for a lateral view of the thorax?
   a. Cranial border of the scapula
   b. Caudal border of the seventh rib
   c. Cranial border of the eighth rib
   d. Caudal border of the scapula

5. When is a lateral view of the thorax with a horizontal beam indicated?
   a. When fluid or free air is suspected in the abdomen
   b. When the patient cannot be properly positioned for a laterally recumbent view on the table
   c. When fluid or free air is suspected in the thorax
   d. When spinal cord injury is suspected

6. Which of the following is true?
   a. During expiration the diaphragm is more cranial than during inspiration.
   b. During inspiration the diaphragm is more cranial than during expiration.
   c. During expiration the diaphragm is more caudal than during inspiration.
   d. Any view of the abdomen should be taken during inspiration.

7. Why is a right lateral view of the abdomen preferred over a left lateral view?
   a. To allow visualization of the descending colon
   b. To allow better separation of the kidneys
   c. So that the fundus of the stomach is closer to the cassette
   d. So that the pylorus is as far away from the cassette as possible

8. What is the preferred exposure time for views of the thorax?
   a. $1/2$ second
   b. $1/30$ second or less
   c. $1/20$ second
   d. $1/10$ second

9. What may help to achieve a long scale of contrast for an abdominal view?
   a. Low kVp and high mAs
   b. High kVp and high mAs
   c. High kVp and low mAs
   d. Contrast media

10. When should an enema be given for a view of the abdomen?
    a. At least 1 hour before radiography
    b. At least 12 hours before radiography
    c. At least 10 minutes before radiography
    d. 24 hours before radiography

SUGGESTED READINGS

Douglas SW, Herrtage ME, Williamson HD: *Principles of veterinary radiography*, ed 4, Philadelphia, 1987, Bailliere Tindall.

Habel RE: *Applied veterinary anatomy*, ed 2, Ithaca, NY, 1978, RE Habel.

Kirk RW: *Current veterinary therapy: small animal practice-thoracic radiography*, Philadelphia, 1986, WB Saunders.

Kleine LJ, Warren RG: *Small animal radiography*, St Louis, 1982, Mosby.

Ryan GD: *Radiographic positioning of small animals*, Philadelphia, 1981, Lea & Febiger.

Schebitz H, Wilkins H: *Atlas of radiographic anatomy of the dog and cat*, Philadelphia, 1986, WB Saunders.

Smallwood JE, Shively MJ: Nomenclature for radiographic views of limbs, *Equine Pract* 1:41-45, 1979.

Ticer JW: *Radiographic technique in small animal practice*, ed 2, Philadelphia, 1984, WB Saunders.

chapter 18

Special Procedures

CHAPTER OUTLINE

Indications
Contrast Media
Patient Preparation

Contrast Studies of the Gastrointestinal Tract
Contrast Studies of the Urinary System
Additional Techniques: A Brief Overview

Angiocardiography: An intravenous radiographic contrast study evaluating the vascular system and chambers of the heart.

Angiography: An intravenous radiographic contrast study evaluating the vascular system.

Antegrade urethrogram: A method of urethrography in which the contrast medium is voided from the urinary bladder.

Arthrography: A radiographic contrast technique evaluating the articular cartilage, joint space, and joint capsule.

Barium sulfate: A common positive-contrast medium that is available in various forms and is often used as a suspension in gastrointestinal evaluations.

Cholecystography: An oral or intravenous radiographic contrast study evaluating the bile ducts and gallbladder.

Contrast medium: A substance that is either radiolucent or radiopaque and can be administered to increase radiographic contrast within an organ or system.

Cystography: Radiographic contrast studies evaluating the urinary bladder.

Double contrast: A radiographic contrast technique that uses a combination of positive- and negative-contrast media simultaneously.

Double-contrast cystogram: A radiographic study of the urinary bladder involving distending the bladder with a gas and then adding a small amount of positive iodinated contrast medium.

Esophagography: A radiographic contrast study performed to evaluate esophageal function and morphology.

Excretory urography: An intravenous radiographic contrast study of the kidneys and ureters.

Fistula: An abnormal tubelike passage within body tissue.

Fistulography: A positive or negative radiographic contrast study used to determine the depth and origin of a fistulous tract.

Gastrography: A radiographic contrast study performed to evaluate the size, shape, position, and morphology of the stomach.

Intravenous pyelogram (IVP): A radiographic contrast study of the kidney structure and collection system.

Intravenous urogram (IVU): A radiographic contrast study of the kidney structure and collection system.

Lower gastrointestinal (LGI) study: Commonly referred to as a *barium enema;* a radiographic contrast study evaluating the rectum, colon, and cecum.

Lymphography: A radiographic contrast study evaluating lymphatic vessels and lymph nodes.

Myelography: A radiographic contrast study evaluating the subarachnoid space surrounding the spinal cord.

Negative-contrast agents: Gases that are more radiolucent to x-rays than are soft tissues and have a black appearance on a radiograph.

Nephrogram: A phase of an excretory urogram characterized by the diffuse opacification of the renal parenchyma.

Parasympatholytic agents: Drugs that eliminate the influence of the parasympathetic nervous system.

Pneumocystogram: A negative-contrast radiographic technique evaluating the urinary bladder.

Pneumoperitoneography: A negative-contrast radiographic study consisting of the introduction of a gas into the peritoneal cavity.

Positive-contrast agents: Substances containing elements of high atomic number that are more radiopaque to x-rays than are tissue and bone and have a white appearance on a radiograph.

Positive-contrast cystogram: A radiographic study of the bladder involving distention of the bladder with positive iodinated contrast medium.

Pyelogram: A phase of an excretory urogram characterized by the opacification of the renal collection system.

Retrograde urethrogram: A method of urethrography by which the contrast medium is infused via a catheter placed at the distal end of the urethra.

Sialography: A radiographic contrast study evaluating the salivary glands and ducts.

Triiodinated compounds: A common component of iodinated positive-contrast media that contains three atoms of iodine per molecule.

Upper gastrointestinal (UGI) study: A radiographic contrast study evaluating the stomach and small intestines.

Urethrography: A radiographic contrast study evaluating the urethra.

Vaginography: A radiographic contrast study evaluating the female reproductive organs.

INDICATIONS

Special radiographic procedures are used to supplement or confirm information garnered from routine survey radiographs. Under normal circumstances, soft tissue structures or organs are difficult or impossible to identify on plain films due to lack of contrast. A **contrast medium** is a substance that is either radiolucent or radiopaque and can be administered to an animal to increase radiographic contrast within an organ or system. With the use of a contrast medium, soft tissue structures can be visualized, and the structure under investigation can be evaluated for size, shape, and position. In addition, defects in the mucosal surface of an organ or its luminal contents can be identified. In some instances it is possible to evaluate organ function or to assess the physiologic condition.

Although contrast studies can be extremely helpful for a complete diagnosis, at no time should a special procedure replace routine survey radiography.

CONTRAST MEDIA

The two basic categories of contrast media are positive and negative. **Positive-contrast agents,** such as barium or iodine compounds, contain high atomic number elements. These agents absorb more x-rays than do soft tissues or bones. Positive-contrast media are radiopaque to x-rays and appear white on a radiograph. These compounds can be used to fill or outline a hollow organ (e.g., urinary bladder, alimentary tract), or they can be injected into a blood vessel (sterile, water-based compounds only) for immediate visualization of the vascular supply or for subsequent excretion evaluation. **Negative-contrast agents** consist of gases (e.g., oxygen, carbon dioxide) that have a low specific gravity. Substances with a low specific gravity are more radiolucent to x-rays than are soft tissues and have a black appearance on a radiograph.

Many different compounds are used as radiographic contrast media. In addition, various manufacturers market identical contrast agents under different names and concentrations. Although it is virtually impossible to become familiar with all of the contrast agents available, it is possible to place them into one of three general categories: (1) positive-contrast iodinated preparations, (2) positive-contrast barium sulfate preparations, and (3) negative-contrast gases. Each category has basic characteristics used to classify contrast agents. These characteristics allow a better understanding of each individual medium.

The majority of agents currently available are intended for human use; however, some products are specifically approved by the U.S. Food and Drug Administration for animals. Contrast agent choice should be made on the basis of the type of study to be performed, the condition of the patient, the possible side effects, and the judgment of the veterinarian that it is the best available product for use.

Iodine Preparations

Iodine compounds are divided into two subcategories: water-soluble agents and viscous/oily agents.

Water-soluble agents.

Water-soluble iodine preparations make up the largest group of contrast agents. Most water-soluble iodine preparations are opaque to x-rays, pharmacologically inert, low in viscosity for rapid intravenous injection, low in toxicity, rapidly excreted by the kidneys, and chemically stable so that no iodine is released in the body.

The choice of radiographic contrast agent is a matter of personal preference. The **triiodinated compounds** are widely accepted because they are well tolerated by the body and provide excellent contrast. Triiodinated compounds contain three atoms of iodine per molecule. They are supplied as sodium or meglumine salts of iothalamic diatrizoic or metrizoic acids or as a mixture of these two salts.

In general sodium salts are less viscous. The meglumine salts reduce toxicity, minimize high sodium concentrations, and lessen tissue irritability. These contrast agents are usually injected into a vascular system for immediate visualization of the system or for subsequent demonstration of the excretory system. In addition, water-soluble agents can be infused into the bladder via a urinary catheter to show the urinary mucosa and bladder shape and size.

Possible toxicity is a concern with any pharmaceutical. The ionic (salt) preparations all have a local irritant effect and should be administered intravascularly or infused into an organ. Because of this property, iodine agents are contraindicated for myelography and arthrography. An intravenous injection of an iodinated contrast agent can cause side effects such as mild discomfort and nausea in an animal patient. Although they are extremely rare, more severe reactions such as cardiac arrest, hypovolemia, and anaphylaxis have been cited in a few clinical cases. In general, sodium salts are more toxic than meglumine salts but are included in the compound to reduce viscosity for easier administration.

Low-osmolar contrast media such as metrizamide, iopamidol, and iohexol are nonionic and reduce adverse side effects resulting from hyperosmolarity. Although expensive, these contrast agents are suitable for both intravascular and myelographic studies.

Water-soluble contrast agents are sometimes indicated for gastrointestinal use in patients with a suspected perforation. If this type of contrast agent were to enter the alimentary tract through a perforation, it would be rapidly absorbed because of its solubility. These agents are not used routinely, however, because of their fast transit time and hypertonicity. The iodine agents lose their contrast because they rapidly absorb fluid in the alimentary tract and become progressively dilute. With these agents, mucosal detail is poor. In some cases, the contrast agent is absorbed into the vascular system and excreted through the urinary system, which causes a confusing radiologic pattern.

Oily/viscous agents.

Oily/viscous agents have little application in veterinary radiography. Their use is limited to lymphography.

Oily contrast media consist of iodized oils. The oil contains a suspension of propyliodone in either water or arachidic oils. Because of their viscous nature and insolubility in water, they are not resorbed in the body and produce fat embolism. The iodized oils cannot be administered intravascularly. In addition, the agent does not mix with cerebrospinal fluid during myelography. The oils tend to coagulate within the spinal canal and fail to outline lesions clearly. Current practice does not include oily media for myelography. If the agent is not removed, the absorption rate within the spinal canal is extremely slow. The absorption rate is estimated at approximately 1 mL/year.

Barium Preparations

Barium sulfate is a positive-contrast suspension and is the medium of choice for radiographic studies of the gastrointestinal tract. Because it is completely insoluble, it is not diluted by alimentary secretions and is not absorbed through the intestines. Barium is available in various forms (e.g., liquid, paste, and powder for reconstitution with water).

The primary disadvantage of barium sulfate is that if it should pass through a perforation in the alimentary tract into the thorax or abdomen, it would not be absorbed or eliminated. The barium can remain in the body indefinitely and could potentially produce a granulomatous reaction. In cases in which a perforation is suspected, it is advisable to use a water-soluble contrast medium. However, if the water-soluble study is negative, a barium study should follow to avoid missing a perforation.

Morbidity and mortality are no worse than those with a leakage of gastrointestinal contents, if the barium is surgically flushed out of the abdominal cavity within 6 to 8 hours. Barium that is inadvertently aspirated into the trachea is usually cleared by coughing. If the medium reaches the small bronchi and alveoli, it is unlikely to be removed.

Negative-Contrast Agents: Gases

Gases used for negative-contrast radiographic studies include air, oxygen, nitrogen, nitrous oxide, and carbon dioxide. Of all the gases available, air, oxygen, and carbon dioxide are most frequently used. Carbon dioxide has an advantage over room air because it is better absorbed into the body when administered into a hollow organ; room air can cause air emboli.

Gases are inexpensive, relatively safe, and easy to administer. Negative-contrast media enhance the contrast between the various soft tissues but produce less mucosal detail than positive-contrast media. Some special procedures call for the use of both negative- and positive-contrast media, or **double contrast.** A double-contrast study gives optimum mucosal detail and avoids masking small anomalies by large volumes of positive-contrast media.

PATIENT PREPARATION

Proper patient preparation is vital to a diagnostic radiographic study. Before the study, the patient's gastrointestinal tract should be emptied by withholding food for 12 to 24 hours and, if necessary, administering a cleansing enema. The presence of any gastrointestinal contents can detract from a quality study and may obstruct the view of certain areas of interest as a result of superimposition. Keep in mind that cathartics and enemas often produce gastrointestinal gas. To reduce the amount of gas present in the gastrointestinal tract during a study, the cathartic should be administered 4 to 12 hours before the radiographic procedure, and a radiographic study should not be administered within 1 hour of enema administration.

Evacuation of the gastrointestinal tract should be as atraumatic as possible, especially when working with an acutely ill patient. When an enema is contraindicated because of the poor condition of the patient, it is usually sufficient to fast the animal. However, if fasting would compromise the patient's health further, mild, nongranular nourishment such as baby food or other commercially available foods (e.g., Hill's a/d, Clinicare) can be given.

Many special radiographic procedures require sedation or anesthesia. Use caution so that the procedure is not compromised by the anesthetic. For example, general anesthesia is contraindicated for a gastrointestinal study due to subsequent slowed motility. If sedation is necessary, it should be limited to the use of a phenothiazine tranquilizer such as acepromazine maleate. Phenothiazine tranquilizers have only minimal effects on gastrointestinal motility or transit time. The use of **parasympatholytic agents** such as atropine should also be avoided for certain studies because of their anticholinergic effect.

CONTRAST STUDIES OF THE GASTROINTESTINAL TRACT

A patient presenting with diarrhea or vomiting is not uncommon in veterinary medicine. If medical management has failed, and survey radiographs are inconclusive, a contrast study may be indicated.

Radiographic studies of the gastrointestinal tract consist of the introduction of contrast media either by oral administration or via an orogastric tube. Radiographs are then taken at intervals to evaluate changes in morphology, the rate of gastric emptying, and small bowel transit time. The studies described here do not include the use of fluoroscopy because the majority of veterinary practices do not have this type of equipment.

Esophagography

Esophagography is performed to evaluate esophageal function and morphology. An esophagogram is indicated for patients with a history of regurgitation of undigested food, acute gagging, or dysphagia. This study consists of administering a positive-contrast medium orally and exposing a number of radiographs during and after the patient swallows the contrast agent. Liquid barium sulfate is usually the contrast medium of choice. Barium sulfate is also available in a thick paste form, which is more difficult to swallow but provides good mucosal coating of the esophagus. Barium can be mixed with canned or hard food, or both, to evaluate the function of the esophagus or for a partial obstruction that may be missed during a plain liquid barium swallow.

Precautions.

When introducing an oral contrast medium, proper care must be taken to minimize the possibility of the patient aspirating the agent into the lungs. If a perforation or rupture is suspected, an iodinated contrast medium should be used rather than a barium compound. Beware of iodinated contrast agents if aspiration is likely. The hypertonicity of these agents, if the ionic variety is used, can cause massive fluid shifts into the lung. The iodinated contrast medium is readily absorbed by the body if it enters the thoracic cavity, whereas barium is not absorbed and can remain in the body indefinitely. A foreign substance such as barium can stimulate granuloma formation within the thoracic cavity.

Upper Gastrointestinal Study

An **upper gastrointestinal (UGI) study** is performed to evaluate the stomach and small intestines. A UGI series may be indicated for patients that have recurrent unresponsive vomiting, abnormal bowel movements, suspected foreign body or obstruction, chronic weight loss, or persistent abdominal pain.

The contrast medium is administered orally (per os or via stomach tube), and radiographs are taken during the passage of the agent. The UGI series is performed in a systematic manner so that the maximum amount of information can be obtained. Both positive- and negative-contrast media can be used if the stomach is the target. However, most studies are performed with a positive-contrast medium such as barium sulfate.

Precautions.

If the patient is suspected of having a gastrointestinal perforation, barium sulfate is contraindicated. If barium were to enter the abdominal cavity, it would not be absorbed and could induce granuloma formation. In the instance of a perforation, an oral iodinated contrast medium should be used. Unfortunately, iodinated contrast media do not produce as much radiographic contrast. Iodine compounds tend to become diluted as they pass through the bowel because they draw extracellular fluid

---

TECHNIQUE OUTLINE

Contrast Media:
70% to 100% barium sulfate (liquid and paste) or iodinated oral contrast agent

Equipment/Supplies:
Optional canned/hard pet food

Patient Preparation:
None necessary

Procedure—Esophagography
I. Expose survey radiographs.
II. Place patient in lateral recumbency on x-ray table.
III. Slowly infuse liquid contrast medium into patient's cheek.
IV. Expose several radiographs of the thorax to monitor the passage of contrast medium. The field of view should include the entire esophagus from the pharyngeal region to the stomach. (NOTE: The first radiograph should be exposed within seconds of swallowing.)
V. Repeat steps III and IV with the patient in dorsal recumbency.
VI. Place the patient in lateral recumbency once again.
VII. Slowly administer barium paste, and expose the radiograph during the swallow (Fig. 18-1).
VIII. If abnormalities still are not detected, mix the liquid contrast medium with canned or hard pet food, or both, and administer per os.

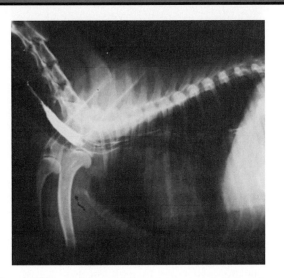

Figure 18-1 *Radiograph of a lateral view of an esophagram immediately after administration of liquid barium.*

IX. Radiographs are repeated; right and left lateral views may be indicated. Ventrodorsal views are contraindicated for patients with a dilated esophagus full of contrast medium. Placing the patient on its back may result in aspiration.

TECHNIQUE OUTLINE

Contrast Media:
30% to 60% liquid barium sulfate or iodinated oral contrast agent

Equipment/Supplies:
60-mL catheter-tip syringes
Orogastric tube

Patient Preparation:
Fast for 12 to 24 hours
Enema if necessary 2 to 4 hours before study
Sedate if necessary

Procedure—UGI Study
I. Expose survey radiographs.
II. Administer barium to distend the stomach with contrast medium.
   A. Route: Per os by placing the positive-contrast medium into the oral cavity and allowing the patient to swallow or via orogastric tube. To ensure correct placement of the orogastric tube, infuse a small amount of water. If the tube is incorrectly placed and is located in the trachea, the patient should cough, signaling incorrect placement.
   B. Dose: 4 to 8 mL/kg body weight.
III. Expose dorsoventral, ventrodorsal, right lateral, and left lateral radiographs immediately after contrast administration (Figs. 18-2 and 18-3).

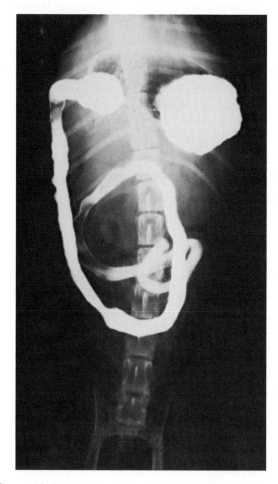

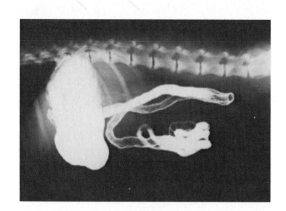

Figure 18-2 *Lateral view of an upper gastrointestinal study exposed 5 minutes after the administration of barium.*

Figure 18-3 *Ventrodorsal view of an upper gastrointestinal study exposed 5 minutes after the administration of liquid barium.*

Continued

from the digestive tract. In addition, because of their osmotic activity, they are not recommended for dehydrated patients.

Gastrography

Gastrography is a relatively quick, simple technique to evaluate the size, shape, position, and morphology of the stomach. A gastrogram is indicated if the patient is experiencing acute or chronic vomiting, blood in the vomitus, or cranial abdominal pain.

The contrast medium is administered orally, and subsequent radiographs are exposed with the animal in various positions. Three different contrast studies can be performed: (1) positive, (2) negative, and (3) double. The positive- and negative-contrast gastrograms are performed primarily to evaluate gastric shape and size. The double-contrast gastrogram is the most diagnostic for examination of the gastric mucosal lining.

Precautions.

A double-contrast gastrogram is not recommended for animals with a history of gastric distention or volvulus. Barium sulfate is contraindicated for a patient with a suspected gastroenteric perforation. In such instances, an oral iodine preparation should be used.

TECHNIQUE OUTLINE—cont'd

IV. Expose right lateral, ventrodorsal, or dorsoventral radiographs at intervals until contrast agent reaches the large bowel (suggested times: 15, 30, 60, and 90 minutes) (Figs. 18-4 and 18-5).

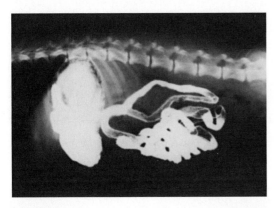

Figure 18-4 *Lateral view of an upper gastrointestinal study exposed 30 minutes after the administration of liquid barium.*

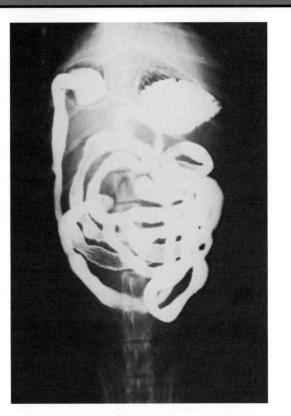

Figure 18-5 *Ventrodorsal view of an upper gastrointestinal study exposed 30 minutes after the administration of liquid barium.*

Lower Gastrointestinal Study

A **lower gastrointestinal (LGI) study (barium enema)** consists of the introduction of contrast medium via a catheter into the rectum, colon, and cecum. This study is indicated when full distention of the large intestine is necessary. Positive-, negative-, and double-contrast studies can be performed to evaluate the large intestine. A positive-contrast barium enema is indicated for a patient with abnormal bowel movements characterized by excessive mucus, bright-red blood in feces, pain during defecation, or diarrhea in high frequency. A barium enema can be used to detect intussusception, rectal mass, abdominal mass, stricture, or colonic obstruction.

Oral administration of a positive-contrast medium does not fully distend the large bowel; therefore rectal administration is necessary. Unfortunately, many animals will not tolerate rectal infusion of contrast medium without the use of chemical restraint. In most circumstances anesthesia is required.

Precautions.

Barium sulfate is contraindicated if the patient has a suspected perforation. In this case, an iodinated contrast medium should be used. Iodine compounds have the advantage of mixing well with colon fluid, coating the mucosa without excessive distention, and allowing finer detail of the intestinal mucosal lining.

It is vital that the patient be properly prepared before the procedure. Any feces or ingestion left in the colon could create a confusing artifact. In addition to fasting the patient and administering a cleansing enema, it may be necessary to administer an oral cathartic such as a stool softener or mineral oil.

All colon examinations such as proctoscopy and rectal palpation should be performed at least 12 hours in advance, and enemas should be given at least 4 hours in advance. Examinations of the rectum and colon induce colonic spasms and gas accumulation. The collection of gas in the gastrointestinal tract can cause radiographic artifacts during a barium enema. The enema solution should consist of warm water or saline to cleanse the colon. Soapy water should not be used because of the irritating effects on the large bowel mucosa.

CONTRAST STUDIES OF THE URINARY SYSTEM

Contrast studies of the upper and lower urinary system are excellent for the evaluation of the kidneys, ureters, bladder, and urethra. Urography and cystography are

TECHNIQUE OUTLINE

Contrast Media:
Barium sulfate (liquid)
Air or carbon dioxide

Equipment/Supplies:
Orogastric tube
60-mL catheter-tip syringes

Patient Preparation:
Fast for 12 to 24 hours or evacuate all stomach contents.
Sedate patient if necessary; suggested sedatives are acepromazine maleate and glucagon (glucagon is a gastrointestinal hypotonic agent that induces gastric hypomotility).

Procedure—Gastrography
I.   Expose survey radiographs.
II. Administer contrast medium orally or via orogastric tube.
   A. Positive-contrast gastrogram.
      1. 4 to 8 mL barium per kilogram.
   B. Negative-contrast gastrogram.
      1. 5 to 8 mL air or carbon dioxide per kilogram.
   C. Double-contrast gastrogram.
      1. 2 mL barium per kilogram.
      2. Air to follow barium: 10 to 20 mL air or carbon dioxide per kilogram.
      3. If patient regurgitates air, add additional air.
      4. Roll patient on its long axis.
III. Expose dorsoventral, ventrodorsal, left lateral, and right lateral radiographs (Figs. 18-6 and 18-7).

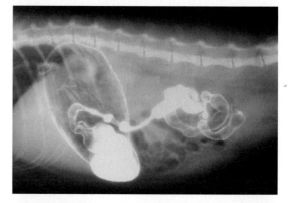

Figure 18-6   *Lateral view of a double-contrast gastrogram.*

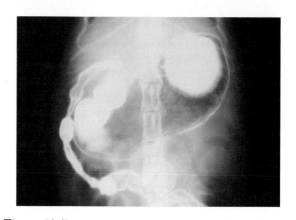

Figure 18-7   *Ventrodorsal view of a double-contrast gastrogram.*

relatively inexpensive and highly diagnostic techniques that can be performed in any veterinary practice with the proper equipment.

A radiographic study of the urinary system may be indicated for a patient with hematuria, proteinuria, crystalluria, polyuria, isosthenuria, or dysuria. The clinical signs of the patient dictate the contrast study that is necessary. Each study has limitations, and a number of different studies may be necessary to evaluate the entire urinary system.

Excretory Urography

Excretory urography consists of an intravenous injection of sterile, water-soluble iodinated contrast medium and exposure of radiographs at subsequent intervals. The iodinated contrast medium circulates through the venous blood, is filtered out of the blood, and collects in the kidneys. An excretory urogram, also referred to as an **intravenous urogram (IVU)** or an **intravenous pyelogram (IVP)**, is a useful radiographic study to evaluate kidney structure and collection system. However, an IVP is not used to evaluate renal function quantitatively.

The excretory urogram is divided into two phases: (1) **nephrogram** and (2) **pyelogram.** Radiographs taken immediately after the injection of contrast medium exhibit the agent uniformly perfused throughout the renal vasculature. The diffuse opacification of the renal parenchyma is characteristic of the nephrogram phase. This phase demonstrates the vascular supply and perfusion of the kidney and documents the presence of functional renal tissue, particularly if it persists beyond the angiographic blush.

As the contrast agent is filtered into the renal collection system with the urine, the renal pelvis and recesses are opacified. This is known as the *pyelogram phase,* which can be accentuated by placing abdominal compression on the caudal abdomen with a compression band or abdominal pressure wrap, resulting in cessation of urine flow to the bladder. This is neither necessary nor recommended

TECHNIQUE OUTLINE

Contrast Media:
30% to 60% barium sulfate or iodinated compound

Equipment/Supplies:
Bardex or Foley balloon-tip catheter
60-mL catheter-tip syringes
Contrast agent reservoir (enema bag or can or commercially available set)
Examination gloves
Lubricant
Hemostat

Patient Preparation:
Low-residue diet 48 hours before study
Fast for 24 hours before study
Enema until clear, 12 hours in advance
Mild oral cathartic if necessary
Anesthesia if necessary

Procedure—LGI Study
I. Expose survey radiographs; ensure that the large bowel is clear of all fecal matter.
II. With the patient in lateral recumbency, gently insert the lubricated catheter tip into the rectum and inflate the balloon so that it is located just inside the internal anal sphincter.
III. Attach the catheter end to the infusion device (bucket or bag) or syringe.
IV. Slowly infuse the contrast medium.
   A. Positive-contrast media should be warmed to body temperature.
   B. Dose is approximately 10 to 15 mL/kg.
V. Clamp catheter with a clamp or hemostat.
VI. With catheter in place, expose lateral radiograph to evaluate distention of the large bowel.
VII. Add more contrast medium if necessary.
VIII. When desired distention of the large bowel is attained, expose ventrodorsal, right, lateral, and left lateral radiographs (oblique views if necessary) (Figs. 18-8 and 18-9).
IX. After study is completed, evacuate the contrast agent from the large bowel as completely as possible. This is accomplished by lowering the contrast reservoir below the patient level and allowing gravity to empty the agent from the bowel.

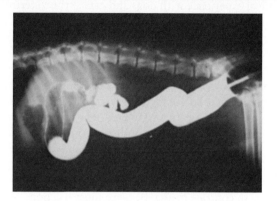

Figure 18-8 *Lateral view of a barium enema.*

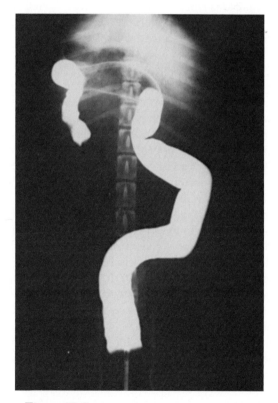

Figure 18-9 *Ventrodorsal view of a barium enema.*

because it can cause transient worsening of renal function under experimental circumstances.

Precautions.
Any urine samples that are necessary for laboratory data should be obtained before injecting the contrast medium. Iodinated contrast agents increase urine-specific gravity to a variable degree and induce a false-positive reaction for protein detected by sulfosalicylic acid.

Because the amount of iodinated contrast medium injected may be quite large, the placement of an indwelling catheter is suggested to assist injection and decrease the possibility of perivascular injection. Sedation usually is not necessary if the patient is cooperative.

Although they are rare, systemic reactions can occur after intravenous injection of iodinated contrast media. In clinical experience with dogs and cats at the Veterinary Teaching Hospital at the University of Minnesota, approximately 1 in 80 intravenous contrast injection procedures resulted in fatality. The incidence of mild reactions is unknown but is probably higher. Most severe, acute reactions occur within the first 5 to 10 minutes and have an unpredictable outcome. They range in severity from mild (requiring no treatment) to fatal. The most frequently observed acute clinical signs in dogs and cats are vomiting, defecation, urination, and hypotension with or without collapse.

Several measures are suggested to prevent adverse reactions to contrast media. Because most reactions occur within minutes, preparation for emergency care should be made before the injection. The animal's disease state should be assessed, and dehydration corrected. An emergency resuscitation kit containing endotracheal tubes, Ambu bag, emergency drugs, and intravenous fluids should be ready before injection. The patient's vital signs should be monitored during and after the injection to observe for any adverse reactions.

Cystography.

Cystography consists of the introduction of contrast medium into the bladder via a urinary catheter. Positive-, negative-, and double-contrast studies can be used for cystography. In addition, a cystogram can be performed in conjunction with an upper urinary tract study. A contrast study of the bladder is beneficial for the investigation of cystic calculi, mural lesions, bladder rupture, and other bladder wall abnormalities.

A cystogram is indicated for an animal exhibiting unresponsive clinical signs such as hematuria, crystalluria, bacturia, dysuria, anuria, and incontinence. At no time should cystography replace a clinical evaluation of the patient history, physical examination, and laboratory data. Radiographic findings from cystography can be used to confirm, refute, or correct diagnoses formulated by earlier clinical evaluation.

Sedation is recommended for cystography because distention of the urinary bladder can be uncomfortable, especially for a patient with cystitis.

Precautions.

Any urine samples that are necessary for laboratory data should be obtained before the injection of contrast medium. Iodinated contrast agents increase urine-specific gravity to a variable degree and induce a false-positive reaction for protein detected by sulfosalicylic acid. Procedures using contrast agents can influence laboratory data obtained from the upper and lower urinary tracts for as long as 24 hours.

Every effort should be made to protect the patient from iatrogenic trauma that can be associated with urinary catheterization. Any induced trauma can predispose an animal to a bacterial infection. A gentle, meticulous technique helps prevent infection or damage to the delicate tissues of the genital tract, the urethra, and the urinary bladder. The smallest-diameter urinary catheter feasible for an objective study should be used. Catheters with flared distal ends are recommended to reduce the risk of catheter migration to a point of no return. The flared tip will also accommodate the tip of the syringe. Keeping a three-way valve (stopcock) on the distal end of the catheter lessens concern about migration. Take care also to ensure that the catheter is not overinserted into the bladder. A sharp-pointed catheter can penetrate the bladder wall if excessive force is used. Pliable catheters can become entangled in the bladder, making removal difficult.

The use of barium sulfate and sodium iodide is contraindicated for cystography. Although they are rare, complications with barium sulfate include barium casts and interstitial fibrosis secondary to vesicoureteral reflux. Barium also serves as a nidus for the formation of uroliths. In addition, granulomatous disease may occur secondary to a rupture of the bladder or urethra. Sodium iodide solution is not recommended for cystography because of its irritating effect on the mucosa of the bladder and urethra. Sodium iodide solution has been known to produce acute hemorrhagic cystitis, epithelial ulcerations, and submucosal hemorrhage. Tri-iodinated ionic compounds are the contrast agents of choice; they are versatile and can be used for excretory urograms, as well as cystourethrograms.

Leakage of urine and contrast medium around or through the catheter may occur during the procedure. It is important that any spill be cleaned off the equipment and patient immediately; contrast contaminants can cause confusing artifacts on a radiograph.

Indications have been made that the injection of room air into the lower urinary tract can cause a fatal air embolism. This has been noted in patients with active bladder hemorrhage. The air can enter the low-pressure venous system via bleeding capillaries. Although this occurrence is rare, carbon dioxide or nitrous oxide should be used for patients with macroscopic hematuria. Carbon dioxide and nitrous oxide are 20 times more soluble in serum than air or oxygen and are better absorbed in the body.

The dose of contrast medium that is necessary to distend an animal's bladder for a cystogram varies according to the size and condition of the bladder. With either an iodinated compound or air, quantities of 10 to 300 mL are usually required to fill the bladder adequately. Distending the bladder moderately is important to avoid artifactual thickening of the bladder wall or folding of the mucosa due to underdistention. In the same respect, the bladder should not be overdistended with contrast medium, which could result in a retrograde reflux of the contrast agent into the ureters and renal pelvis or even cause a bladder rupture (Fig. 18-13).

TECHNIQUE OUTLINE

Contrast Media:
Water-soluble iodinated compound

Patient Preparation:
Fast 12 to 24 hours
Cleansing enema (administer 4 hours before study to minimize gas artifact)

Procedure—Excretory Urography
I. Expose survey radiographs.
II. Place intravenous indwelling catheter in cephalic or saphenous vein.
III. Place the patient in dorsal recumbency.
IV. Infuse contrast medium.
   A. Concentration: 300 to 400 mg iodine per milliliter is suggested.
   B. Dose: 3 mL/kg (90 mL maximum).
   C. Injection rate: rapid bolus (1 to 3 minutes for entire injection).
V. Expose ventrodorsal projection immediately after rejection for nephrogram phase (Fig. 18-10).

VI. Subsequent lateral and ventrodorsal films are taken at 5, 10, and 20 minutes to show the pyelogram and drainage phases (Figs. 18-11 and 18-12). (If a compression band is used, remove it before exposing the 20-minute drainage phase radiograph.)
VII. Cystography can be performed at this time.

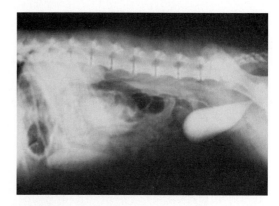

Figure 18-11 *Lateral view of the pyelogram and drainage phase of an intravenous pyelogram.*

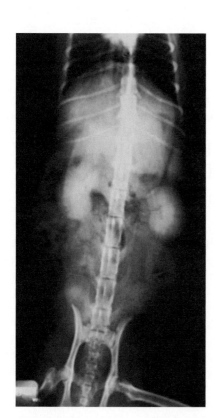

Figure 18-10 *Ventrodorsal view of the nephrogram phase of an intravenous pyelogram.*

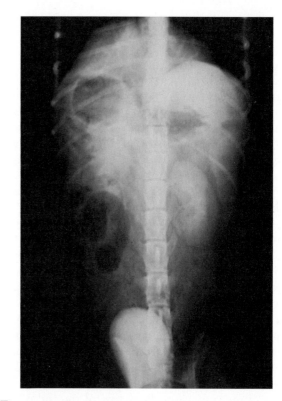

Figure 18-12 *Ventrodorsal view of the pyelogram and drainage phase of an intravenous pyelogram.*

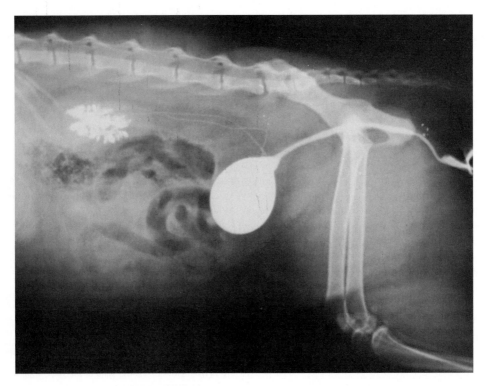

Figure 18-13 *Lateral view of a cystogram showing overdistention of the bladder, resulting in ureteral reflux of contrast medium.*

Urethrography

Urethrography consists of filling the urethra with contrast medium to detect urethral trauma, stricture, obstruction, and other pathologic disturbances such as tumor invasion. Filling the urethra can be done with either retrograde or antegrade infusion of contrast medium. A **retrograde urethrogram** can be performed with either positive- or negative-contrast media. An **antegrade urethrogram** is best done with positive-contrast media.

Precautions.

Sedation is recommended for urethrography because there is slight patient discomfort. The retrograde study of the urethra requires the use of a balloon-tip catheter such as a Swan-Ganz. Placing the balloon tip just inside the urethral orifice so that the majority of the urethra can be examined is important. A sufficient amount of contrast agent must be injected to fully distend the urethra; otherwise, it can mimic a stricture lesion or other mucosal impingement. It is best to make the exposure during the infusion of the contrast medium, toward the end of the injection. For male dogs, the bladder should be filled with the actual urethral injection.

Antegrade urethrography can be conveniently performed after a positive-contrast cystogram. Distending the bladder is important to create pressure to induce micturition. However, excessive pressure should never be placed on the urinary bladder because it could induce a bladder rupture. If a voiding urethrogram cannot be obtained, retrograde urethrography should be performed.

ADDITIONAL TECHNIQUES: A BRIEF OVERVIEW

Arthrography

Arthrography is a technique in which a contrast agent is injected through a needle into a true joint space, and radiographs are subsequently exposed. A contrast medium placed within a joint cavity demonstrates the articular surfaces and outlines the joint capsule. This type of study may be necessary for a patient that is lame or has pain associated with a joint, when survey radiographs provided insufficient information. An arthrogram can be used to evaluate a ruptured joint capsule, the presence of a cartilaginous flap, meniscal injuries, or the necessity for surgery.

The positive or negative arthrogram can be performed with a water-soluble iodine compound or air (carbon dioxide or nitrous oxide). The iodinated contrast agent should be diluted with sterile saline to a 20% to 40% solution. Use of more concentrated contrast solutions can completely obliterate the intracapsular ligaments or damaged cartilage.

An arthrogram is contraindicated if there is an infection of the soft tissues surrounding the joint. In this

TECHNIQUE OUTLINE

Contrast Media:
Any of the triiodinated contrast agents

Equipment/Supplies:
$3\frac{1}{2}$ to 5 French sterile polypropylene or red rubber urinary catheter (metal catheters are not recommended for female dogs because their rigid structure frequently causes trauma to the urethra or bladder)

Three-way valve (stopcock)

Syringes ranging from 3 to 60 mL in volume

Sterile aqueous lubricant or sterile lidocaine gel to reduce discomfort and risk of iatrogenic trauma caused by urethral spasms

Germicidal soap and water

Gauze pads

Sterile gloves

Otoscope speculum (to aid in visualizing the urethral opening in female patients)

Patient Preparation:
Fast 12 to 24 hours

Cleansing enema (administer 4 hours before study to minimize gas artifact)

Procedure—Cystography

I. Expose survey radiographs.

II. Cleanse adjacent structures external to the urethral orifice with germicidal soap and water.

III. Gently insert the lubricated catheter so that the tip is positioned in the trigone of the bladder.

IV. Gently aspirate all urine out of the bladder.
   A. Note the amount of urine withdrawn to give an estimate of the amount of contrast medium that is necessary.

V. If blood clots are present in the bladder, they should be flushed out with saline.

VI. Infuse 5 to 10 mL of 2% lidocaine into the bladder, if necessary, to decrease spasticity. Unless spasticity is reduced, it may be difficult or impossible to distend the bladder.

VII. Negative-contrast cystogram (pneumocystogram) (Fig. 18-14).
   A. Slowly infuse negative-contrast agent into the bladder via the urinary catheter.
      1. Dose: Approximately 10 mL air per kilogram.
         a. The dose varies with the size of the animal; smaller dogs usually require a larger amount per kilogram than larger dogs to fill the bladder. Always palpate the bladder during infusion and stop when it is moderately turgid.
   B. Expose lateral and ventrodorsal radiographs of the caudal abdomen.

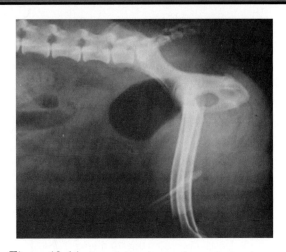

Figure 18-14 *Lateral view of a negative-contrast cystogram.*

1. An oblique view may be necessary, especially of male dogs, because of the superimposing penis over the bladder on the ventrodorsal projection.

VIII. Double-contrast cystogram (Fig. 18-15).
   A. This study can follow a negative-contrast cystogram, or the bladder should be distended with a negative-contrast agent.
      1. Dose: Approximately 10 mL air per kilogram.
         a. The dose varies with the size of the animal; smaller dogs usually require a larger amount per kilogram than larger dogs to fill the bladder.
   B. Infuse a small amount of positive (triiodinated) contrast medium via the catheter into the bladder.

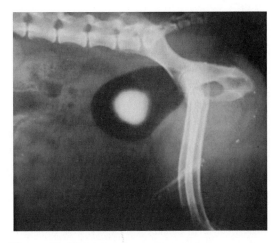

Figure 18-15 *Lateral view of a double-contrast cystogram.*

Continued

TECHNIQUE OUTLINE—cont'd

1. Cat: 1 to 2 mL into the bladder.
2. Dog: 1 to 3 mL into the bladder.
   a. Amount depends on size of the animal and residual volume of the catheter.
C. Expose lateral and ventrodorsal radiographs of the caudal abdomen.
   1. An oblique view may be necessary, especially of male dogs because of the superimposing penis over the bladder on the ventrodorsal projection.
IX. Positive-contrast cystogram (Fig. 18-16).
   A. Slowly infuse 50% positive- (triiodinated) contrast medium diluted with saline into the bladder until distended.
      1. Dose: Approximately 10 mL/kg.
         a. The dose varies with the size of the animal; smaller dogs usually require a larger amount per kilogram than larger dogs to fill the bladder. Always palpate the bladder during infusion, and stop when it is moderately distended.
   B. Expose lateral and ventrodorsal radiographs of the caudal abdomen.

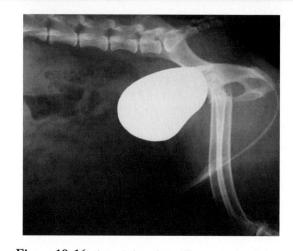

Figure 18-16 *Lateral view of a positive-contrast cystogram.*

1. An oblique view may be necessary, especially of male dogs, because of the superimposing penis over the bladder on the ventrodorsal projection

---

circumstance, insertion of the needle into a joint capsule could result in an injected joint. This could lead to severe infection of the joint. The use of air for a negative-contrast arthrogram may result in an air embolism. Carbon dioxide or nitrous oxide may be appropriate rather than air for a pneumoarthrogram.

Angiography and Angiocardiography

Angiography consists of a bolus injection of iodinated positive-contrast medium into a vascular system (e.g., cardiac, extremity), which is immediately followed by radiographic exposures. An angiogram may be used to demonstrate occlusion of a particular blood vessel, to demonstrate pathologic lesions of the vascular system, or to provide evidence of a tumor that was indefinable on survey radiographs.

A water-soluble iodine compound is the contrast medium of choice for angiography. For most procedures (e.g., angiography, **angiocardiography**), the contrast medium can be injected into a blood vessel proximal to the region of interest. Because circulating blood rapidly transports the contrast agent away from the area under examination, it is necessary to expose the radiographs during or immediately after the injection.

Ideally, the progress of a bolus injection of contrast medium should be followed by a series of radiographs exposed in rapid succession. This can be accomplished with a commercially available rapid film changer, or in a small veterinary practice, it can be conveniently done with a sheet of sturdy clear plastic and a number of loaded cassettes (Fig. 18-19). The sheet of clear plastic is positioned on top of small wood blocks, and the patient is centered on top of the glass sheet. The cassettes are numbered, placed under the plastic sheet, and positioned in a single-file line, with each cassette abutting the next. As the contrast medium is injected, the exposures are taken. The cassettes are advanced as each exposure is made.

Cholecystography

Cholecystography consists of oral or intravenous administration of a positive-contrast medium that is excreted through the biliary system. The degree of opacification of the gallbladder and bile ducts can be useful in evaluating gallbladder function and health. Nonvisualization of the gallbladder after injection of the contrast medium indicates possible gallbladder disease, biliary obstruction, gallstones, hepatocellular dysfunction, or failure to absorb the contrast agent if orally administered. Although opinions vary, the intravenous route of administration is most predictable and most rapid.

Injectable contrast cholecystographic agents are recommended for dogs because the oral preparations have variable absorption and do not always provide a satisfactory study.

TECHNIQUE OUTLINE

Contrast Media:

Water-soluble iodinated contrast agent or air, carbon dioxide, or nitrous oxide

Equipment/Supplies:

12- to 20-mL syringes
Balloon-tip urinary catheter
Sterile lubricant

Patient Preparation:

Fast 12 to 24 hours
Cleansing enema (administer 4 hours before study to minimize gas artifact)

Procedure—Urethrography

I. Expose survey radiographs.
II. Place the patient in lateral recumbency.
III. Retrograde urethrogram (Fig. 18-17).

A. Fill the lumen of the catheter with contrast medium before placement into the urethra.
B. Insert the lubricated tip of the catheter 1 to 3 cm into the urethral orifice and inflate the balloon.
C. Inject 3 to 20 mL of contrast medium into the urethra (amount of agent needed varies with size of patient).
D. Make the exposure during infusion, toward the end of the injection.
E. Repeat the injection for ventrodorsal and oblique projections, if necessary.
IV. Antegrade (voiding) urethrogram (Fig. 18-18).
A. With the bladder distended with a positive-contrast agent, place gentle pressure on the bladder with a paddle or wooden spoon.
B. Exposure is taken when urine is noted at the urethral orifice.

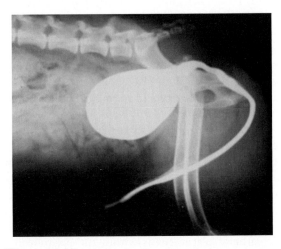

Figure 18-17 *Lateral view of a retrograde cystourethrogram.*

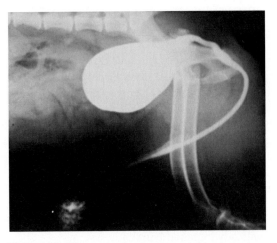

Figure 18-18 *Lateral view of an antegrade cystourethrogram.*

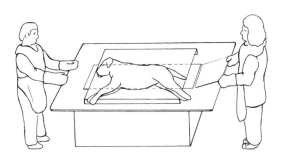

Figure 18-19 *Simple cassette tunnel system for a nonselective cardioangiogram. A sheet of plastic is propped a couple of inches off the table with wood or foam blocks. The cassettes are placed on the table and advanced after each exposure.*

After injection of the cholecystographic agent, radiographs should be taken at intervals of 15, 30, 60, and 120 minutes. The time required for complete opacification of the gallbladder varies with each patient. Once the gallbladder is identified radiographically, a small, preferably fatty, meal may be given to the patient and a second set of radiographs obtained. Feeding the patient a small meal allows evaluation of the emptying of the gallbladder.

Fistulography

Fistulography consists of injection of a positive- or negative-contrast medium into a fistula to determine the depth and origin of the tract. A **fistula** is any abnormal, tubelike passage within the body tissue. The occurrence of a fistula is usually the result of an injury or congenital deformity. The presence of a draining wound of undetermined origin may indicate a fistulous tract and the need for a fistulogram. Often, the site of the wound is far removed from the site of the drainage.

The contrast medium of choice for a fistulogram is any water-soluble iodinated agent. The contrast agent is infused into the fistulous tract with a syringe and flexible catheter, preferably with a balloon tip. After the contrast medium is infused, radiographs of the area are taken to document the flow of the agent.

Lymphography

Lymphography demonstrates the lymphatic system with the use of an injectable positive-contrast medium. This type of study may be indicated to evaluate the cause of edema in the forelimb or hind limb of an animal.

Lymphography is usually limited to areas of the extremities, head, and cervical region due to the inaccessibility of the lymphatic vessels in other areas of the body. The procedure involves identification and surgical exposure of a lymphatic duct and direct introduction of contrast medium into that duct. Radiographs of the area are obtained immediately after the injection of the contrast agent.

The contrast medium used for lymphography is either a water-soluble or an oily iodinated agent. The advantage of the oily agent is that it remains within the lymph nodes for up to 1 month, which allows for repeated radiographic studies. Unfortunately, the oily iodinated compounds can also cause local irritation and may be contraindicated for a patient with lymphedema. Oily compounds could aggravate an already impaired lymphatic system.

Myelography

Myelography consists of the introduction of a positive-contrast medium into the subarachnoid space of the spine, after which radiographs of the opacified region of the spine are taken. A myelogram is indicated to highlight a lesion that is undetectable on survey radiographs. Positive contrast in the subarachnoid space can be used to identify spinal cord compression resulting from a mass, protruding disk, vertebral abnormality, or spinal cord swelling.

General anesthesia is required for myelography because of the sensitive nature of a subarachnoid injection. The site of injection should be surgically prepared, after which a spinal needle is introduced into the cisternal or lumbar space. The contrast medium is then slowly injected into the subarachnoid space. A proper dose of contrast agent is determined by patient size and the area under examination. After injection, radiographs are taken of the areas

of interest. Personnel should be familiar with injection sites, techniques of injection, and caveats (which are beyond the scope of this text) before administering myelography.

A number of contrast agents have been used for myelography in the past, but many have posed considerable problems. Because of the extreme sensitivity of the spinal tissues and the irritating effects of conventional ionic contrast agents, some patients suffered convulsions and death after subarachnoid injection of these media. Oily iodinated contrast agents have also been used but do not mix well with the spinal fluid; they tend to coagulate and have an extremely slow absorption time. Currently, a low-osmolar, nonionic, water-soluble contrast medium is the standard choice for myelography.

Pneumoperitoneography

Pneumoperitoneography consists of the introduction of a negative-contrast agent (gas) into the peritoneal cavity to obtain better contrast within the abdomen. This type of study is beneficial for the evaluation of the liver, spleen, stomach, distal colon, kidneys, urinary bladder, uterus, and abdominal wall.

Carbon dioxide and nitrous oxide are the preferred gases for pneumoperitoneography because of their rapid absorption in the body. Room air does not absorb as readily, and its use results in an increased incidence of air embolism.

This study usually requires a sedated patient. Any gas in the peritoneal cavity can be uncomfortable and may cause the patient to struggle. An injection site on the midline halfway between the umbilicus and the pubis should be surgically prepared. A plastic or metal catheter with a stylet is inserted into the peritoneal cavity, and the stylet is withdrawn. With a syringe, a test aspiration is made to ensure that catheter placement is within the peritoneal cavity. Once the placement is confirmed, a negative contrast agent is injected until the abdominal wall is moderately distended. Abdominal distention can be evaluated by thumping the abdominal wall. A dull thud or the sound of a flat bongo drum indicates proper distention. Standard projections of the abdomen are then obtained.

Sialography

Sialography involves injection of a positive-contrast medium into the salivary ducts and glands. This type of study is beneficial for evaluating salivary duct patency and gland morphology. The parotid, zygomatic, mandibular, and sublingual salivary ducts can be examined with this technique. The most frequent use of sialography in veterinary radiography is for confirmation of a salivary mucocele.

The procedure requires that the patient be sedated. A blunt-ended needle is inserted into the salivary duct, and a small amount of water-soluble contrast medium is infused. Lateral and dorsoventral radiographs of the skull are obtained to visualize the salivary system.

Vaginography

Vaginography consists of introducing a positive-contrast medium into the vagina and cervix. The uterus and fallopian tubes may opacify if the cervix is open, as in estrus. This study can be used to evaluate the morphology of the vaginal vault and possibly the reproductive tract. A vaginogram may be indicated for a female patient to investigate infertility or a possible mass lesion.

A vaginogram is performed on an anesthetized patient. A balloon-tip syringe is inserted into the vulva, and the cuff is inflated just inside the vaginal vault. Once the catheter is in the correct position, a water-soluble iodinated contrast medium is infused into the vagina until back pressure is felt on the syringe. The amount necessary to distend the vagina varies according to patient size. Lateral and ventrodorsal abdominal radiographs are taken to record the infusion of the contrast medium.

KEY POINTS

1. All iodine agents have local irritant effects and are contraindicated for myelography and orthography.
2. Barium sulfate is contraindicated if an upper gastrointestinal perforation is suspected.
3. Using room air as a negative control agent can cause air emboli; alternatively, carbon dioxide is absorbed by the body and is safer to use.

REVIEW QUESTIONS

1. What is the disadvantage of using low-osmolar contrast media?
   a. Expense
   b. Short shelf life
   c. Can be used for myelography but not intravascularly
   d. Can be used intravenously but not for myelography

2. This positive-contrast medium is completely insoluble in the gastrointestinal tract and is not absorbed by the abdomen or thorax if leakage occurs.
   a. Iohexol
   b. Propyliodone
   c. Barium sulfate
   d. Metrizamide

3. Which of the following are true statements?
   a. All patients who will receive a gastrointestinal contrast study must receive an enema.
   b. General anesthesia and atropine are contraindicated for gastrointestinal contrast studies because of the degree to which they alter gastrointestinal motility.
   c. If an enema is administered, the contrast radiograph should not be taken until at least 1 hour postadministration.
   d. Both b and c are correct.

4. Which view is contraindicated during an esophagography and why?
   a. Dorsoventral; contrast agent in the esophagus superimposed over the heart
   b. Left lateral; potential for aspiration
   c. Ventrodorsal; potential for aspiration
   d. Right lateral; contrast agent in the esophagus superimposed over the heart
   (NOTE: The potential for aspiration should always be considered in any view, especially if the animal is sedated.)

5. Preparing a patient for an upper gastrointestinal study includes all of the following except:
   a. an enema 4 hours before the procedure as needed.
   b. fasting the patient for 12 to 24 hours.
   c. sedation as needed.
   d. administration of oral emetic such as hydrogen peroxide.

6. What is the most diagnostic examination of the gastric mucosal lining?
   a. Double-contrast gastrogram
   b. Double-contrast upper gastrointestinal study
   c. Positive-contrast gastrogram
   d. Negative-contrast gastrogram

7. Which of the following is a suitable agent to use as an enema before a lower gastrointestinal study?
   a. Barium sulfate
   b. Warm water
   c. Soapy water
   d. Mineral oil

8. Which of the following are recommended for performing intravenous pyelography?
   a. Placement of indwelling urinary catheter
   b. Fast 12 to 24 hours before
   c. Placement of abdominal pressure wrap during procedure
   d. Obtain urinary samples immediately after procedure

9. Which of the following is the safest combination of agents to use for a cystogram?
   a. Barium sulfate and carbon dioxide
   b. Sodium iodide and nitrous oxide
   c. Triiodinated ionic compounds and carbon dioxide
   d. Triiodinated ionic compounds and room air

10. What additional view can be helpful for assessing a positive-contrast cystogram, especially in a male patient?
    a. Lateral view with a horizontal beam
    b. Lateral cubitus
    c. Dorsoventral
    d. Oblique

Suggested Readings

Allan GS, Dixon RT: Cholecystography in the dog: the choice of contrast media and optimal dose rates, *JAVRS* 16:98-103, 1975.

Feeney DA, Walter PA, Johnston GR: The effect of radiographic contrast media on the urinalysis. In Kirk RW, editor: *Current therapy IX: Small animal practice,* Philadelphia, 1986, WB Saunders.

Harvey CE: Sialography in the dog, *JAVRS* 10:18-27, 1969.

Lavin-Cunliffe LM: Feline cystography and urethrography: technical use in practice, *Vet Tech* 10:364-373, 1989.

Morgan JP, Silverman S: *Techniques in veterinary radiography,* ed 4, Ames, Iowa, 1987, Iowa State University Press.

Osborne CA, Jessen CR: Double-contrast cystography in the dog, *J Am Vet Med Assoc* 154:1100, 1971.

Park RD: Contrast studies of the lower urinary tract, *Vet Clin North Am* 4:863, 1974.

Prior JE, Schaffer B, Skelly JF: Direct lymphangiography in the dog, *J Am Vet Med Assoc* 140:943-946, 1962.

Suter PF, Carb AV: Shoulder arthrography in dogs: radiographic anatomy and clinical application, *J Small Anim Dis* 10:407-413, 1969.

Ticer JW: *Radiographic techniques in small animal practice,* ed 2, Philadelphia, 1984, WB Saunders.

Webbon PM, Clark KW: Bronchography in normal dogs, *J Small Anim Dis* 18:327-332, 1972.

chapter 19

Large Animal Radiography

CHAPTER OUTLINE

Special Considerations
Distal Phalanx (Pedal Bone)
Navicular Bone
Proximal Phalanges
Fetlock Joint
Metacarpus/Metatarsus
Carpus Joint
Tarsus Joint

Elbow Joint
Shoulder Joint
Stifle Joint
Pelvis
Skull
Cervical Spine
Additional Areas: A Brief Overview

INTRODUCTION

Working with large animal patients requires much patience and time. Any procedure performed must be well thought out before it is started. The radiographer must also expect the unexpected. Successful large animal radiography is the result of forming a plan before the examination, teamwork during the examination, and patience throughout.

Although the differences between large and small animals are great, the principles of radiography are essentially the same. All directional terms and positions that apply to a dog and a cat apply to a horse and a cow. The two major differences are size and posture. In large animal radiography, unless the animal is young or small enough to be placed on an x-ray table, the patient is in a standing position. The size and posture of the patient necessitate special consideration in the areas of patient restraint, equipment, patient preparation, radiation safety, and positioning devices.

SPECIAL CONSIDERATIONS

Patient Restraint

A large animal is often startled by unfamiliar objects, especially those brought close to its body. A good prelude to a radiographic examination of a large animal is an official introduction of the patient to the x-ray machine. Allowing the horse or cow to gently sniff the machine and cassette may eliminate fear of the unknown. Always avoid sudden movements or loud noises, which may startle the animal. Continually reassure the patient in a calm voice.

In a standing position, the large animal patient is relatively unrestrained. Because of this, there is a greater risk of injury to personnel and to the x-ray machine. The x-ray tube is particularly vulnerable because it must be positioned close to the animal's leg and is liable to be kicked.

Several methods can be used to restrain a large animal for a radiographic examination including a twitch, stocks, and sedation. Sedation is a common method of restraint. The patient is given a small amount of chemical sedative to allow the radiographer freedom to move the x-ray machine without startling the animal, which would result in movement. If sedation is not possible or if the patient is restless, movement can be restricted if an attendant holds up one of the animal's legs. When attempting to radiograph a limb, the opposite limb is raised. Rarely, it may be necessary to place the patient under general anesthesia. Many attendants are required to manipulate the patient and to position the equipment when the large animal is anesthetized. The veterinarian must assess the situation and determine the type of restraint necessary.

Equipment

The radiographic machinery required for large animals must have adequate power and easy maneuverability. The x-ray tube must be able to move horizontally around the standing patient and vertically to expose an area as low as the level of the floor. The x-ray machines used for radiography of large animals fall into three categories: (1) small portable units, (2) mobile units, and (3) mounted units.

The portable unit is commonly used by equine and bovine veterinary practitioners who make "house calls." The portable unit is small and light enough that it can easily be moved from one location to another (see Fig. 2-4). The average power capacity of a portable unit is limited to a maximum milliamperage (mA) setting of 20 and a maximum kilovoltage (kVp) of 90. Due to the low mA capability, exposure times of 0.1 second or longer usually are necessary. However, long exposure times increase the likelihood of motion during exposure. Because line voltage varies from barn to barn, exposures are not always consistent with portable units. The collimation on a portable unit also varies, and the collimator may not always have a light to visualize the field of exposure. Therefore it is often easy to expose an area larger than necessary. This can pose a special problem with radiation safety (i.e., the exposure of personnel to excessive radiation).

Mobile units have the advantage of more power. The capacity of an average mobile unit ranges from 100 to 300 mA and up to 120 kVp. The higher mA capacity allows for shorter exposure times. The main disadvantage of this unit is its weight and consequent lack of maneuverability. The mobile unit has large wheels to allow ambulation but tends to be cumbersome and difficult to move on uneven floor surfaces (see Fig. 4-2).

Large, permanently mounted x-ray units are commonly used by veterinary specialty and referral practices. The power capacity may exceed 1000 mA. For large animal radiography, these units are commonly mounted on the ceiling with a series of overhead rails, which allow the x-ray tube to be moved vertically and horizontally around the patient (see Fig. 2-19, *B*). Unfortunately, ceiling units that have overhead rails can be noisy and distracting to a fearful patient. In addition, the size of the x-ray tube housing may limit its use for studies of the feet. Even if the tube is on the floor, the focal spot may be 6 to 8 inches off the floor, resulting in obliquity of the views.

Patient Preparation

Careful preparation of the patient is necessary for an artifact-free radiograph. For all examinations, the hair coat should be brushed or washed to remove obvious dirt, bedding, and other surface artifacts. The areas of interest also should be wiped dry with a towel to remove any water or other remaining liquid contaminants. For radiography of the equine foot, a number of steps are necessary to prevent extraneous radiographic shadows over the areas under examination. The first step is to remove the shoe of the patient and trim back any overgrown portions of the hoof. Next, the sole and clefts should be picked and scrubbed clean. The final step is to pack the sole of the foot with a radiolucent material such as methylcellulose, softened soap, or Play-Doh. Packing the sole prevents the appearance of an air artifact superimposed over the areas of interest.

Radiation Safety

All rules of radiation safety discussed in Part 1 of this text also apply to large animal radiography. A few extra rules of safety must be considered, however, because of the size and posture of the patient and the considerably high exposure factors needed.

The attendants holding the patient and holding the cassette next to the anatomy must be wearing appropriate lead attire. Because the attendants' attention is focused on the patient rather than the x-ray beam, it is the responsibility of the radiographer to ensure that all personnel are a safe distance from the primary beam. Cassette-holding devices help reduce exposure to the attendants. The device usually consists of a clamp that is attached to the cassette and held at length by a handle (Fig. 19-1).

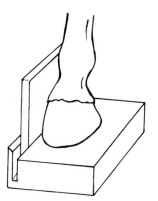

Figure 19-2 *For equine pedal radiography, it may be necessary to raise the patient's foot off the ground to radiograph that area. A wood block is commonly used for this purpose. The wood block pictured here has a slot designed to hold a cassette next to the limb of interest.*

Positioning Devices

At times, it may be necessary to raise the animal's foot because the x-ray tube cannot be dropped to the level of the floor. A positioning block can be used to raise the foot into position and to serve as a cassette holder (Fig. 19-2). The block is usually constructed of wood built to suit the particular x-ray unit. A slot can be cut into the wood to serve as a cassette holder. The foot of the patient can be placed directly onto the block to raise it into position next to the cassette, or the cassette can be placed beside the block.

Another device that is often necessary is a cassette tunnel. A tunnel can be constructed of a radiolucent wood or hard plastic, but it must be durable enough to withstand the weight of the patient. For a dorsopalmar/dorsoplantar oblique view of the coffin or navicular bone, the patient must be standing on top of the cassette. A cassette cannot withstand such weight without sustaining damage. A tunnel device can make the examination possible without damaging the equipment (Fig. 19-3).

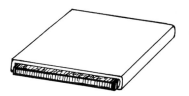

Figure 19-3 *A cassette tunnel.*

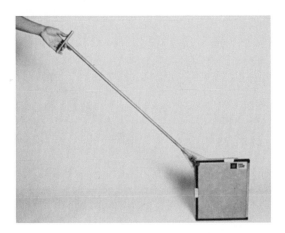

Figure 19-1 *A cassette holder used for equine radiography.*

DISTAL PHALANX (PEDAL BONE)

Lateral View

The patient's foot is placed on a wood block to elevate it to a level at which the central x-ray beam can be directed horizontally toward the pedal bone. The placement of the foot must be as close to the edge of the block as possible so that the cassette is as close to the medial aspect of the foot as possible (Figs. 19-4 and 19-5). The object–film distance must be minimal. To prevent motion, it may be helpful to have an attendant hold the patient's leg of interest over the carpus or elevate the opposite limb so that the limb being examined is completely weight bearing. The cassette is placed on the medial side of the foot, either directly on the floor or in the cassette groove in the wood block. The field of view should include the entire hoof. (NOTE: This same position is used to examine the lateral navicular bone. In that case, the beam center is directed at the palmar aspect of the coronary band.)

BEAM CENTER: Over hoof wall just below coronary band

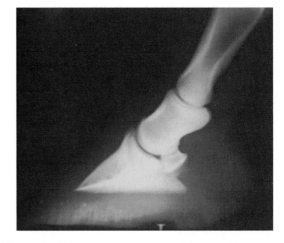

Figure 19-5 *Radiograph of the lateral view of the distal phalanx.*

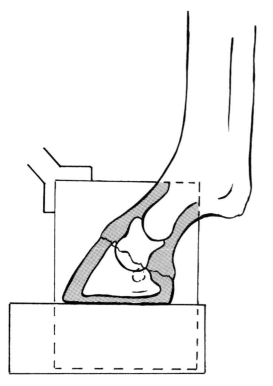

Figure 19-4 *Correct positioning for the lateral view of the distal phalanx.*

DISTAL PHALANX (PEDAL BONE)—*cont'd*

Dorsopalmar/Dorsoplantar View

The patient's foot is placed on a wood block so that it is elevated to the level of the horizontal central x-ray beam. The heel of the foot should be placed on the edge of the block or cassette groove. The cassette is placed directly behind the foot on the floor or in the cassette groove and held perpendicular to the floor (Figs. 19-6 and 19-7). It may be helpful to raise the opposite limb so that full weight is placed on the limb of interest. This decreases the possibility of motion. The field of view should include the entire hoof.

BEAM CENTER: Over middle of pedal bone just below coronary band

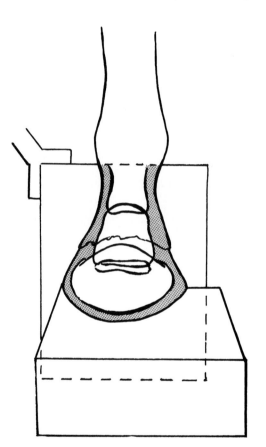

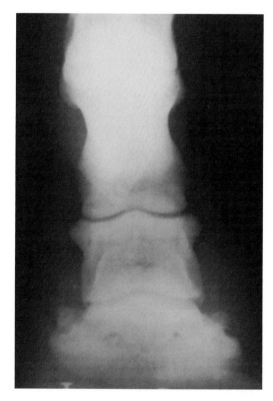

Figure 19-7 *Radiograph of the dorsopalmar view of the distal phalanx.*

Figure 19-6 *Correct positioning for the dorsopalmar/dorsoplantar view of the distal phalanx.*

DISTAL PHALANX (PEDAL BONE)—*cont'd*

Dorsopalmar/Dorsoplantar Oblique View

The cassette is placed in a tunnel cassette holder, and the foot of the patient is positioned on top of the tunnel. The foot should be in the center of the cassette so that the entire hoof and pedal bone are included in the field of view (Figs. 19-8 and 19-9). It may be necessary to raise the opposite limb so that the limb of interest is weight bearing. The x-ray tube is angled 45 degrees to the ground and directed at the hoof wall. (NOTE: This same view can be used to visualize the navicular bone. Because of superimposition of the navicular bone over the second phalanx, higher exposure factors are necessary to visualize this area, and an angle of 65 degrees off horizontal should be used.)

BEAM CENTER: Over middle point of hoof wall just below coronary band

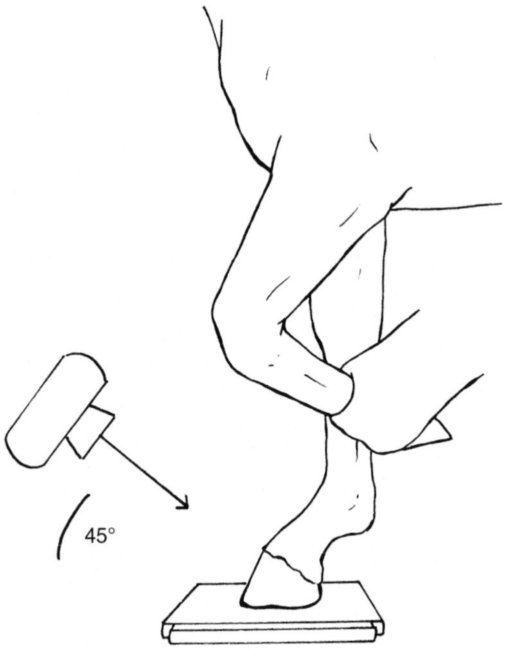

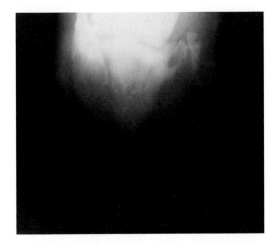

Figure 19-9 *Radiograph of the dorsopalmar oblique view of the distal phalanx.*

45°

Figure 19-8 *Correct positioning for the dorsopalmar/dorsoplantar oblique view of the distal phalanx.*

NAVICULAR BONE

Dorsopalmar/Dorsoplantar Oblique View

The patient's foot can be placed (1) on a cassette within a cassette tunnel, as shown for the dorsopalmar/dorsoplantar oblique view of the distal phalanx, or (2) on a block with specially designed grooves that hold the hoof at an angle (Figs. 19-10 through 19-12). With the patient standing on the cassette, the x-ray beam is angled 65 degrees toward the middle of the second phalanx. When the block is used, the toe of the hoof is placed in a vertical groove so that the dorsal wall of the hoof is positioned vertically. The cassette is placed behind the heels in a cassette groove. The opposite leg must bear the majority of the patient's weight. The x-ray beam is directed parallel to the ground, and the field of view should include the second and third phalanges. With the foot on the block in this vertical position, a 45- to 65-degree angle view of the navicular bone is projected onto the x-ray film.

BEAM CENTER: Over center of second phalanx just above coronary band

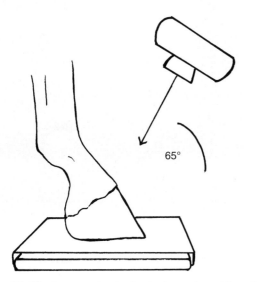

Figure 19-10 *Correct positioning for the dorsopalmar oblique view of the navicular bone with the patient standing on a cassette tunnel.*

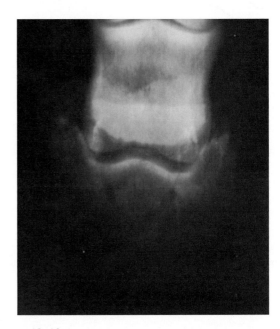

Figure 19-12 *Radiograph of the dorsopalmar oblique view of the navicular bone.*

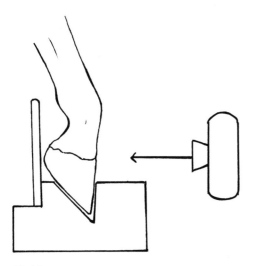

Figure 19-11 *Correct positioning for the dorsopalmar oblique view of the navicular bone with the dorsal wall of the hoof held in a vertical position with the use of a wood block.*

NAVICULAR BONE—*cont'd*

Flexor View

The foot of the patient is placed on top of a cassette within a cassette tunnel (Figs. 19-13 and 19-14). If possible, the patient should be stepping back slightly so that the fetlock is in an extended position. The first phalanx is almost perpendicular to the ground in this position, allowing better visualization of the navicular bone. The x-ray tube is positioned directly behind the foot and angled approximately 65 degrees to the floor. Great care must be taken with the x-ray tube in this position immediately behind the limb. It may be necessary to reduce the source–image distance (SID) when placing the x-ray tube under the belly of a horse for views of the front navicular bone.

BEAM CENTER: Over middle of heel bulbs

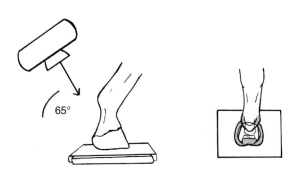

Figure 19-13 *Correct positioning for the flexor view of the navicular bone.*

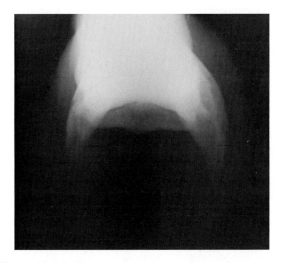

Figure 19-14 *Radiograph of the flexor view of the navicular bone.*

PROXIMAL PHALANGES

Lateral View (Short and Long Pastern)

The foot of the patient is placed on a wood block so that it is elevated slightly off the floor. The cassette is placed next to the medial aspect of the foot and should be on and perpendicular to the floor. The limb of interest should be weight bearing (Figs. 19-15 and 19-16). It may be necessary to raise the opposite limb to eliminate motion. The x-ray beam is directed horizontally toward the phalanx. The field of view should include the first and second phalanges for a general projection of the area.

BEAM CENTER: Over area of interest

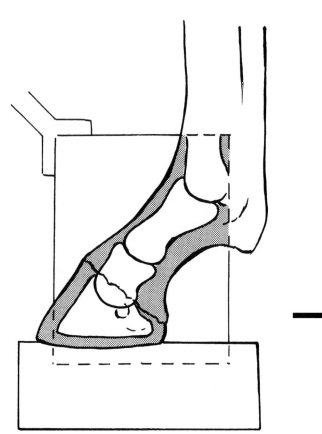

Figure 19-15 *Correct positioning for the lateral view of the proximal phalanges.*

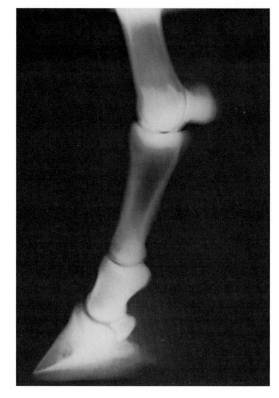

Figure 19-16 *Radiograph of the lateral view of the proximal phalanges.*

PROXIMAL PHALANGES—*cont'd*

Dorsopalmar/Dorsoplantar View

The patient is positioned so that the limb under examination is weight bearing. The cassette is placed behind the limb parallel to the phalanges (Figs. 19-17 and 19-18). It may be necessary to elevate the opposite limb to minimize motion. Depending on the angle of the foot and the placement of the cassette, it may be necessary to direct the x-ray tube at a 30- to 45-degree angle to the floor. The x-ray beam must be perpendicular to the cassette. The field of view should include the first and second phalanges.

BEAM CENTER: Over area of interest

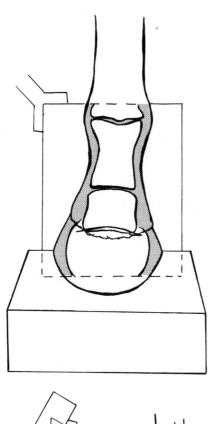

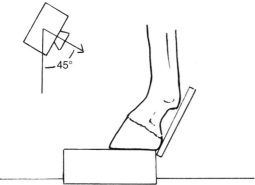

Figure 19-17 *Correct positioning for the dorsopalmar view of the proximal phalanges.*

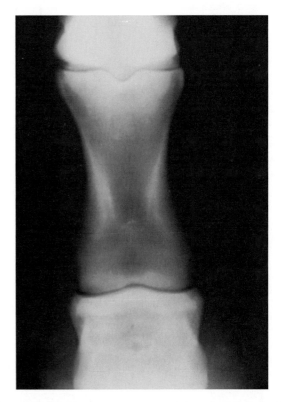

Figure 19-18 *Radiograph of the dorsopalmar view of the proximal phalanges.*

FETLOCK JOINT

Dorsopalmar/Dorsoplantar View

The foot of the patient is placed with full weight on the floor directly under the body. The cassette is positioned on the floor directly behind the foot, touching the palmar or plantar aspect of the digit. The cassette should be held perpendicular to the floor (Figs. 19-19 and 19-20). The opposite limb may be elevated if necessary to control the patient. The field of view should include the entire fetlock joint and a small portion of the bones that are proximal and distal to the joint. (NOTE: Aiming the x-ray beam at a slight tilt downward minimizes the sesamoid superimposition on the joint surfaces.)

BEAM CENTER: Through joint at right angle to cassette

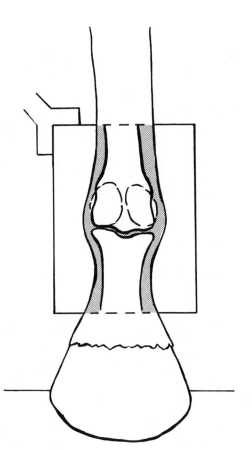

Figure 19-19 *Correct positioning for the dorsopalmar view of the fetlock joint.*

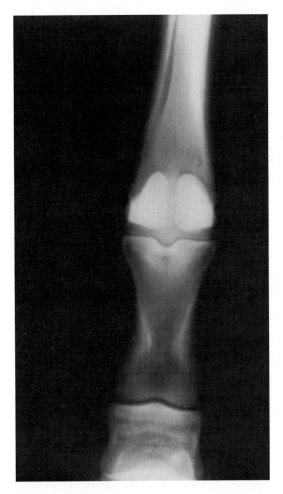

Figure 19-20 *Radiograph of the dorsopalmar view of the fetlock joint.*

FETLOCK JOINT—*cont'd*

Lateral View

The foot of the patient is placed in a weight-bearing position directly under the body. The cassette is placed on the floor on the medial side of the foot of interest. The cassette should remain perpendicular to the floor (Figs. 19-21 and 19-22). Raising the opposite limb may be necessary to control the patient. The field of view should include the fetlock joint and a small portion of the bones proximal and distal to the joint.

BEAM CENTER: Through joint at right angle to cassette

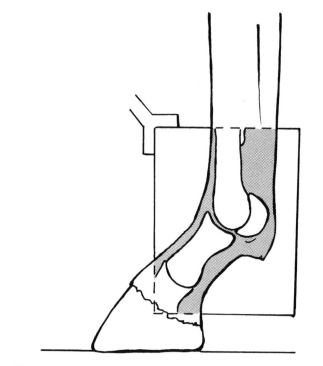

Figure 19-21 *Correct positioning for the lateral view of the fetlock joint.*

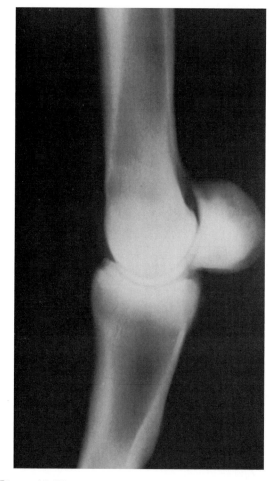

Figure 19-22 *Radiograph of the lateral view of the fetlock joint.*

FETLOCK JOINT—*cont'd*

Flexed Lateral View

The limb of interest is elevated, and the fetlock joint is flexed. The attendant holding the limb must be properly protected with lead gloves and apron. The cassette is positioned against the medial aspect of the joint. The cassette must remain perpendicular to the floor (Figs. 19-23 and 19-24). The limb should remain under the patient's body and not be abducted laterally. The x-ray beam is directed horizontally and parallel with the floor toward the cassette. The field of view should include the fetlock joint and a portion of the bones proximal and distal. The primary x-ray beam should be collimated so that the attendants' hands holding the limb are not exposed.

BEAM CENTER: Through joint at right angles to cassette

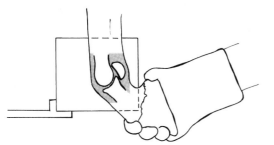

Figure 19-23 *Correct positioning for the flexed lateral view of the fetlock joint.*

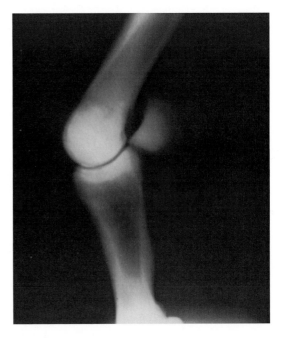

Figure 19-24 *Radiograph of the flexed lateral view of the fetlock joint.*

FETLOCK JOINT—*cont'd*

Oblique Views (Lateral and Medial)

The foot of the patient is placed in a normal weight-bearing position under the body. Depending on the oblique view desired, the x-ray tube is angled 30 to 45 degrees to either side of the dorsal midline of the foot (Figs. 19-25 and 19-26). The precise tube angle varies with the patient and the area under investigation. The cassette is placed on the floor against the palmar or plantar aspect of the foot. The cassette is positioned so that the front of the x-ray beam is directed at a right angle to the cassette front. This view of the fetlock allows visualization of the medial and lateral sesamoid bones on the palmar/plantar aspect of the limb.

BEAM CENTER: Through middle of joint at 30-to 45-degree angle from dorsal midline of joint

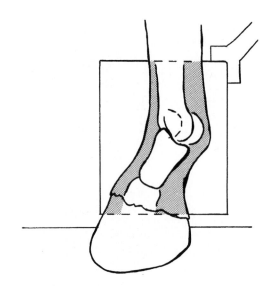

Figure 19-25 *Correct positioning for the lateral or medial oblique view of the fetlock.*

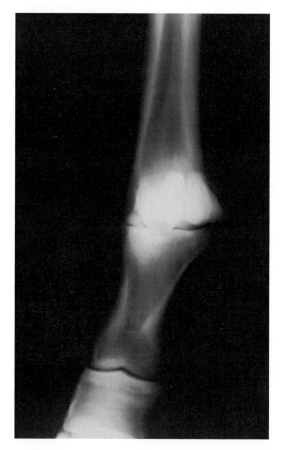

Figure 19-26 *Radiograph of the lateral or medial oblique view of the fetlock.*

METACARPUS/METATARSUS

Dorsopalmar/Dorsoplantar View

The patient is allowed to stand in a normal position, bearing weight on the limb under investigation. The cassette is placed against the palmar or plantar aspect of the limb and is held perpendicular to the floor (Figs. 19-27 and 19-28). The x-ray beam is directed parallel to the ground and at a right angle to the cassette. The cassette should be large enough that the field of view includes the joints proximal and distal to the metacarpus or metatarsus (a 7- × 17-inch cassette is recommended).

BEAM CENTER: Over midpoint of metacarpus or metatarsus

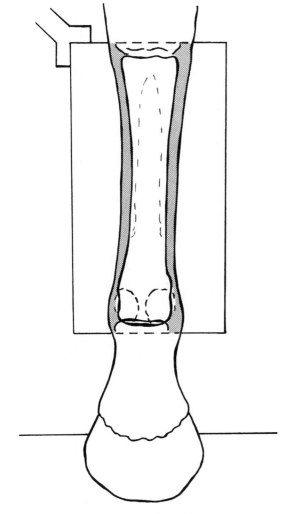

Figure 19-27 *Correct positioning for the dorsopalmar view of the metacarpus.*

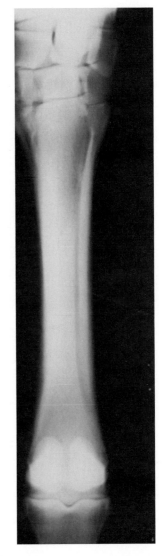

Figure 19-28 *Radiograph of the dorsopalmar view of the metacarpus.*

METACARPUS/METATARSUS—*cont'd*

Lateral View

With the patient standing in a natural weight-bearing position, the cassette is placed medially against the limb (Figs. 19-29 and 19-30) and should remain perpendicular to the floor. The x-ray tube is positioned laterally, and the x-ray beam is directed at a right angle to the cassette. The cassette should be large enough that the field of view includes the joints proximal and distal to the metacarpus or metatarsus.

BEAM CENTER: Over midpoint of metacarpus or metatarsus

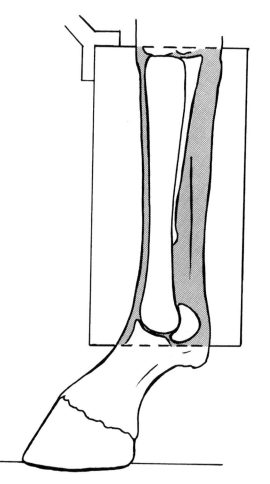

Figure 19-29 *Correct positioning for the lateral view of the metacarpus.*

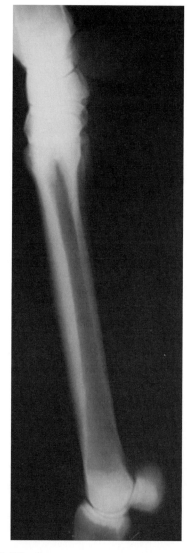

Figure 19-30 *Radiograph of the lateral view of the metacarpus.*

METACARPUS/METATARSUS—*cont'd*

Oblique Views (Lateral and Medial)

For an unobstructed examination of the splint bones (second and fourth metacarpals/metatarsals) of the horse, oblique views are necessary. The patient is allowed to stand normally, bearing weight on the limb of interest. The cassette is placed either medial or lateral to the palmar or plantar aspect of the limb (Figs. 19-31 and 19-32).

For visualization of the lateral splint bone, the cassette is positioned at an approximate 45-degree angle medially. For the medial splint bone, the cassette is positioned laterally approximately 45 degrees. The field of view should include the metacarpus or metatarsus and the joints proximal and distal.

BEAM CENTER: At middle of metacarpus/metatarsus, approximately 45 degrees lateral or medial to a true dorsopalmar/dorsoplantar projection

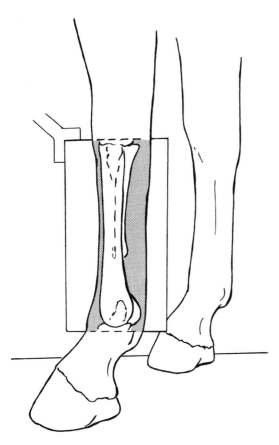

Figure 19-31 *Correct positioning for the oblique view of the metacarpus for visualization of the splints.*

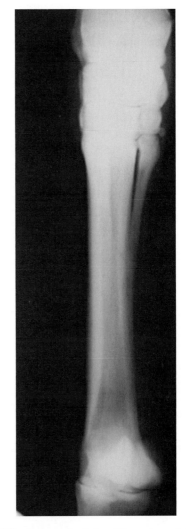

Figure 19-32 *Radiograph of the oblique view of the metacarpus (splints).*

CARPUS JOINT

Dorsopalmar View

The patient should be standing in a normal position with full weight placed on the limb of interest. The cassette is placed against the palmar aspect of the carpus and held perpendicular to the floor (Figs. 19-33 and 19-34). It may be necessary to elevate the opposite limb to eliminate patient motion. The x-ray beam is directed perpendicular to the cassette. The field of view should include the entire carpus joint and a portion of the bones proximal and distal.

BEAM CENTER: Over middle of carpus joint at true dorsopalmar plane. A helpful guideline for determining a true dorsopalmar direction is to draw an imaginary line from the middle of the hoof wall to the radius. Center the beam on that imaginary line

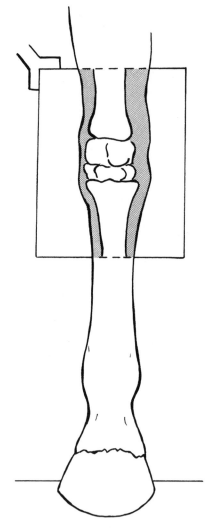

Figure 19-33 *Correct positioning for the dorsopalmar view of the carpus.*

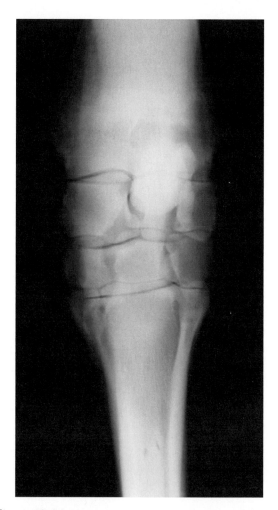

Figure 19-34 *Radiograph of the dorsopalmar view of the carpus.*

CARPUS JOINT—*cont'd*

Lateral View

The patient is placed in a normal position with full weight placed on the limb to be examined. The cassette is placed against the medial aspect of the carpus and held perpendicular to the floor (Figs. 19-35 and 19-36). The x-ray beam is directed perpendicular to the cassette. The field of view should include the carpus joint and a small portion of the bone proximal and distal.

BEAM CENTER: Over lateral aspect of limb in middle of carpus joint

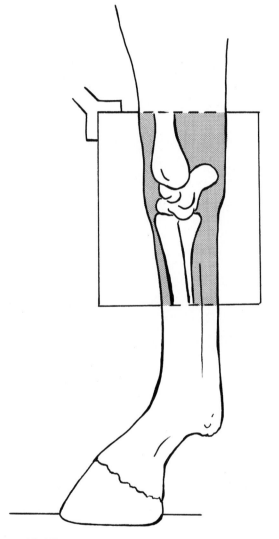

Figure 19-35 *Correct positioning for the lateral view of the carpus.*

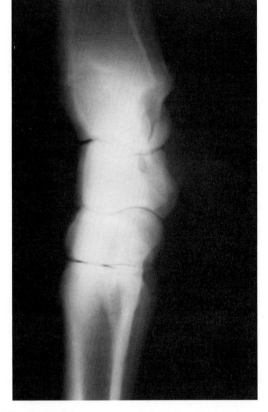

Figure 19-36 *Radiograph of the lateral view of the carpus.*

CARPUS JOINT—*cont'd*

Flexed Lateral View

The limb of interest is elevated, and the carpus is flexed. The attendant holding the limb should be properly attired in lead and out of line of the primary beam. The cassette is placed against the medial aspect of the carpus and held perpendicular to the floor (Figs. 19-37 and 19-38). It is important to prevent abduction of the limb and to keep the carpus directly under the body. The x-ray beam is directed perpendicular to the cassette; the field of view should include the entire carpus joint.

BEAM CENTER: Over lateral aspect of limb in middle of carpus joint

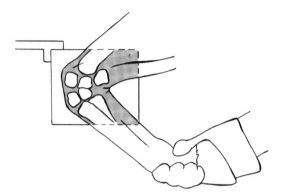

Figure 19-37 *Correct positioning for the flexed lateral view of the carpus.*

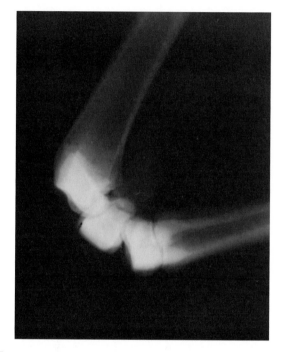

Figure 19-38 *Radiograph of the flexed lateral view of the carpus.*

CARPUS JOINT—*cont'd*

Oblique Views (Lateral and Medial)

The patient is placed in a normal weight-bearing posture. The cassette is positioned against the palmar aspect of the carpus toward the medial or lateral side. The cassette must be held perpendicular to the surface of the floor, with the carpus centered to the cassette (Figs. 19-39 and 19-40). The x-ray beam is directed perpendicular to the cassette. The field of view should include the entire carpus and a portion of the adjacent bones distal and caudal.

BEAM CENTER: Through middle of carpus angled approximately 45 degrees from dorsal midline of joint

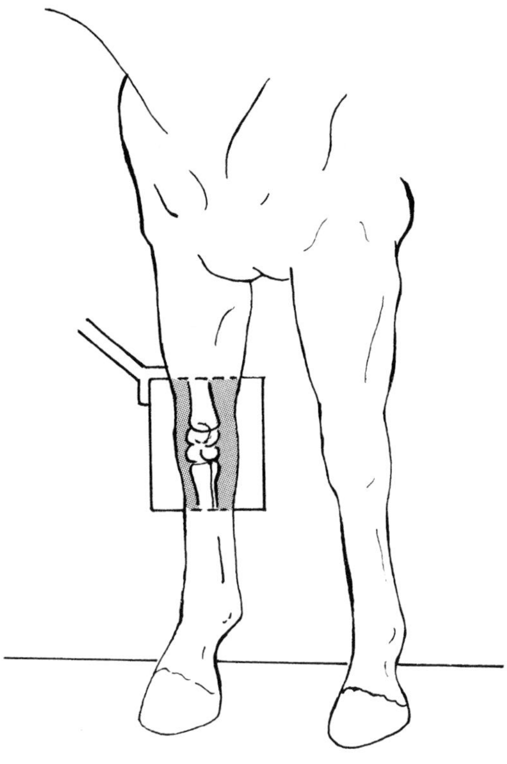

Figure 19-39 *Correct positioning for the lateral or medial oblique view of the carpus.*

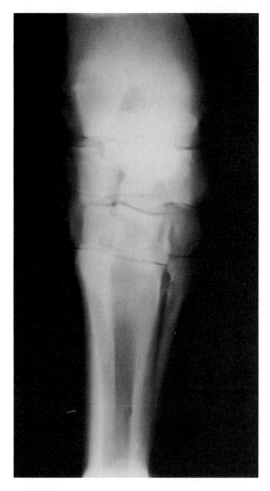

Figure 19-40 *Radiograph of the lateral or medial oblique view of the carpus.*

CARPUS JOINT—*cont'd*

Skyline View

The patient's limb is elevated, and the carpus joint is flexed so that the metacarpus is parallel with the floor. The cassette is placed firmly against the dorsal surface of the proximal metacarpal region (Figs. 19-41 and 19-42) and should be as nearly parallel with the floor as possible. The x-ray beam is directed toward the dorsal surface of the carpus. The angle of the x-ray beam varies according to the row of carpal bones under examination. It is directed at a near-perpendicular angle to the cassette to highlight the proximal row of carpal bones. To highlight the distal row, the beam is angled approximately 30 degrees to the cassette. The field of view should include the dome of the carpus.

BEAM CENTER: Through row of carpal bones of interest

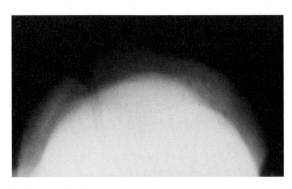

Figure 19-42   *Radiograph of the skyline view of the carpus.*

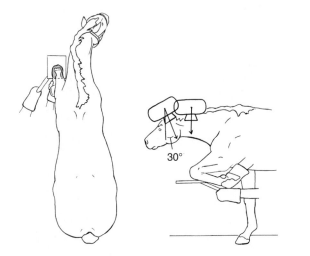

Figure 19-41   *Correct positioning for the skyline view of the carpus.*

TARSUS JOINT

Dorsoplantar View

The patient is placed in a normal standing posture, bearing weight on the limb of interest. The limb should be rotated slightly lateral ("toe out") so that the x-ray tube does not need to be positioned directly under the body. The cassette is placed firmly against the plantar aspect of the tarsus and held perpendicularly to the floor (Figs. 19-43 and 19-44). Great care must be taken when working around the rear legs of large animals. Never stand directly behind the patient; instead, stand off to the side when holding the cassette in place. To prevent patient motion, the front limb of the opposite side can be elevated. The x-ray beam is directed perpendicularly to the cassette, and the field of view should include the entire tarsus and a portion of the adjacent bones distal and proximal.

BEAM CENTER: Through middle of joint at a true dorsoplantar plane. A guideline for determining a true dorsoplantar direction is to draw an imaginary line from the middle of the hoof wall to the tibia. Center the beam on this imaginary line

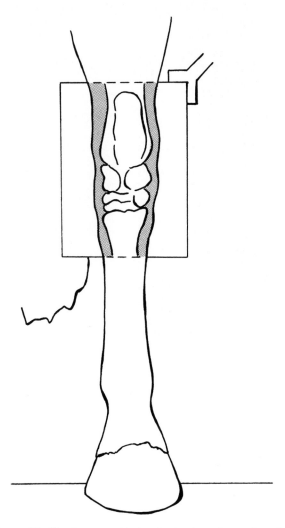

Figure 19-43 *Correct positioning for the dorsoplantar view of the tarsus.*

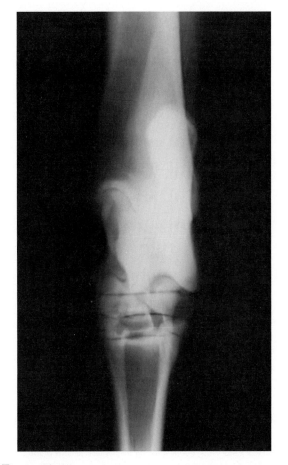

Figure 19-44 *Radiograph of the dorsoplantar view of the tarsus.*

TARSUS JOINT—*cont'd*

Lateral View

The patient should be standing in a normal weight-bearing position. The cassette is placed against the medial aspect of the tarsal joint and held perpendicularly to the floor (Figs. 19-45 and 19-46). The tarsal joint should be centered to the cassette, and the x-ray beam directed perpendicularly to the cassette. The field of view should include the entire tarsal joint and a small portion of the adjacent bones distal and proximal.

For an alternative lateral projection of the tarsus, the joint can be elevated and flexed. The x-ray beam is directed in the manner just described. This view allows better visualization of the tibiotarsal joint.

BEAM CENTER: Over middle of tarsal joint approximately 4 inches distal to calcaneal tuberosity

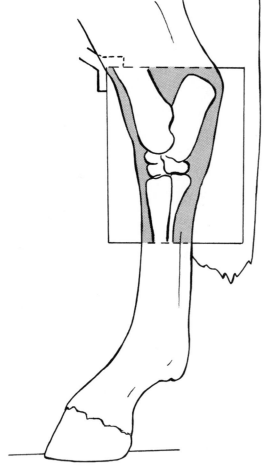

Figure 19-45 *Correct positioning for the lateral view of the tarsus.*

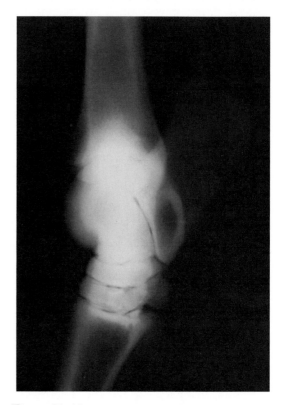

Figure 19-46 *Radiograph of the lateral view of the tarsus.*

TARSUS JOINT—*cont'd*

Oblique Views (Lateral and Medial)

The patient is placed in a normal weight-bearing stance. The cassette is held firmly against the medial or lateral aspect of the plantar surface of the tarsus (Figs. 19-47 and 19-48). The x-ray tube is positioned in front of the limb of interest, and the x-ray beam is angled approximately 45 degrees lateral or medial from the dorsal midline. The field of view should include the entire tarsal joint and a small portion of the bones distal and proximal.

BEAM CENTER: Over middle of tarsal joint approximately 4 inches distal to calcaneal tuberosity

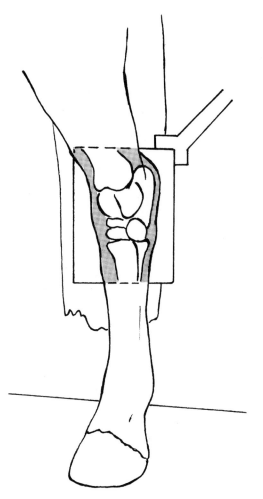

Figure 19-47 *Correct positioning for the lateral or medial oblique view of the tarsus.*

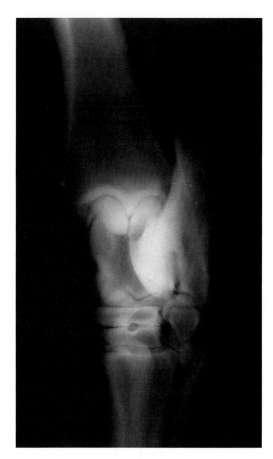

Figure 19-48 *Radiograph of the lateral or medial oblique view of the tarsus.*

ELBOW JOINT

Craniocaudal View

The elbow joint is difficult to radiograph while the animal is in a standing position because of its proximity to the ventral body wall. Although it is not always feasible, use of general anesthesia is preferred. With the patient anesthetized and placed in lateral recumbency, the limb can be abducted and extended away from the body wall for radiography.

With the patient in a standing position, the affected limb should be extended as far cranial as possible. The long edge of the cassette is pressed firmly against the thorax at the caudal aspect of the elbow (Figs. 19-49 and 19-50). With the cassette pressed into the rib cage, the medial portion of the elbow should be in the field of view. The x-ray beam is directed through the cranial aspect of the joint, perpendicular to the cassette.

BEAM CENTER: Over middle of joint over cranial midline

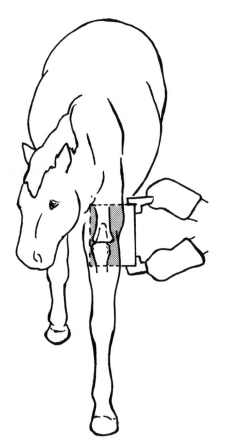

Figure 19-49 *Correct positioning for the craniocaudal view of the elbow.*

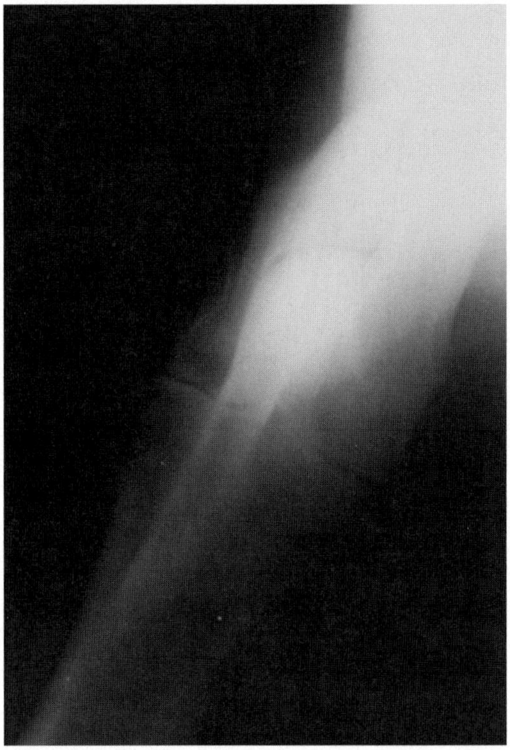

Figure 19-50 *Radiograph of the craniocaudal view of the elbow.*

ELBOW JOINT—*cont'd*

Lateral View

With the patient in a standing position, the limb of interest should be extended as far cranially as possible. To achieve full extension, the limb should be elevated and manually pulled forward. The success of this view depends on the extension of the limb. The cassette is placed firmly against the lateral aspect of the limb, with the elbow joint centered to the cassette (Figs. 19-51 and 19-52). The cassette should remain perpendicular to the floor, and the x-ray beam is directed horizontally toward the medial side of the joint. The field of view should include the entire elbow joint.

BEAM CENTER: Over middle of elbow joint

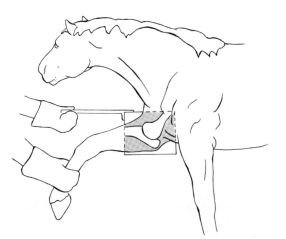

Figure 19-51 *Correct positioning for the lateral view of the elbow.*

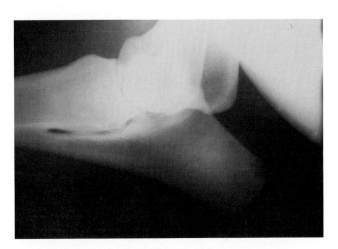

Figure 19-52 *Radiograph of the lateral view of the elbow.*

SHOULDER JOINT

Lateral View

To attain a quality projection of the shoulder joint, using general anesthesia and placing the patient in lateral recumbency are recommended. Because general anesthesia is not always practical, a standing lateral view is possible if the patient will allow the necessary manipulation of the limb.

With the patient standing, the affected limb is elevated and pulled cranially (Figs. 19-53 and 19-54), which pulls the shoulder joint away from the ventral body wall. The cassette is placed firmly against the lateral aspect of the shoulder joint. The x-ray beam is directed horizontally toward the medial side of the joint and perpendicularly to the cassette.

BEAM CENTER: Over shoulder joint

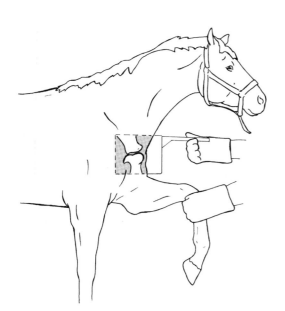

Figure 19-53 *Correct positioning for the lateral view of the shoulder.*

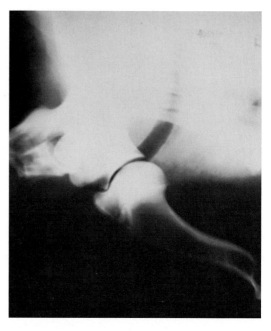

Figure 19-54 *Radiograph of the lateral view of the shoulder.*

STIFLE JOINT

Caudocranial View

Radiography of the stifle joint is difficult because of the thickness of the surrounding tissue. Because of the depth of the muscle in the femoral region, the caudocranial projection demonstrates little above the joint space.

The patient should be in a natural standing posture, and the x-ray tube positioned caudally to the stifle joint. If possible, the limb of interest should be stepped back in a caudally extended, weight-bearing position (Figs. 19-55 and 19-56). Extension of the limb assists placement of the cassette. The cassette is placed cranially to the stifle and tilted so that the long edge is snug against the body wall. The x-ray beam is directed perpendicularly to the cassette.

Great care must be taken because of patient sensitivity in this region of the body. The attendant holding the cassette and the radiographer positioning the x-ray tube should be prepared to move if the patient becomes agitated. It may be helpful to elevate the opposite limb to minimize motion and the risk of being kicked. Sedation is highly recommended.

BEAM CENTER: Over stifle joint, approximately 4 inches distal to patella

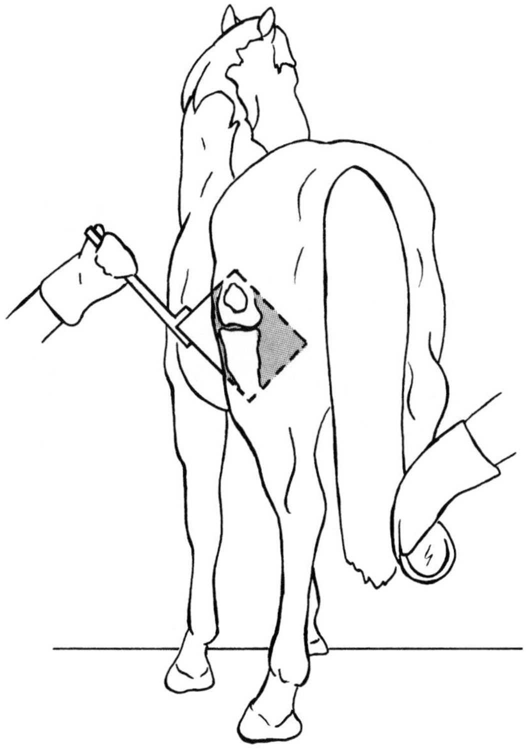

Figure 19-55 *Correct positioning for the caudocranial view of the stifle joint.*

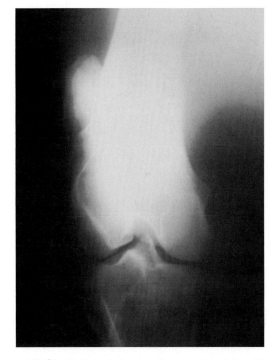

Figure 19-56 *Radiograph of the caudocranial view of the stifle joint.*

STIFLE JOINT—*cont'd*

Lateral View

With the patient in a natural standing posture, the cassette is angled and cautiously placed against the medial side of the stifle joint (Figs. 19-57 and 19-58). Gentle force should be used to push the flat edge of the cassette as far into the flank as possible. Most patients object to this cassette placement, and it may be necessary to elevate the opposite limb to prevent motion. The x-ray tube is positioned laterally to the stifle, and the x-ray beam is directed perpendicularly to the cassette.

BEAM CENTER: Over stifle joint space, approximately 4 inches distal to patella

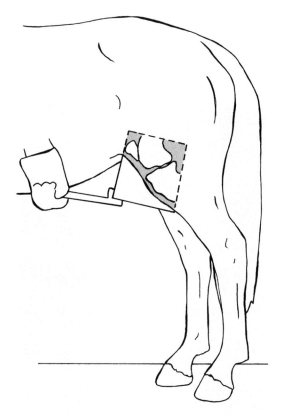

Figure 19-57 *Correct positioning for the lateral view of the stifle joint.*

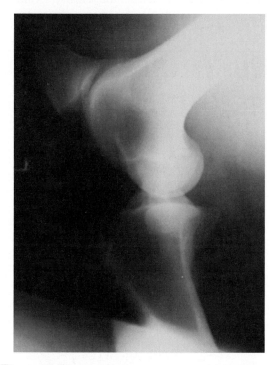

Figure 19-58 *Radiograph of the lateral view of the stifle joint.*

PELVIS

Ventrodorsal View

General anesthesia is required for this radiographic study of a large animal patient. Because of the thickness of this area, the use of a grid is suggested. The mA and kVp necessary for this region require the use of a high-powered x-ray machine such as a mobile or ceiling-mounted unit.

The patient is placed in dorsal recumbency with the hind limbs flexed in a "frog-leg" position (Figs. 19-59 and 19-60). The cassette is positioned under the patient, with the pelvis centered on the cassette. Exposing the pelvis in two or three sections may be necessary. The use of a cassette tunnel eases changing the cassettes. The x-ray tube is positioned over the ventral region of the pelvis and centered on the cassette. A 5:1 crisscross grid is also helpful, provided that the x-ray machine output is adequate.

BEAM CENTER: Over area of interest. If more than one projection is necessary, each centering point should be marked with a felt pen or tape. Marking the centering points allows adjustments to be made from the previously exposed site

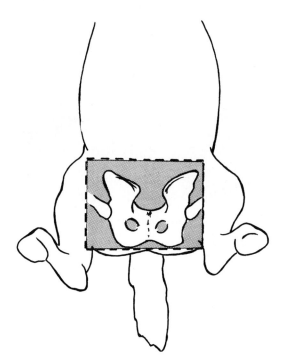

Figure 19-59 *Correct positioning for the ventrodorsal view of the pelvis.*

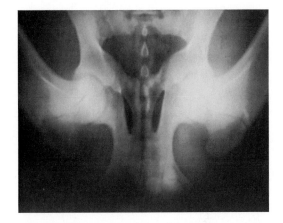

Figure 19-60 *Radiograph of the ventrodorsal view of the pelvis.*

SKULL

Lateral View

Before beginning the examination, the patient's halter should be checked. If it has any metal on it, it should be removed and replaced with a rope halter. A rope halter usually does not have metal clips and buckles, which could impose radiographically on an area of interest.

The patient is positioned in a natural standing posture, and the head is held without rotation. The cassette is placed against the side of the skull with the lesion (Figs. 19-61 and 19-62). The x-ray tube is positioned on the opposite lateral side. The x-ray beam is directed perpendicularly to the cassette.

BEAM CENTER: Over area of interest

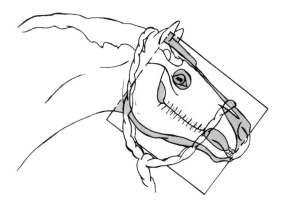

Figure 19-61 *Correct positioning for the lateral view of the skull.*

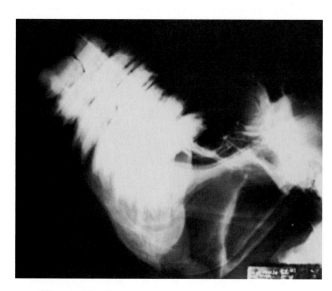

Figure 19-62 *Radiograph of the lateral view of the skull.*

GUTTURAL POUCH/LARYNX/PHARYNX

Lateral View

The positioning of the caudal skull and laryngeal region is essentially the same as for the routine skull views. The fundamental difference is the placement of the cassette and the x-ray beam center point (Figs. 19-63 and 19-64). The cassette is placed on the lateral side of the skull, with the caudal skull centered on the cassette, and the x-ray tube is positioned on the opposite lateral side of the skull.

BEAM CENTER: Caudal to vertical ramus of mandible (over guttural pouch region)

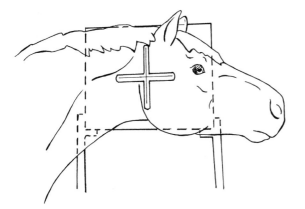

Figure 19-63 *Correct positioning for the lateral view of the guttural pouch, larynx, and pharynx.*

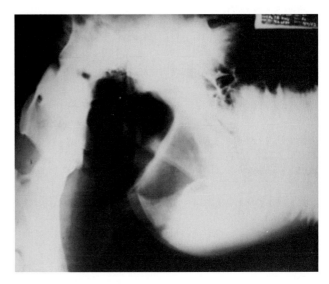

Figure 19-64 *Radiograph of the lateral view of the guttural pouch, larynx, and pharynx.*

GUTTURAL POUCH/LARYNX/PHARYNX—*cont'd*

Dorsoventral View

Sedation is highly recommended for this view of the skull. With the patient in a normal standing posture, the head is lowered as far as possible. The cassette is placed against the ventral side of the skull under the mandible. The x-ray tube is positioned over the head with the x-ray beam directed perpendicularly to the cassette (Figs. 19-65 and 19-66).

BEAM CENTER: At midline of skull over area of interest

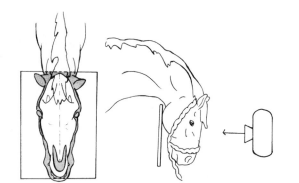

Figure 19-65 *Correct positioning for the dorsoventral view of the skull.*

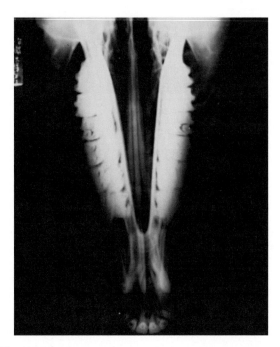

Figure 19-66 *Radiograph of the dorsoventral view of the skull.*

TEETH (MANDIBULAR AND MAXILLARY)

Oblique views

Cheek teeth are difficult to visualize on the routine lateral and ventrodorsal views because of superimposition of the opposite arcade. An oblique view is necessary to isolate the arcade of interest.

The patient is positioned as for the lateral view, with the cassette placed against the lateral side of interest (Figs. 19-67 through 19-69). The cassette remains perpendicular to the floor, and the x-ray beam is angled. For visualization of the maxillary teeth, the x-ray tube is angled down approximately 30 degrees from the parallel plane of the floor and centered over the teeth of interest. For the mandibular teeth, the x-ray tube is angled up approximately 45 degrees from the parallel plane and centered over the area of the lesion.

Views of the incisors can be made by placing the cassette inside the mouth. The x-ray tube is positioned either above or below the head for the corresponding view, and the x-ray beam is centered over the area of interest. Sedation is required for intraoral radiography.

BEAM CENTER: Over area of interest

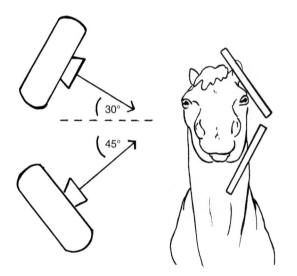

Figure 19-67 *Correct positioning for the lateral oblique view of the cheek teeth.*

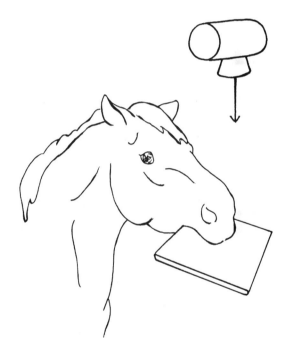

Figure 19-69 *Correct positioning for the intraoral projection of the incisor teeth.*

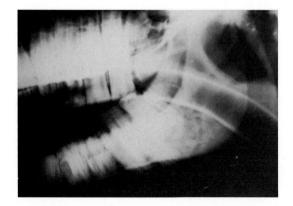

Figure 19-68 *Radiograph of the lateral oblique view of the cheek teeth.*

CERVICAL SPINE

Lateral View

In most circumstances cervical spine radiography can be performed with the patient standing, provided the x-ray machine output is adequate. Because of the size of the patient, the cervical spine must be exposed in three views: (1) base of the skull, C-1, C-2, and C-3; (2) C-3, C-4, and C-5; and (3) C-5, C-6, and C-7 (Figs. 19-70 and 19-71).

The cassette is placed against the side of the cervical region. The x-ray tube is positioned on the opposite side of the patient with the x-ray beam directed perpendicularly to the cassette. Remember that the cervical spine runs along the ventral portion of the neck. Many times the spine is "missed" by centering the x-ray beam too far dorsally.

BEAM CENTER: Area 1: Over C-2
Area 2: Over C-4
Area 3: Over C-5

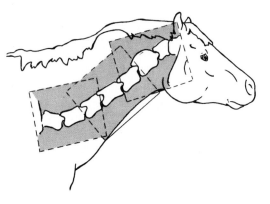

Figure 19-70 *Correct positioning for the lateral view of the cervical spine.*

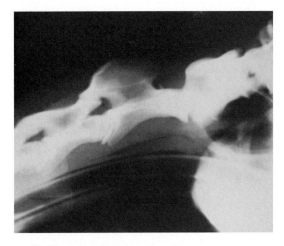

Figure 19-71 *Radiograph of the lateral view of the cranial cervical spine.*

ADDITIONAL AREAS: A BRIEF OVERVIEW

Areas of the body such as the thorax, abdomen, and thoracic spine can be radiographed only with special high-powered equipment. The ability to radiograph such areas is usually limited to highly specialized veterinary hospitals.

Thorax

Because of patient size, four views of the thorax are usually required: (1) craniodorsal lateral, (2) caudodorsal lateral, (3) cranioventral lateral, and (4) caudoventral lateral. The thorax can be radiographed with the patient standing. The cassette is placed in a standing mechanical cassette holder that has a built-in grid, which is necessary because of the high kVp used. Centering the x-ray beam on the grid before walking the patient into position is important. The SID is usually increased to 80 inches. The patient is walked between the x-ray tube and the cassette. The lateral side of the patient should be as close to the cassette as possible. However, it is possible to radiograph the caudodorsal region with low-output equipment, short SID, and fast intensifying screens (Figs. 19-72 and 19-73).

Abdomen

The same equipment and preparation are required for the abdomen as for the thorax. An abdomen can be radiographed with the patient in a standing position as well. A series of radiographs are recommended, starting cranioventral and extending caudodorsal (Fig. 19-74).

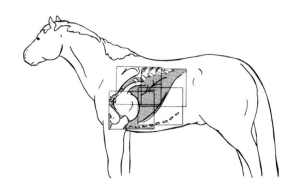

Figure 19-73 *The four views of the lateral thorax.*

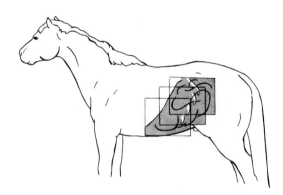

Figure 19-74 *The three views of the lateral abdomen.*

Thoracic Spine

A lower-powered unit can be used to visualize the dorsal spinous processes (withers) of the thoracic spine. If the ventral portion of the thoracic vertebrae must be examined, higher exposure factors are necessary to penetrate the thick tissues of this area. With a high-powered x-ray apparatus and a grid, it is possible to radiograph the thoracic spine. Patient positioning is similar to that for radiographs of the thorax except that the x-ray beam is centered over the thoracic spine.

KEY POINTS

1. General anesthesia is required to radiograph the equine pelvis.
2. The equine cervical spine is positioned along the ventral neck. A common mistake is to radiograph too far dorsally.
3. When attempting to radiograph an equine limb, it may be helpful to elevate the opposite limb to prevent movement.

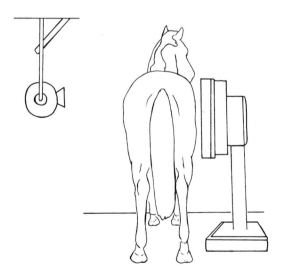

Figure 19-72 *Drawing showing the placement of the cassette and x-ray tube for the lateral view of the thorax. A standing cassette holder with grid is used, with the patient standing in front of the cassette.*

REVIEW QUESTIONS

1. What device can be used to protect the assistant during a lateral view of the distal phalanx?
   a. Cassette tunnel
   b. Wood block with slot to hold cassette
   c. Cassette holder with a clamp and long handle
   d. Both b and c are correct.

2. What is the advantage of raising the limb opposite to the limb being radiographed?
   a. Restricts patient's movement
   b. Causes fractures to be more readily apparent on film
   c. Allows kVp to be reduced
   d. Increases pressure on limb of interest and improves visualization of cartilage pathology

3. What angle is required for a dorsopalmar/dorsoplantar oblique view of the third phalanx?
   a. 40-degree angle to the hoof wall directed at the ground
   b. 45-degree angle to the hoof wall directed at the ground
   c. 65-degree angle to the ground directed at the hoof wall
   d. 45-degree angle to the ground directed at the hoof wall

4. What x-ray tube angle is required for a dorsopalmar/dorsoplantar oblique view of the navicular bone with the animal standing on the cassette?
   a. 45 degrees to the ground directed at the hoof wall
   b. Parallel to the ground
   c. 45- to 65-degree angle to the ground directed at the hoof wall
   d. 65-degree angle directed toward the middle of the second phalanx

5. What is the difference between the dorsopalmar/dorsoplantar view and the lateral view of the proximal phalanges?
   a. The limb of interest must be completely weight bearing for the lateral but not for the dorsopalmar/dorsoplantar view.
   b. The x-ray beam is directed horizontally toward the proximal phalanx for the dorsopalmar/dorsoplantar view and at approximately a 30- to 45-degree angle for the lateral view.
   c. The x-ray beam is directed at approximately a 30- to 45-degree angle for the lateral view and horizontally toward the proximal phalanx for the dorsopalmar/dorsoplantar view.
   d. The limb of interest must be on a wooden block for the lateral but not for the dorsopalmar/dorsoplantar view.

6. Which statement is true?
   a. For a flexed lateral view of the fetlock, the cassette is placed against the medial aspect of the limb, perpendicularly to the floor.
   b. For a lateral view of the fetlock, the cassette is placed against the lateral side of the limb, perpendicularly to the floor.
   c. For a dorsopalmar/dorsoplantar view of the fetlock the cassette is placed medial to the limb, perpendicularly to the floor.
   d. For a flexed lateral view of the fetlock, the cassette is placed against the medial aspect of the limb, parallel with the floor.

7. What view is taken to study the medial sesamoid bone of the right front fetlock? (see Fig. 12-2 for assistance)
   a. Dorsomedial-palmarolateral oblique view
   b. Dorsolateral-palmaromedial oblique view
   c. Lateral view
   d. Dorsopalmar view

8. What are the splint bones also known as?
   a. First and fifth metacarpals/metatarsals
   b. Second and fourth metacarpals/metatarsals
   c. Second and third metacarpals/metatarsals
   d. Third and fourth metacarpals/metatarsals

9. In order to determine the true dorsopalmar direction for a dorsopalmar view of the carpus, the radiographer can view the following imaginary line:
   a. Middle of hoof to ulna
   b. Middle of hoof to tarsus
   c. Radius to middle of carpus
   d. Middle of hoof to radius

10. Where is the beam centered for a skyline view of the carpus?
    a. Through the row of carpal bones of interest
    b. Distal radius
    c. Distal ulna
    d. Patella

11. Where is the cassette placed for a craniocaudal view of the elbow?
    a. Palmar aspect of the elbow joint
    b. Plantar aspect of the elbow joint
    c. Cranial aspect of the joint
    d. Caudal aspect of the joint

12. Where should the beam be centered for views of the stifle joint?
    a. 4 inches proximal to the patella
    b. 4 inches distal to the patella
    c. At the level of the patella
    d. 4 inches distal to the tarsus

13. Why are oblique views necessary for dental arcades?
    a. To avoid the increased amount of soft tissue on the head
    b. To avoid superimposition of the guttural pouch
    c. To avoid superimposition of the frontal sinuses
    d. To avoid superimposition of the opposite arcade

14. Which statements are true regarding views of the incisors?
    a. Oblique views are required.
    b. The cassette must be in the mouth.
    c. The patient must be sedated.
    d. Both b and c are correct.

15. In order to prevent an air artifact superimposed over the area of interest when radiographing the equine foot, which of the following materials can be used to pack the foot?
    a. Play-Doh
    b. Sand
    c. Styrofoam
    d. Plaster

Suggested Readings

Dik KJ, Gunsser I: *Atlas of diagnostic radiology of the horse: Parts I-III*, Philadelphia, 1988, WB Saunders.

Douglas SW, Herrtage ME, Williamson HD: *Principles of veterinary radiography*, ed 4, Philadelphia, 1987, Bailliere Tindall.

Koblik PD, Toal R: Portable veterinary x-ray support systems for field use, *J Am Vet Med Assoc* 199:186-188, 1991.

Morgan JP, Silverman S: *Techniques in veterinary radiography*, ed 4, Ames, Iowa, 1987, Iowa State University Press.

Phillips DF: Radiology in your practice: choosing the right equipment, *Vet Med* 587-598, 1987.

Smallwood JE, Shively MJ: Nomenclature for radiographic views of limbs, *Equine Pract* 1:41-45, 1979.

chapter 20

Avian and Exotic Radiography

CHAPTER OUTLINE

Special Considerations
Avian Radiography
Rodent Radiography

Reptile Radiography
Fish Radiography

INTRODUCTION

Birds and exotic pets including rodents, reptiles, and fish have become popular in recent years. Consequently, veterinary practitioners have experienced increased demand for diagnostic and therapeutic care of these animals. Radiography is a valuable diagnostic technique because it is noninvasive and available for rapid interpretation. All principles pertaining to companion animal radiography can be applied to avian and exotic radiography. A few minor differences in equipment and technique are noted in this chapter.

SPECIAL CONSIDERATIONS

Equipment

The equipment necessary for avian and exotic radiography is essentially the same as for domestic animals. New high-detail film-screen systems enable most practitioners to radiograph exotic pets. Nonscreen film was advocated in the past for radiographic studies of smaller exotic animals. Although nonscreen film produces high-detail radiographs, it is impractical at times because of the need for a long exposure time.

A high-milliamperage (mA) x-ray machine such as a 200- or 300-mA unit, is recommended to allow the use of a short exposure time. Exposure times of $^1/_{40}$ second or less are preferred to decrease the chance of a motion artifact on the radiograph. If the output of the machine is less than 200 mA, it may be necessary to decrease the source–image distance (SID) to compensate for the decreased output of the x-ray machine.

Maximum kilovoltage (kVp) is less important for avian and exotic radiography than for domestic animal radiography. Rather, the x-ray machine must have a low kVp setting and the ability to make small, incremental changes in kVp. A grid is not usually necessary. Scatter radiation must be minimized by the use of a beam-limiting device to collimate the x-ray beam to the smallest area possible. Because of the comparatively small patient size, negligible amounts of scatter radiation can greatly reduce the quality of a radiographic image.

Exposure Factors

Avian and exotic patients usually are not measured with a caliper to calculate the exposure. Normally, exposure factors are chosen according to the species and general size of the patient. Keep in mind that the exposure factors required for birds are less than those necessary for reptiles of the same thickness. Soaring (flying) birds have thin cortices and tubular bones. Compared with mammals, avian long bones have significantly less calcium and ossification, which makes them more radiolucent. Slight exposure variations can produce marked alterations in radiographic images of birds.

The exposure factors listed in Table 20-1 can be used for an ultradetail rare-earth screen/medium (par)-speed film system. If a Plexiglas sheet is used for avian radiography, add 2 to 4 kVp to the exposure factors listed.

Patient Restraint

Three types of restraint are used for avian and exotic patients during radiography: (1) manual, (2) physical, and (3) chemical. Regardless of the species and restraint device used, the methods of restraint are similar. The head and torso are restrained first, then the wings (in the case of a bird), and the legs last. With larger rodent mammals, it is possible to use the same restraint methods as for a dog or cat.

Manual restraint involves an attendant (wearing lead attire) who holds the animal in position while the exposure is taken. This method results in increased exposure to personnel and may be illegal in some states. Manual restraint should be avoided if at all possible.

Physical restraint involves such devices as a Plexiglas sheet, ropes, sandbags, and radiolucent adhesive tape. Birds can be restrained directly on a cassette; however, it is recommended that they be positioned on an intermediate surface, especially if several views of the same projection are scheduled. A thin radiolucent sheet of Plexiglas slightly larger than the cassette often serves as an intermediate surface. The avian patient can be placed in position and secured with tape on the radiolucent sheet, which can then be placed directly on the cassette (Fig. 20-1). The type of tape used for physical restraint is important. Scotch tape and cloth medical tape should be avoided because they can damage or remove feathers, fur, or scales.

Plexiglas tubes have been used for the restraint of rodents and other laboratory animals. However, this method is not ideal for radiography because it is difficult to position a patient accurately in a tube. For example,

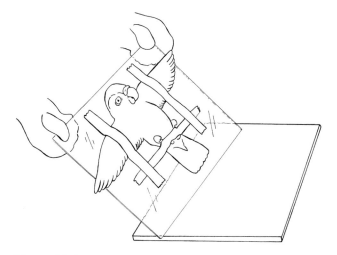

Figure 20-1 *Example of restraint used for avian radiography. The bird is placed on a radiolucent sheet (clear plastic) and secured in position with adhesive tape. The radiolucent sheet is then placed onto the cassette.*

TABLE 20-1

AVIAN AND EXOTIC EXPOSURE FACTORS

PATIENT	kVp	mA	EXPOSURE TIME (SEC)	SID (INCHES)	mAs
PSITTACINE					
Finch	42	300	$1/60$	40	5
Canary	44	300	$1/60$	40	5
Budgerigar	46-50	300	$1/60$	40	5
Cockatiel	50-55	300	$1/40$	40	7.5
Parrot	55-65	300	$1/40$	40	7.5
RAPTOR					
Small	50-65	300	$1/40$	40	7.5
Kestrel					
Saw-whet owl					
Screech owl					
Medium	55-60	300	$1/30$	40	10
Barred owl					
Red-tailed hawk					
Great horned owl					
Large	60-65	300	$1/20$	40	15
Eagle					
Extra Large	66	300	$1/15$	40	20
Trumpeter swan					
RODENTS					
Small	42-46	300	$1/40$	40	7.5
Mouse					
Gerbil					
Hamster					
Medium	46-52	300	$1/40$	40	7.5
Rat					
Dwarf rabbit					
Ferret					
Large	54-60	300	$1/40$	40	7.5
Rabbit					
Guinea pig					
REPTILES					
Snake (small)	40-44	300	$1/40$	40	7.5
Snake (large)	45-55	300	$1/40$	40	7.5
Lizard	40-45	300	$1/40$	40	7.5
Turtle (small)					
Lateral/DV	50-55	300	$1/40$	40	7.5
Craniocaudal	55-60	300	$1/40$	40	7.5
Turtle (large)					
Lateral/DV	65-70	300	$1/30$	40	10
Craniocaudal	70-75	300	$1/30$	40	10

it is not practical to expect a diagnostic radiograph of a rodent thorax if the front limbs are superimposed over the thoracic cavity.

Both manual and physical restraint methods have limitations. Physical restraint may result in excessive patient stress and possible injury from struggling. Injectable sedatives and inhalant anesthetics have greatly increased the feasibility and safety of radiographic procedures involving birds and exotic animals; in fact, they have become the safest methods in use. Chemical restraint is most often used in combination with other positioning techniques to obtain a properly positioned radiograph.

Patients must be evaluated individually to determine the appropriate restraint necessary. Manual or physical restraint should be used only with animals that are not prone to struggle and self-trauma. Supportive therapy such as a heat lamp may be helpful when using anesthesia to keep the patient warm during and after the radiographic examination. Another technique to keep the avian patient warm during recovery is to gently roll the bird into a towel. This technique not only keeps the patient warm but prevents thrashing and possible injury during anesthesia recovery. Careful judgment must be used with a critically ill patient. In some cases it may be necessary to postpone radiography until the patient is stable.

AVIAN RADIOGRAPHY

Whole-Body Ventrodorsal View

The avian patient is positioned on its back so that the sternum is superimposed over the spine. The wings are extended laterally and secured. If manual restraint is used, one hand grasps the head from the back, holding the mandibular articulation between the thumb and the forefinger. The other hand takes the feet and carefully extends them caudally. The wings should be abducted slightly from the body and held down by adhesive tape (Fig. 20-2).

Physical restraint for avian radiography is preferred. The patient is placed in dorsal recumbency as described, except that the head is secured with adhesive tape. The neck is gently extended in a cranial direction and secured to the cassette with adhesive tape (Figs. 20-3 and 20-4). Care must be taken that the airway is not compromised by the tape across the neck region. The wings are abducted laterally and taped to the cassette in full extension. The legs are extended caudally, positioned symmetrically, and fastened to the cassette with masking tape. The tip of the tail can be secured to the cassette to provide additional restraint, if necessary.

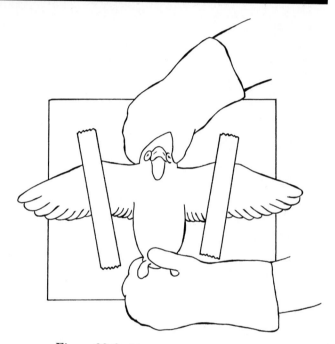

Figure 20-2 *Manual restraint of an avian patient.*

BEAM CENTER: Over midline at caudal tip of sternum

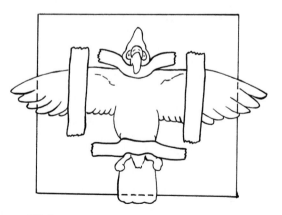

Figure 20-3 *Correct physical restraint and positioning for the ventrodorsal view of the entire body of a bird.*

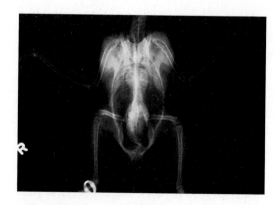

Figure 20-4 *Radiograph of the whole-body ventrodorsal view of a bird.*

AVIAN RADIOGRAPHY—*cont'd*

Whole-Body Lateral View

The patient is placed in lateral recumbency, and the neck is secured to the cassette with masking tape. (NOTE: Right lateral views are taken to maintain consistency with comparable anatomic reference material.) The wings are extended dorsally directly above the body of the patient. The wing that is down on the cassette is positioned cranial to the other wing, and both are secured with adhesive tape (Figs. 20-5 and 20-6). The legs are extended ventrally away from the body wall and fastened with tape. The dependent leg is positioned cranial to the other leg. The limb closest to the cassette is always cranial to the contralateral limb so that each limb is identifiable on a lateral radiograph. The tail and body of the patient can be secured with tape if additional restraint is necessary.

BEAM CENTER: Over middle of body between spine and sternum at level of caudal tip of sternum

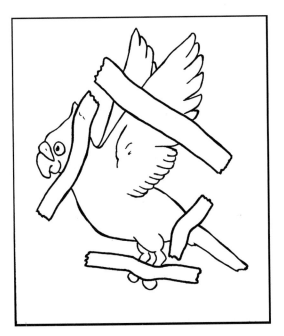

Figure 20-5 *Correct positioning for the whole-body lateral view of a bird.*

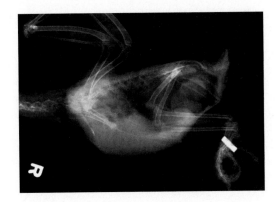

Figure 20-6 *Radiograph of the whole-body lateral view of a bird.*

AVIAN RADIOGRAPHY—*cont'd*

Wing-Caudocranial View

Manual positioning is necessary for the caudocranial view of the wing because of the awkward position required of the patient. Lead gloves are worn, and the bird is held upside down so that the body is perpendicular to the cassette. The tip of the wing feathers is held gently, and the wing of interest is extended away from the body. The cranial edge of the wing is placed on the cassette. In order for the edge of the wing to be in contact with the cassette, it is helpful to allow the head of the patient to hang over the edge of the cassette (Fig. 20-7). Exposure factors required for this view are approximately the same as those required for the entire body.

BEAM CENTER: Over area of interest

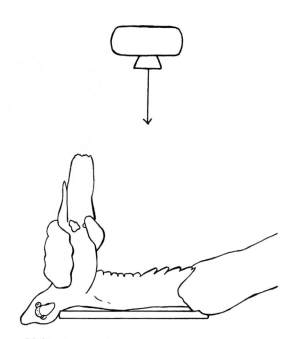

Figure 20-7 *Correct positioning for the caudocranial view of a bird's wing.*

Gastrointestinal Contrast Study

A contrast study of the gastrointestinal tract can be valuable to the avian practitioner. Because visualization of many abnormalities on routine survey radiographs is difficult, the use of contrast media can be helpful in defining the location and size of a lesion. For example, because birds love to chew, they often suffer from gastrointestinal foreign bodies. In addition, stasis of the gastrointestinal tract is a common consequence when a bird is ill. Without the use of contrast media, diagnosis of such problems may be difficult or impossible.

TECHNIQUE OUTLINE

Contrast Media

20% to 30% barium sulfate (Gastrografin is indicated if a perforation is suspected but is not routinely used due to its local mucosal irritant effect and rapid absorption through the intestinal walls)

Patient Preparation

Fast approximately 4 hours (because of the high metabolic rate of a bird, fasting longer than 4 hours could compromise the health of the patient)

Procedure-Avian Gastrointestinal Contrast Study

I. Draw contrast medium into a syringe, warmed to approximately 80°F.

II. Administer contrast agent to bird with a small feeding tube or urinary catheter.

   A. Force the patient's mouth open, and insert the feeding tube into the crop.

   B. For birds without a crop, pass the feeding tube into the midesophageal region.

   C. Verify the position of the tube by palpation before injecting contrast medium because it is possible for it to be inadvertently placed into the trachea.

   D. To fill the gastrointestinal tract, administer 25 mL/kg of barium sulfate. For a small bird such as a parakeet, 0.5 to 1.5 mL is adequate. Larger birds such as parrots may require up to 10 mL of contrast medium.

III. Expose lateral and ventrodorsal radiographs immediately after the administration of contrast medium (Figs. 20-8 and 20-9). By 10 minutes after administration, the contrast agent should have moved past the crop and into the stomach. Radiographs normally are obtained in 30-minute intervals until the contrast medium has reached the cloaca. The amount of time it takes the barium to travel from the crop to the cloaca (transit time) varies according to the size, species, and pathology of the patient. The average time ranges from 30 to 240 minutes. Small psittacines have the fastest transit time.

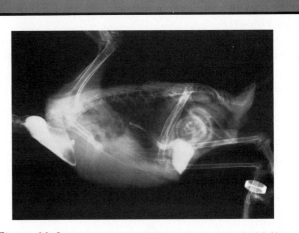

Figure 20-8 *Lateral view of a barium series on a cockatiel. Note the small amount of barium aspiration in the trachea. All precautions should be taken to prevent this occurrence.*

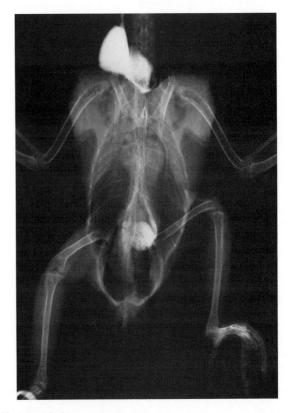

Figure 20-9 *Ventrodorsal view of a barium series on a cockatiel. Note the small amount of barium aspirated in the trachea. All precautions should be taken to prevent this occurrence.*

RODENT RADIOGRAPHY

Rat

Whole-body dorsoventral view.

Positioning for a dorsoventral projection can be performed in two ways: (1) by placing the small patient in a radiolucent tube or (2) by securing the patient to the cassette with adhesive tape. For whole-body radiographs of larger rodents (guinea pigs and rabbits), the animal can be placed in the same positions as a small domestic animal (dog).

The radiolucent tube with the patient inside is placed on top of the cassette so that the animal is in sternal recumbency. The x-ray beam is directed vertically through the back of the rodent, and the field of view should include the entire body. A tube has disadvantages, however. A quality radiograph is compromised by superimposition of the legs under the body of the patient and by rotation. Superimposition and rotation decrease visualization of the thoracic and abdominal cavities.

Adhesive tape is the preferred method of restraint for a rodent because the extremities can be extended and rotation of the body can be eliminated. The patient is placed on top of the cassette in sternal recumbency. The head and legs are extended away from the body and secured with adhesive tape (Figs. 20-10 and 20-11). The patient must be in a true dorsoventral position, with the sternum superimposed over the spine. The x-ray beam is directed vertically through the back of the rodent, and the field of view should include the entire body.

BEAM CENTER: Over thoracolumbar spinal junction

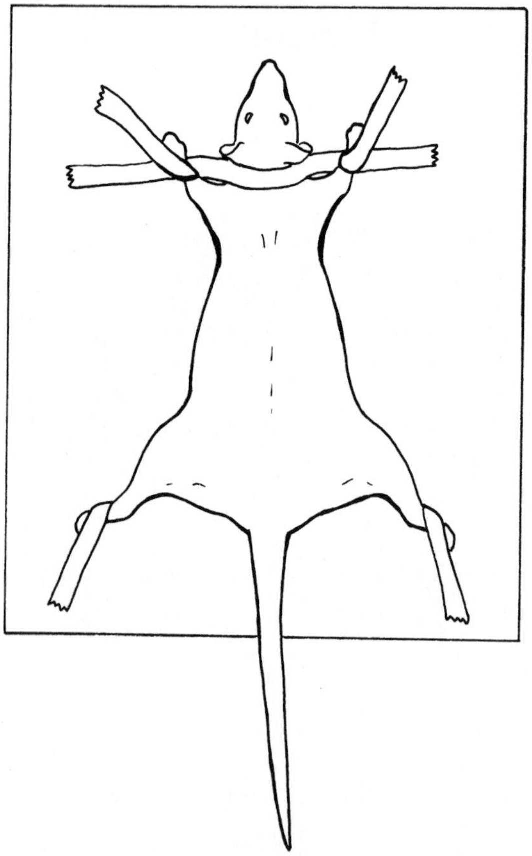

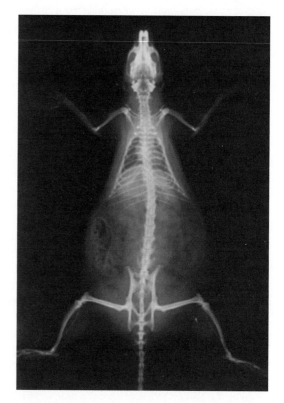

Figure 20-11 *Radiograph of the whole-body dorsoventral view of a rat.*

Figure 20-10 *Correct positioning for the whole-body dorsoventral view of a rodent.*

RODENT RADIOGRAPHY—*cont'd*

Whole-Body Lateral View

The advantage of using a radiolucent tube for small rodent radiography is that both the lateral and the ventrodorsal views can be obtained without manipulating the patient. With the patient positioned in the tube, the x-ray beam is directed horizontally toward the left side of the tube. The cassette is placed against the right side of the animal in the tube. Elevate the radiolucent tube so that the entire body of the rodent can be visualized on the radiograph. Unfortunately, the tube technique may compromise a quality radiograph because of the superimposition of the legs over the thoracic and abdominal cavities (Fig. 20-12).

The best method of restraint is adhesive tape. The patient is placed in right lateral recumbency on top of the cassette. The front limbs and rear limbs are extended cranially and caudally, respectively, and secured (Figs. 20-13 and 20-14). It may be necessary to place a length of adhesive tape over the neck if the patient is struggling. If manual restraint is used, string or small forceps can be used to extend the limbs to decrease exposure to the attendants. The x-ray beam is directed vertically toward the rodent, and the field of view should include the entire body.

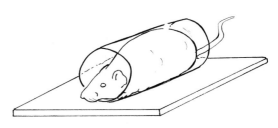

Figure 20-12 *Correct use of a radiolucent tube for rodent radiography.*

BEAM CENTER: Over thoracolumbar spinal junction

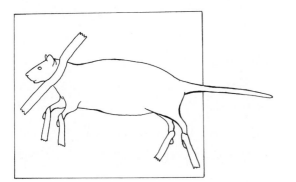

Figure 20-13 *Correct positioning for the whole-body lateral view of a rodent.*

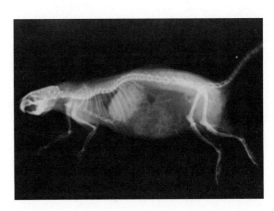

Figure 20-14 *Radiograph of the whole-body lateral view of a rat.*

REPTILE RADIOGRAPHY

Turtle

Whole-body dorsoventral view.

Radiographic examination of turtles can be difficult because of the presence of a shell. A number of views may be necessary to view the internal anatomy of the turtle adequately. The three routine views include (1) dorsoventral, (2) lateral, and (3) craniocaudal.

Under most circumstances, turtles are slow and docile. Normally, radiographic studies can be performed without sedation. Movement can be restricted by use of restraint devices such as adhesive tape or a radiolucent plastic box in which the turtle is placed. In the case of a snapping turtle, sedation may be warranted if the patient becomes uncooperative.

To prepare a turtle for dorsoventral radiography, the patient is turned on its back. Just before the exposure is to be made, the patient is turned back on its ventral side. The turtle requires a few moments to become reoriented and will naturally extend its legs and head from the shell (Figs. 20-15 and 20-16). At this moment, the exposure should be made. The field of view should include the entire body.

BEAM CENTER: Over center of shell

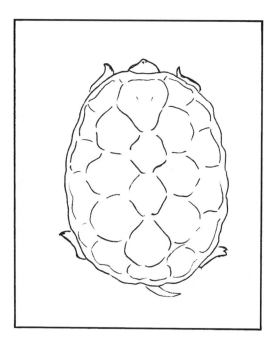

Figure 20-15 *Correct positioning for the whole-body dorsoventral view of a turtle.*

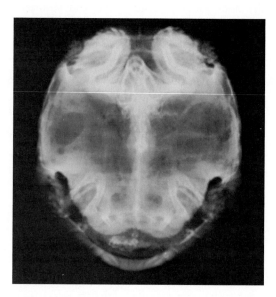

Figure 20-16 *Radiograph of the whole-body dorsoventral view of a turtle.*

REPTILE RADIOGRAPHY—*cont'd*

Whole-body lateral view.
The turtle is attached to a wood or plastic rack with adhesive tape. The ventral aspect of the body is in contact with the rack, and tape is wrapped around the circumference of the shell and rack (Fig. 20-17). The rack is elevated into a vertical position so that the turtle is on its right side on top of the cassette. The x-ray beam is directed parallel to the rack through the patient from left to right.

With x-ray machines that have the capability of horizontal x-ray beam radiography, a lateral view can be taken with the patient in ventral recumbency (Figs. 20-18 and 20-19). The turtle is placed on top of a sponge or wood block and secured with adhesive tape. The cassette is positioned vertically against the right side of the patient. The x-ray beam is directed parallel to the sponge or block through the patient from left to right.

BEAM CENTER: Over center of body

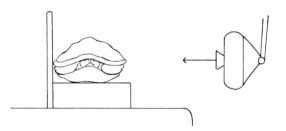

Figure 20-18 *Correct positioning for the whole-body lateral view of a turtle with the use of a horizontal x-ray beam.*

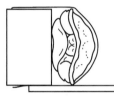

Figure 20-17 *Correct positioning for a whole-body lateral view of a turtle with the use of a rack.*

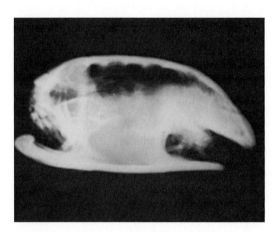

Figure 20-19 *Radiography of the whole-body lateral view of a turtle.*

REPTILE RADIOGRAPHY—*cont'd*

Whole-body craniocaudal view.
The turtle is placed in ventral recumbency and fixed to a wood or plastic rack with adhesive tape. With the cassette on the table in horizontal position, the rack is elevated into a vertical posture. The caudal aspect of the turtle is placed against the cassette, and the head is pointed toward the x-ray tube. The x-ray beam is directed toward the head and should pass through the body from the head to the tail (Fig. 20-20).

The craniocaudal view can also be performed with horizontal beam radiography. The patient is positioned in ventral recumbency on a sponge or wood block and secured with adhesive tape. The cassette is placed in vertical position against the caudal aspect of the patient, and the x-ray beam is directed horizontally to the sponge through the body from the head to the tail (Figs. 20-21 and 20-22).

BEAM CENTER: Through middle of head

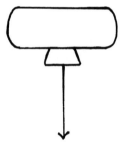

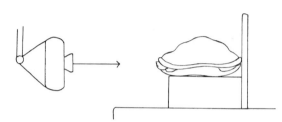

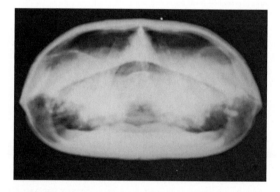

Figure 20-21 *Correct positioning for the whole-body craniocaudal view of a turtle using a horizontal x-ray beam.*

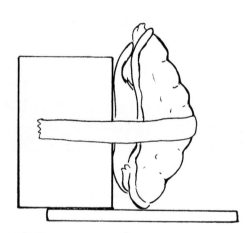

Figure 20-20 *Correct positioning for the whole-body craniocaudal view of a turtle using a rack.*

Figure 20-22 *Radiograph of the whole-body craniocaudal view of a turtle.*

REPTILE RADIOGRAPHY—*cont'd*

Lizard

Whole-body dorsoventral view.

The size and disposition of a lizard determine the type of restraint necessary. Calm and docile reptiles can be secured with adhesive tape, whereas restless or fractious reptiles require further restraint measures (Fig. 20-23). Aggressive lizards and crocodiles should be radiographed with the snout tied to prevent injury to personnel. Smaller lizards usually require chemical or physical restraint, or both. Larger lizards usually can be restrained manually. Sometimes it is sufficient to cover the animal with both hands and withdraw them just before the exposure is taken. For most species of lizards, it is necessary to restrain the tail as well.

The patient is placed in sternal recumbency on the cassette. The body is gently stretched, and the limbs are extended laterally and secured to the cassette. If necessary, the tail is secured with a length of adhesive tape. The patient must be in a true dorsoventral position, with the sternum superimposed over the spine. The x-ray beam is directed vertically through the back of the patient, and the field of view should include the entire body.

BEAM CENTER: Over middle of body, to include thorax, abdomen, and entire skeletal system

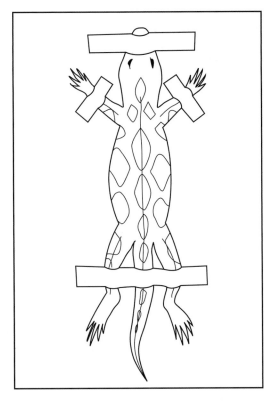

Figure 20-23 *Correct positioning for the whole-body dorsoventral view of a lizard.*

REPTILE RADIOGRAPHY—*cont'd*

Whole-body lateral view.
Restraint considerations are the same as for the whole-body dorsoventral view of the lizard.

The patient is placed in right lateral recumbency against the cassette. The head and front limbs are extended cranially and secured either manually or with tape. The rear limbs are extended in a caudal direction and secured (Fig. 20-24). If manual restraint is used, a firm grip may be necessary at first but can be relaxed after a few seconds. The x-ray beam is directed vertically through the left side of the patient, and the field of view should include the entire body.

BEAM CENTER: Over middle of body, to include thorax, abdomen, and vertebral column

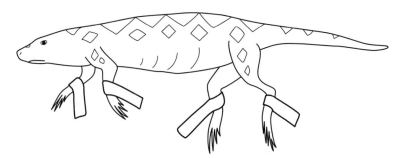

Figure 20-24   *Correct positioning for the whole-body lateral view of a lizard.*

REPTILE RADIOGRAPHY—*cont'd*

Snake

Whole-body dorsoventral view.

Radiography of snakes can be difficult because of their unique anatomy. In most cases the entire body can be radiographed with the dorsoventral view. Small, non-poisonous snakes can be placed directly on the cassette. If the patient is active, it can be placed in a double-open-ended cardboard or radiolucent plastic box. The box is then placed on top of the cassette, and the exposure is taken. A restless snake can also be secured in a long radiolucent tube. If directed, the snake will usually crawl into the tube on its own. The ends of the tube can be plugged with porous cork or other suitable material. In the case of a restless or even fractious (poisonous) snake, sedation may be warranted.

Often the patient can be allowed to lay in a natural coiled position on the cassette without any restraint (Figs. 20-25 and 20-26). With the patient in a coiled position, the entire body can be radiographed. If necessary, the patient can be placed in a plastic radiolucent tube and radiographed in segments. When radiographing a snake in segments, it is important to number or label each projection so that they can be viewed in proper sequence.

BEAM CENTER: Over area of interest

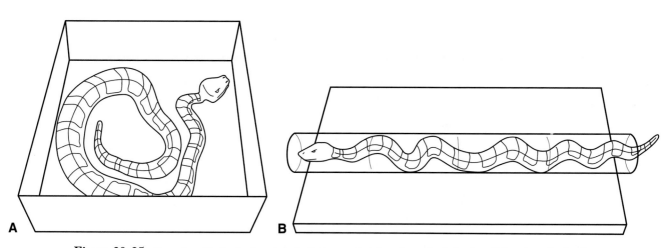

Figure 20-25   *Correct positioning for the whole-body dorsoventral view of a snake. **A**, In a box. **B**, In a clear plastic tube.*

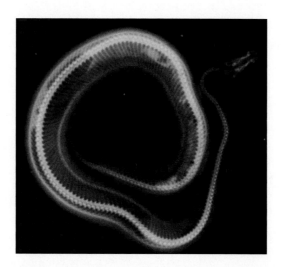

Figure 20-26   *Radiograph of the whole-body dorsoventral view of a snake.*

REPTILE RADIOGRAPHY—*cont'd*

Whole-body lateral view.
For longer snakes, radiograph the patient in segments or concentrate on a certain segment of the body (Figs. 20-27 and 20-28). As mentioned earlier, when radiographing a snake in segments, it is important to number or label each projection so that they can be viewed in proper sequence. In either case it is possible to fix the patient in position on the cassette with either manual or physical restraint. If a radiolucent tube is used, it is necessary to rotate the tube until the patient is in lateral recumbency.

BEAM CENTER: Over area of interest

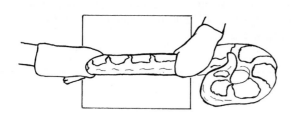

Figure 20-27 *Correct positioning for a lateral view of a portion of a snake.*

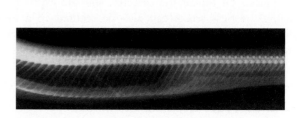

Figure 20-28 *Radiograph of lateral view of a portion of a snake.*

FISH RADIOGRAPHY

Dorsoventral and Lateral Whole-Body View

Radiography of a fish can be challenging because the patient needs water to breathe. A dorsoventral view of a fish can be obtained by placing the patient in a sealable plastic bag with enough water to allow respiration. The plastic bag is placed directly on top of the cassette, and the exposure is made when the fish is stationary (Fig. 20-29).

A lateral view can be exposed in one of two ways. The first method requires the use of a horizontal x-ray beam. The plastic bag containing the fish and water is suspended beside the cassette, which is placed in a vertical position. The x-ray beam is directed horizontally at the fish in the bag, and the field of view should include the entire body (Fig. 20-30). To reduce and equalize the amount of water surrounding the fish, the bag can be compressed with a thin sheet of Plexiglas.

An alternative method of obtaining a lateral view requires rapid preparation and exposure by the radiographer. The fish is wrapped in a wet paper towel and placed in lateral recumbency on the cassette (Figs. 20-31 and 20-32). The exposure is taken quickly so that the patient can be returned to the water.

(NOTE: For amphibians, the same radiographic techniques as for other exotics are suitable.)

BEAM CENTER: Over middle of body

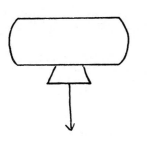

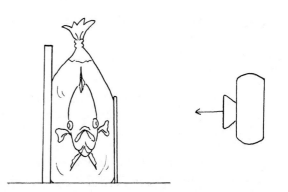

Figure 20-30 *Correct positioning for a whole-body lateral view of a fish with the use of a bagful of water placed next to a cassette in a vertical position. A horizontal x-ray beam is used.*

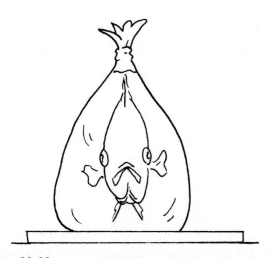

Figure 20-29 *Correct positioning for a whole-body dorsoventral view of a fish with the use of a bagful of water placed on a cassette.*

Continued

BEAM CENTER: Over middle of body—cont'd

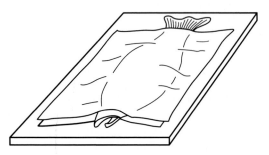

Figure 20-31 *Correct positioning for a whole-body lateral view of a fish with the use of a wet paper towel wrapped around the fish.*

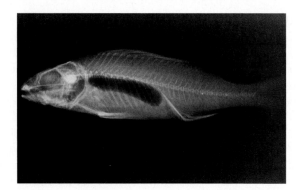

Figure 20-32 *Radiograph of a whole-body lateral view of a fish.*

*K*ey *P*oints

1. As with other species, at least two radiographic views at 90-degree angles to each other are recommended.
2. If Plexiglas is used for avian radiography, increase the kVp by 2 to 4.
3. Scotch tape and cloth medical tape should not be used to restrain because they can cause feather, fur, and scale loss.

*R*eview *Q*uestions

1. What is the preferred exposure time for radiographs of avian and exotic animals?
   a. $^1/_{20}$ second or less
   b. 1 second or less
   c. $^1/_{50}$ or less
   d. $^1/_{40}$ or less

2. Birds require smaller exposure factors than reptiles and mammals because:
   a. birds' cortices are thinner.
   b. birds' tubular bones are much thicker.
   c. birds' long bones have more calcium.
   d. reptiles' cortices and tubular bones are much thinner than those of birds and mammals.

3. What method of restraint of avian and exotic animals is generally safest for the animal and personnel?
   a. Physical
   b. Manual
   c. Chemical
   d. Manual and physical

4. Which of the following statements is true regarding avian radiography?
   a. The left lateral whole body view is preferred over the right lateral.
   b. The wing closest to the cassette should be positioned caudal to the other wing.
   c. The leg closest to the cassette should be positioned cranial to the other wing.
   d. The right lateral whole body view is preferred over the left lateral.

5. How long should a bird be fasted before administering contrast media for a gastrointestinal study?
   a. 2 hours
   b. No longer than 4 hours
   c. 24 hours
   d. 30 minutes

6. What is an advantage of using a radiolucent tube to radiograph rodents?
   a. Superimposition of legs under the body
   b. Shorter exposure times can be used
   c. No manipulation is required for whole body views
   d. A lower kVp can be used

7. Where should the beam be centered for a whole-body view of a rodent?
   a. T11
   b. TL junction
   c. L1
   d. LS junction

8. Which statement is false?
   a. Fish can survive for up to 15 minutes out of water during radiography.
   b. A lateral whole-body view can be taken while a fish is in a plastic bag filled with water.
   c. A dorsoventral view can be taken while the fish is in a plastic bag filled with water.
   d. Fish may be radiographed out of water if the radiograph is taken quickly and the fish is wrapped in wet paper towels.

9. Over what must the sternum be superimposed for a true dorsoventral whole-body view of a lizard?
   a. Heart
   b. Stomach
   c. Ribs
   d. Spine

10. What is the average transit time of barium to travel from the gizzard to the cloaca in birds?
    a. $\frac{1}{2}$ to 1 hour
    b. $\frac{1}{2}$ to 4 hours
    c. 10 minutes to 1 hour
    d. 1 to 24 hours

Suggested Readings

Douglas SW, Herrtage ME, Williamson HD: *Principles of veterinary radiography*, ed 4, Philadelphia, 1987, Bailliere Tindall.

Harrison GJ, Harrison LR: *Clinical avian medicine and surgery*, Philadelphia, 1986, WB Saunders.

McMillan MC: Avian gastrointestinal radiography, *Compend Cont Educ* 5:273-278, 1983.

McMillan MC: Diseases of cage and aviary birds. In Petrak ML, editor: *Avian radiology*, ed 2, Philadelphia, 1982, Lea & Febiger.

Morgan JP, Silverman S: *Techniques in veterinary radiography*, ed 4, Ames, Iowa, 1984, Iowa State University Press.

Rubel GA, Isenbugal E, Wolvekamp P: *Atlas of diagnostic radiology of exotic pets*, Philadelphia, 1991, WB Saunders.

Silverman S: Avian radiographic technique and interpretation. In Kirk R, editor: *Current Veterinary Therapy VII*, Philadelphia, 1980, WB Saunders.

$\mathcal{A}$lternative $\mathcal{I}$maging $\mathcal{T}$echnologies

Patricia A. Walter

CHAPTER OUTLINE

Ultrasonography
Computed Tomography
Nuclear Scintigraphy

OBJECTIVES

Upon completion of this chapter, the reader should do the following:

- Be familiar with basic principles of ultrasonography, nuclear scintigraphy, and computed tomography.

- Appreciate clinical indications for performing ultrasound, nuclear, and computed tomographic scanning.

GLOSSARY

Acoustic impedance: Relationship between density or stiffness of tissue and the velocity of sound within the tissue. Differences in acoustic impedance of adjacent tissues determine the intensity of reflected sound.

Acoustic shadow: Ultrasound artifact. Echo-free zone created distal to the imaged organ when sound waves hit a highly reflective tissue that prevents sound from being transmitted to greater depths.

Anechoic: No echoes are detected, and the area is black. Typically associated with fluid-filled structures such as the urinary bladder.

Attenuation: Reduced intensity of radiation caused by absorption or scattering, or both, during passage through tissue. Sound is also attenuated as it passes through tissue and the intensity is reduced.

B-mode (brightness-mode) ultrasonography: Intensity of returning echoes is expressed as brightness in the display.

Computed tomography (CT) number: Number converted to gray scale in the final image, which represents the attenuation of the x-ray beam in tissue within a voxel. The number is also referred to as a *Hounsfield number,* named for the inventor of CT scanning.

Curie (Ci): A unit of activity (3.7×10^{10} disintegrations per second).

Distant enhancement: Ultrasound artifact. Increased sound intensity beyond a fluid-filled, anechoic area, created by absence of attenuation of the sound beam as it passes through the fluid.

Doppler shift: Difference between transmitted and received sound frequencies. The greater the Doppler shift, the greater the flow velocity.

Echogenicity: Intensity of reflected echoes.

Half-life ($t_{1/2}$): Time in which the initial activity of a radionuclide is reduced to one half. Biologic half-life includes excretion, as well as the characteristic half-life of the isotope.

Hyperechoic: Echoes produced are brighter than in surrounding tissue.

Hypoechoic: A few echoes are detected, and the area is low-level gray compared with adjacent tissues. Usually seen with solid homogeneous tissues or complex fluid containing cells such as blood.

Labeled compound: A compound whose molecule is tagged with a radionuclide.

Linear array probe: Ultrasound probe containing multiple in-line transducers that create a rectangular-shaped image.

Long-axis view: Echocardiographic image showing the heart from base to apex in a longitudinal or sagittal plane.

M-mode (motion-mode) ultrasonography: Information is displayed as depth versus time on a graph. Used for echocardiography.

Pixels (picture elements): Tiny squares making up the image matrix; represent voxels.

Radiopharmaceutical: A radioactive drug that can be administered for diagnostic or therapeutic purposes.

Sector probe: Ultrasound probe with multiple rotating or oscillating transducers that produce a wedge-shaped image.

Short-axis view: Echocardiographic image showing the heart in transverse plane.

Target organ: The organ intended to be imaged and expected to receive the greatest concentration of administered radioactivity.

Voxel (volume element): Three-dimensional box represented on an image matrix by the two-dimensional pixel.

INTRODUCTION

The foundation of diagnostic imaging in veterinary practice has always been radiography. With advancements of the computer age, other modalities have assumed prominence, especially for the diagnosis of diseases that are often difficult to see on radiographs. These imaging techniques are complementary to radiography, which is still recognized as an essential part of the diagnostic work-up. Ultrasonography, computed tomography (CT), and nuclear scintigraphy enhance the quality of practice; they make it possible for clinicians to image noninvasively and to make earlier and more accurate diagnoses. The purpose of this chapter is to familiarize the reader with alternative imaging technologies and to identify the most common clinical indications for use of these imaging methods.

ULTRASONOGRAPHY

Ultrasonography has been an important imaging modality in veterinary medicine since the 1980s. Ultrasound can provide information about organ architecture independent of organ function. It is especially helpful in debilitated or young patients, in which the contrast agents used in special procedures or exploratory surgery may be contraindicated. Ultrasonographic findings are not necessarily specific for histopathologic diagnoses. However, the ability to distinguish solid masses from those containing fluid and to determine the distribution of lesions in organs allows the sonographer to focus differential diagnoses and to formulate management plans.

Technical Aspects

The ultrasound beam is created by a piezoelectric crystal that oscillates at several million Hertz per second (MHz) within a transducer (probe). When the sound wave interacts with tissues in the body, it is reflected, and the echo is received by the transducer. The received impulse is converted to an electronic signal and processed through a computer to become part of a composite of signals that make up the final image of the organ. Differences among organs are identified on a survey radiograph because of the different x-ray attenuating properties that tissues have. With ultrasound, returning signals have different intensities because tissues have different acoustic properties or **acoustic impedance.** Elasticity of the tissue determines the way sound interacts with the tissue: reflection, transmission, or refraction (Fig. 21-1). Air scatters sound. Water transmits sound with little **attenuation** or reflection. This lack of attenuation creates **distant enhancement,** an ultrasound artifact that indicates the presence of fluid. Minerals and metals are highly reflective. Sound cannot penetrate bone. This results in **acoustic shadowing,** which is a lack of echoes beyond the reflecting object. The **echogenicity** of tissues is an indication of the liquid or solid composition of the tissue. **Anechoic** tissues reflect few, if any, echoes. A full urinary bladder is anechoic. **Hypoechoic** tissues reflect few echoes. The medullary papillae of the kidney are hypoechoic. **Hyperechoic** tissues reflect bright white echoes. A bladder stone is hyperechoic.

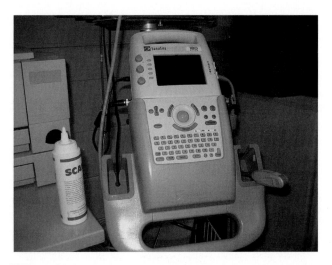

Figure 21-2 *Portable ultrasound machine (Ausonics Microimager) showing the variety of probes available for different applications.*

Ultrasound machines display images in real time. Sector probes or linear array probes are applicable for small and large animals; typically, 5- and 7.5-MHz transducers are used. A large animal practice may also require lower-frequency probes such as 3- or 2.5-MHz (Fig. 21-2). The frequency of the probe is tailored to the size of the animal and to the depth of the organ or area to be imaged. A higher-frequency probe provides better resolution and detail. However, the depth to which the sound can penetrate is limited to areas closer to the surface. A 7.5-MHz transducer is effective in cats and small dogs or for equine reproductive and tendon work. A 5-MHz transducer is used for medium- to large-breed dogs and for equine reproductive scanning. To penetrate at greater depths, a lower-frequency transducer is used. The detail in the image, however, is not as sharp.

Many sonographers use a videotape recorder to record images. The advantage of the videotape is the ability to capture real-time images for review. Organ motion can be assessed. This is especially useful for echocardiography. Thermal printers produce high-quality paper images that can be included in the medical record.

Clinical Applications

Echocardiography

M-mode (motion-mode) and two-dimensional **B-mode (brightness-mode)** echocardiography are used to evaluate cardiac disease (myocardial and valvular disease, as well as congenital anomalies). To perform an echocardiogram, there is no specific preparation. Restraint of the patient is necessary to protect personnel and equipment, and sedation is rarely necessary. An area of chest wall over the heart is clipped. Acoustic gel is applied to conduct sound from the transducer to the thoracic wall. The left and right cardiac windows, located just caudal to the elbow,

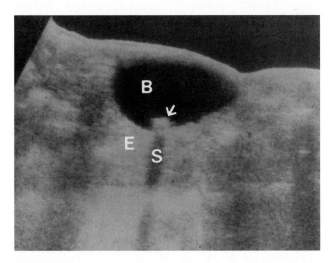

Figure 21-1 *Ultrasound scan of a urinary bladder in a dog with signs of lower urinary tract infection to show ultrasound principles and artifacts. The bladder (B) is filled with anechoic urine. There is a hyperechogenic stone (arrow) with acoustic shadowing beneath it (S) and distant enhancement (E) on either side of the shadow, distal to the bladder.*

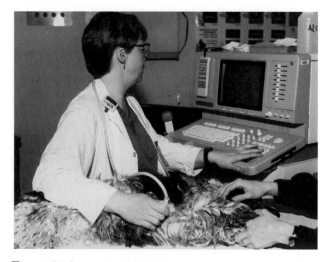

Figure 21-3 *Echocardiography performed on a dog showing position-ing for the right parasternal approach to the heart.*

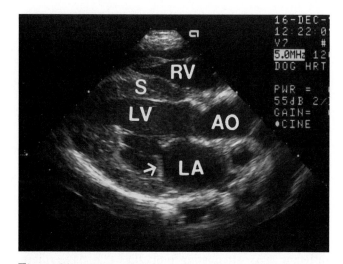

Figure 21-4 *Echocardiogram of a normal dog. Two-dimensional long-axis view showing left ventricle **(LV)**, left atrium **(LA)**, mitral valve (arrow), aorta **(AO)**, interventricular septum **(S)**, and right ventricle **(RV)**.*

are used. The forelimb on the side to be imaged is pulled forward to permit directional freedom of the transducer and to prevent superimposition of bone or muscle over the window (Fig. 21-3). If the ribs are so close together that the transducer head cannot make contact with the chest wall, or if the available window is too narrow (which is often the case in cats), a pillow, rolled-up towel, or sponge wedge may be placed beneath the patient to spread the ribs. In the normal approach, the transducer is directed downward toward the chest wall, which is on the upper side of the patient. The patient may also be approached from the dependent side by directing the transducer upward from beneath table level. Imaging of a patient in sternal or in standing position is also an option, especially in large-breed dogs. Echocardiography is especially difficult in deep-chested breeds such as the Irish wolfhound or the Borzoi and in barrel-chested breeds such as the bulldog because of their conformation.

Two-dimensional echocardiography improves understanding of cardiac and regional mediastinal anatomy. Several standard views are obtained in both the **long-axis** and the **short-axis** directions (Figs. 21-4 through 21-7). Long-axis scans should include the left atrium, mitral valve, interventricular septum, and left ventricular free wall. By slightly tipping the transducer, the aortic valve and aortic root can be seen. In cats the right atrium and right ventricle are difficult to see on the long-axis view when approached from the right parasternal position because the right side of the cat heart is so close to the thoracic wall, and this side of the heart is often outside of the focal zone of the transducer. In dogs the right heart chambers are usually seen on the long-axis view from this position. Short-axis scans should include structures from the base to the apex of the heart. The aortic valve, pulmonary trunk, pulmonic valve, and left atrium are seen at the base of the heart. The mitral valve is the next structure to be seen as the transducer is directed more toward

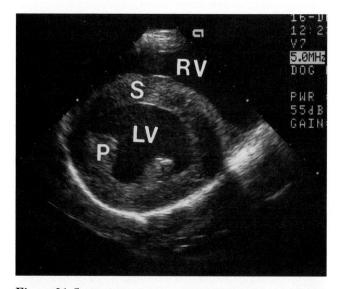

Figure 21-5 *Echocardiogram of a normal dog. Two-dimensional short-axis view through the left ventricle **(LV)** below the level of the mitral valve. Papillary muscles **(P)**, interventricular septum **(S)**, and right ventricle **(RV)** are also seen.*

the apex of the heart. Below the mitral valve level are the left ventricle, interventricular septum, and right ventricle. The four-chamber view shows the left and right atria, the mitral and tricuspid valves, and the right and left ventricles. This view is obtained from the left parasternal position.

A quick overview of the anatomy and function of the heart allows a rapid assessment of functional compromise and detection of obvious chamber size abnormalities (Figs. 21-8 and 21-9). Two-dimensional scans are helpful in identifying cardiac abnormalities such as pleural and pericardial effusion, cardiac masses, and congenital anomalies such as defects in the interventricular septum. An M-mode examination is optimal to detect abnormal

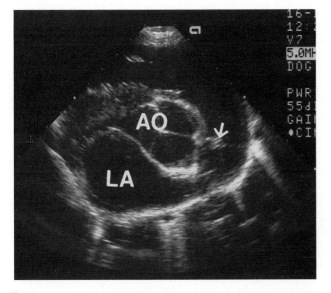

Figure 21-6 *Echocardiogram of a normal dog. Short-axis view of the base of the heart showing the aorta* **(AO)**, *left atrium* **(LA)**, *and pulmonic valve (arrow).*

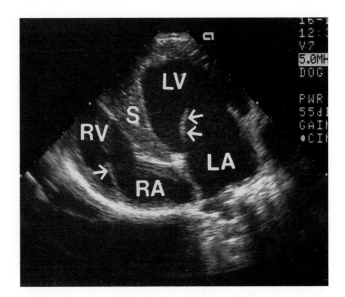

Figure 21-7 *Echocardiogram of a normal dog showing a four-chamber view. This is the best view to see a ventricular septal defect or a right atrial mass. Right atrium* **(RA)**, *right ventricle* **(RV)**, *tricuspid valve (single arrow), interventricular septum* **(S)**, *left ventricle* **(LV)**, *left atrium* **(LA)**, *and mitral valve (double arrow) are seen.*

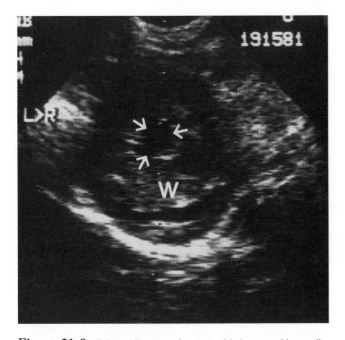

Figure 21-8 *Echocardiogram of a cat with hypertrophic cardiomyopathy. Notice the small left ventricular lumen (arrows) and thickened wall* **(W)** *on the two-dimensional short-axis view.*

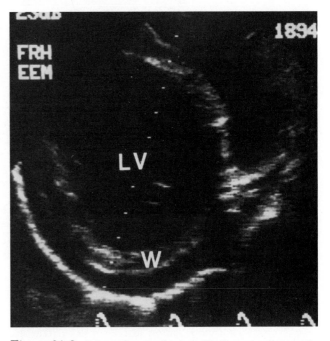

Figure 21-9 *Echocardiogram of a dog with dilatory cardiomyopathy shows a dilated left ventricle* **(LV)** *and thin ventricular wall* **(W)** *on the short-axis two-dimensional view.*

valvular motion such as fluttering, prolapse, or insufficient closure and to accurately measure chamber size and wall thickness. M-mode ultrasound displays cardiac wall and valvular movement as a graph over a period of time (Fig. 21-10). The graph represents the distance of structures from the transducer on the vertical axis and allows the investigator to measure the thickness of the interventricular septum, left ventricular and atrial chamber size, left ventricular wall thickness, and the aortic outflow track (Figs. 21-11 and 21-12). Aortic and mitral valvular motion and thickness can also be assessed. The right thoracic wall is approached to obtain the M-mode views used for measurements. Cardiac function is determined from the dimensions of the left ventricular lumen in systole and diastole to calculate fractional shortening (contractility).

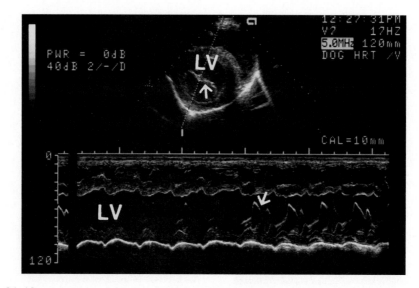

Figure 21-10 *Echocardiogram of a normal dog showing the two-dimensional image with the cursor through the left ventricle (LV) at the level of the mitral valve (arrow). The corresponding M-mode graph is seen below.*

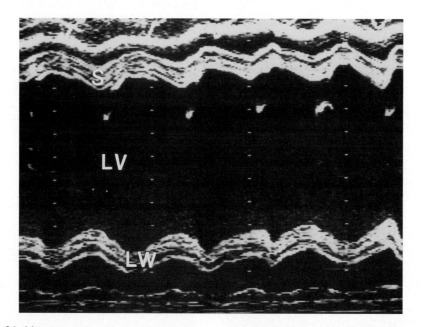

Figure 21-11 *Echocardiogram of a dog with dilatory cardiomyopathy shows a dilated left ventricle (LV), poor contractility (fractional shortening) of the interventricular septum (S), and the left ventricle wall (LW) on the M-mode image.*

Horses are scanned in a standing position, usually confined in stocks. Indications for echocardiography of the horse are congenital heart disease and acquired valvular disease. Ventricular septal defect (VSD) is the most commonly diagnosed lesion (Fig. 21-13). Acquired valvular disease is commonly seen in middle-aged to older horses. Myocardial disease and pericardial effusion are uncommon in the horse.

Doppler echocardiography is an important part of a cardiac evaluation to assess turbulence and velocity of red blood cells within a vessel by measuring the **Doppler shift.** Indications for Doppler studies are pulmonic, aortic, mitral, and tricuspid valvular insufficiencies and stenosis and congenital heart defects such as VSD and persistent ductus arteriosus (PDA). Most recent advances have computerized the Doppler signals so that color is added to better detect subtle abnormalities.

Abdominal Ultrasound

To prepare a small animal for abdominal scan, nonemergency patients may be fasted for 12 hours to reduce the amount of intestinal gas. A full urinary bladder is optimal for scanning the bladder or prostate. The hair coat is clipped around the margins of the costal arch, along the flank, and caudally to the bladder. Coupling gel

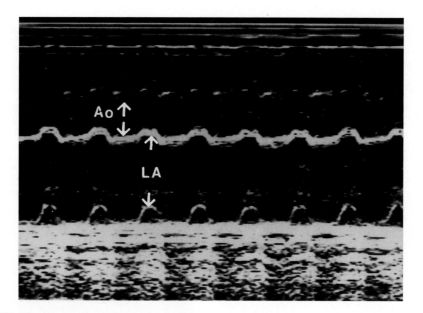

Figure 21-12 *Echocardiogram of a cat with hypertrophic cardiomyopathy shows a dilated left atrium (**LA**) compared with the aortic width (**Ao**) on the M-mode image.*

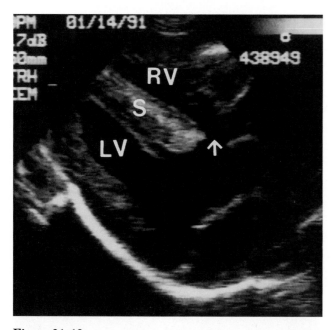

Figure 21-13 *Echocardiogram of a foal with a heart murmur showing a defect (arrow) in the interventricular septum (**S**) between the left ventricle (**LV**) and right ventricle (**RV**).*

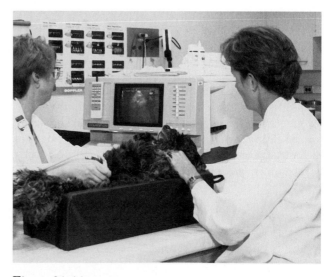

Figure 21-14 *Abdominal ultrasound of a dog in ventrodorsal position.*

is applied. The animal is positioned in ventrodorsal or lateral recumbency; several different positions may be used to obtain optimal B-mode images (Fig. 21-14).

Liver and biliary tract.   Survey radiographs are superior to ultrasound for assessing liver volume. On an ultrasound, the normal liver has a uniform but slightly coarse echotexture; it is less echogenic than the spleen and more echogenic than the renal cortex. Typically, the larger vessels and the gallbladder are visible. The normal gallbladder has a smooth wall and anechoic contents (Fig. 21-15). Visibility of the common bile duct is variable in animals. The portal veins are clearly defined by echogenic walls resulting from adjacent fat. Hepatic veins, in contrast, have poorly defined walls. Bile ducts and hepatic arteries are not well visualized in small animals, and in normal animals, separate lobes cannot be identified. Primary indications for liver scanning are abnormalities seen on survey radiographs (hepatomegaly or a mass in the area of the liver). Elevations in liver enzymes, ascites, or suspected hepatic metastases also indicate a liver scan.

Ultrasound-guided biopsy or fine-needle aspiration is often performed in conjunction with liver scanning. Heavy sedation or general anesthesia is required for biopsy, but for fine-needle aspiration, sedation is not required unless

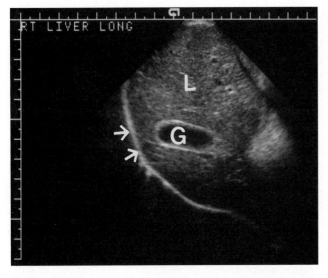

Figure 21-15 *Abdominal ultrasound of a normal dog shows the liver (L) and gallbladder (G) in sagittal plane. The diaphragm (arrows) is an echogenic landmark.*

the patient is active. For this procedure the animal is placed in dorsal or lateral recumbency, and the area is surgically prepared. A local analgesic may be placed in the skin and muscle layer. The lesion of interest is identified on the ultrasound monitor and positioned to be in line with the predicted track of the needle. The biopsy needle is inserted through a biopsy guide attached to the probe, or a freehand technique is used (Fig. 21-16). The needle can be clearly seen within the organ (Fig. 21-17). Because hemorrhage is a potential complication, a clotting profile is recommended before biopsy to identify animals at risk.

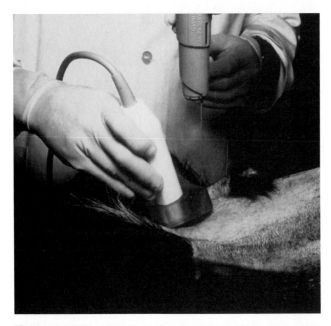

Figure 21-16 *An ultrasound-guided biopsy is performed by inserting the needle through a plastic guide attached to the probe.*

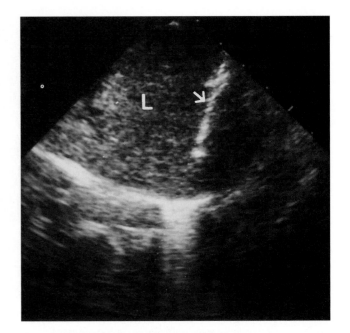

Figure 21-17 *The hyperechogenic needle (arrow) is easily seen during ultrasound-guided biopsy of the liver (L).*

Spleen. The normal spleen is elliptic, flat, and smoothly contoured. Echogenically, it is homogeneous, finely grained, and more echogenic than the liver (Fig. 21-18). Small vessels are seen at the hilus. Indications for scanning are a mass, diffuse enlargement or an abnormal position of the spleen identified on survey radiographs or during abdominal palpation. Abdominal trauma with hemorrhage, acute abdominal pain, or signs of anemia and collapse also indicate a splenic scan. In cases of splenic mass (hemangiosarcoma) (Fig. 21-19), the liver is scanned to search for metastases.

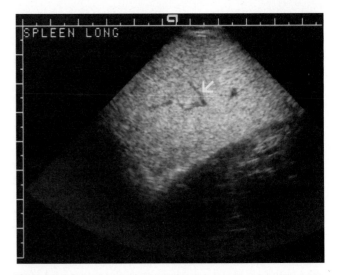

Figure 21-18 *Abdominal ultrasound of a normal dog shows the spleen. The echotexture is homogeneous and finely grained. A vessel is also seen (arrow).*

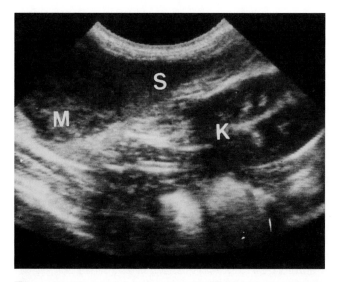

Figure 21-19 *Abdominal ultrasound of a dog with a history of collapse and anemia. There is a 3- × 3-cm hypoechogenic mass (M) (hemangiosarcoma) in the spleen. The body of the spleen (S) appears to be normal. The left kidney (K) is also seen.*

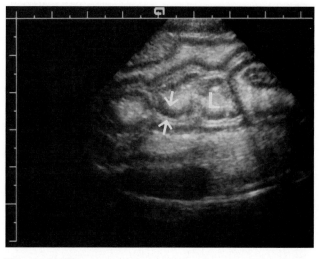

Figure 21-20 *Abdominal ultrasound of the abdomen in a normal dog shows loops of small intestines with hyperechogenic lumen (L) and hypoechogenic wall (between arrows).*

Pancreas. The normal pancreas is narrow, smoothly marginated, and hypoechoic. The right pancreatic lobe is imaged best from the right side of the abdomen with the animal in left lateral recumbency. Identifying the descending duodenum is important because the right limb of the pancreas lies along it. The left pancreatic lobe is more difficult to image because of gas in the adjacent stomach and transverse colon. Usually the animal is placed in right lateral recumbency. Landmarks include a triangular area bounded by the caudal margin of the stomach, the cranial margin of the left kidney, and the area medial to the spleen. Pancreatitis is the most common indication for scanning. Neoplasms, cysts, and abscesses are rare.

Gastrointestinal tract. Gastrointestinal sonography can be difficult due to variable amounts of gas within the lumen, which reflect sound and prevent imaging of deeper structures. In addition, feces within the colon cause shadows. The normal bowel has distinguishable layers (lumen, mucosal surface and mucosa, submucosa, muscularis, and subserosa-serosa; Fig. 21-20). The normal intestinal wall is about 3 mm thick. Ultrasound can be used to identify gastrointestinal mural masses, assess bowel peristalsis, locate intraluminal masses and foreign bodies, and confirm intussusception.

Kidneys and adrenal glands. To prepare for renal and adrenal scanning, the abdomen is clipped wide enough in the flank area to allow easy visualization. The left kidney is mobile, especially in cats. The normal kidney has a hyperechogenic capsule. The cortex is less echogenic than liver or spleen (Fig. 21-21) and more echogenic than the almost anechoic medullary papillae (Fig. 21-22). The renal sinus area is hyperechogenic due to fat and vascular interfaces. The renal pelvis is not identified as an anechoic

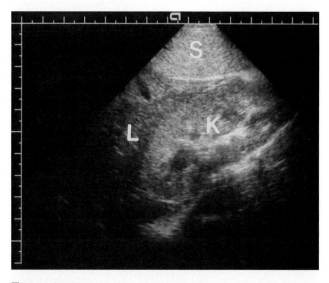

Figure 21-21 *Abdominal ultrasound of a normal dog showing comparative echogenicity of the liver (L), spleen (S), and right kidney (K). The kidney is hyperechogenic to the liver. The spleen is hyperechogenic to the kidney.*

cavity except when dilation is present. Evaluation of renal size based on sonographic assessment is less accurate than size determined by radiographs because of falloff of the sound beam at the rounded edges of the cranial and caudal poles.

Sonography is used to identify kidneys not visualized on survey radiographs, characterize a mass seen on radiographs, assess location and distribution of disease in enlarged kidneys, determine the location of mineralizations, and confirm pelvic and perinephric fluid accumulations (Fig. 21-23). Ultrasonography does not assess kidney function unless Doppler technique is applied. Sonography in renal disease is helpful to identify fluid-

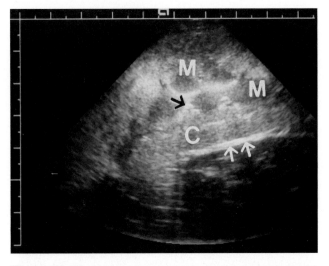

Figure 21-22 *Abdominal ultrasound of a normal dog shows the left kidney. The cortex (**C**) is hyperechogenic compared with the medullary papillae (**M**). The bright echoes are from the diverticula (single arrow) and the capsule (double arrow).*

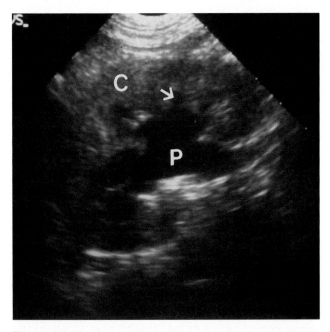

Figure 21-23 *Abdominal ultrasound in a dog with an enlarged kidney noticed on radiographs. There is anechoic fluid dilatation of the renal pelvis (**P**) and renal pelvic recesses (arrow), indicating hydronephrosis caused by distal obstruction. The renal cortex (**C**) is normal.*

filled, cystlike lesions or solid masses (Fig. 21-24). Ultrasonographic findings for diffuse infiltrative disease are not specific, and biopsy is usually necessary to confirm the diagnosis.

Normal adrenal glands are small (<1 cm in height) and are located in perirenal fat medial to the cranial pole of each kidney. The left adrenal gland has a dumbbell-like shape with widened cranial and caudal poles, whereas the right one is more triangular in shape, and the cranial third of the gland is widened. Indication for imaging is to deter-

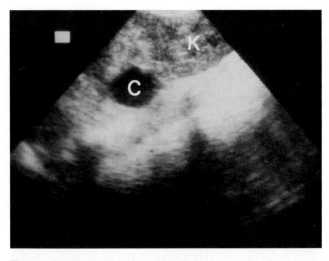

Figure 21-24 *Abdominal ultrasound shows a solitary anechoic cyst (**C**) in the cranial pole of the right kidney (**K**) of a dog.*

mine bilateral or unilateral enlargement. In pituitary-dependent hyperadrenocorticism, both glands become symmetrically enlarged and there is no change in shape. An adrenal mass such as adenocarcinoma, adenoma, or pheochromocytoma is usually unilateral and alters the shape of the gland.

Prostate. The normal prostate gland has homogeneous echogenicity and fine texture. Ultrasound is indicated in cases of prostatomegaly, signs of lower urinary tract disease, constipation, or caudal abdominal pain. Prostatic and paraprostatic cysts, focal and multifocal masses, and sublumbar lymph nodes can be identified. Ultrasound is not specific enough to differentiate benign prostatic hyperplasia from neoplasia or infection, and biopsy is recommended.

Urinary bladder. The normal urinary bladder contains anechogenic urine. The bladder mucosa is smooth, and the thickness of the bladder wall is uniform (Fig. 21-25). Indications for bladder scanning are signs of lower urinary tract disease. Calculi, blood clots, and masses arising from the bladder wall can be identified (Fig. 21-26). Scanning with the bladder filled is necessary. Tumors in the bladder neck area can be difficult to see, and urethral masses are not visible because of their intrapelvic location.

Reproductive tract. The normal, nonpregnant reproductive tract is not commonly seen in small animals. Indications for ultrasound are to diagnose pregnancy, pyometra, stump granuloma, or ovarian neoplasia. The optimal time for pregnancy detection in small animals is 30 days after the last breeding (Fig. 21-27). At that time gestational sacs with viable embryos can be identified. Ultrasound is not accurate for determining numbers of fetuses because of the superimposition of bowel gas and also because only a small segment of the uterus can be

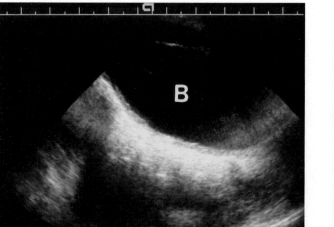

Figure 21-25 *Abdominal ultrasound of a normal dog shows the urinary bladder (**B**). The urine is anechoic, and bright echoes beneath the bladder (far enhancement) indicate that the sound is being transmitted through the fluid without being attenuated (reflected).*

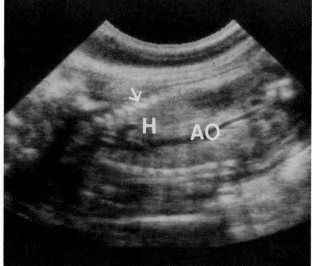

Figure 21-27 *Ultrasound of a fetus at approximately 30 days' gestation in a dog. The ribs (arrow), heart (**H**), and aorta (**AO**) are clearly seen.*

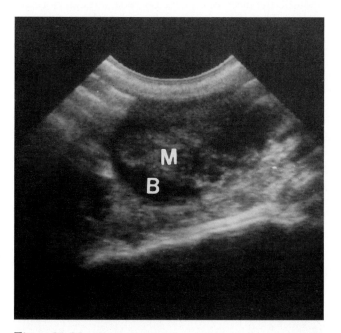

Figure 21-26 *Ultrasound of the urinary bladder of a dog with hematuria. An irregular hyperechogenic and hypoechogenic mass (**M**) projects into the bladder lumen (**B**). This was determined at surgery to be a blood clot.*

imaged at one time. However, ultrasound is effective in detecting enlargement of the uterine horn in cases of pyometra. Ultrasonography is also an important tool to evaluate the reproductive tract of the mare; the optimal time to detect pregnancy is day 11 of gestation.

Ultrasound Examination of the Eyes

A 7.5-MHz transducer may be placed directly on the cornea after application of topical anesthetic. It can also be placed on the eyelid, although with this technique the hair must be clipped or coupling gel must be applied liberally. The cornea, anterior chamber, ciliary body and lens, vitreous chamber, optic disc, optic nerve, extraocular muscle, and retrobulbar fat can be seen. Indications for scanning the orbital region are intraocular masses such as melanoma or ciliary body tumors. Intraocular hemorrhage and inflammatory masses may also be seen.

Ultrasound Examination of the Extremities

Ultrasound examination of extremities has focused primarily on the equine limb below the carpus and tarsus (Fig. 21-28). Sonography plays an important role in the diagnosis of traumatic injury, infection, and inflammation of the equine extremities. Indications in thoroughbred horses are "bowed tendons," tenosynovitis, and suspensory ligament tear. Monitoring the healing process of the acute injury and determining when the horse can begin rehabilitation and return to work are important. Consistently identified structures are skin, superficial and deep digital flexor tendons, inferior check ligament, and suspensory ligament including medial and lateral branches. The intersesamoidean ligaments also are easily identified. The inferior check ligament and the suspensory ligament are the most echogenic because of their dense fibrous composition. The superficial and deep flexor tendons have a medium echogenicity but are distinguishable from one another because of a slight difference in echo intensity and also because of their differing shapes.

COMPUTED TOMOGRAPHY

CT, which is available at most academic institutions and in some veterinary specialty practices, is one of the most expensive diagnostic tests in veterinary medicine. Its

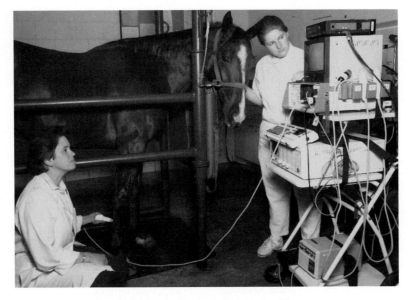

Figure 21-28   *Ultrasound of the flexor tendons on the distal front leg of a horse.*

major advantage is the ability to acquire information not available from radiographs, contrast studies, or ultrasound examinations. The primary indications for CT are central and peripheral nervous system diseases of the brain, spinal cord, and lumbosacral spine. It is also useful for obscured masses in the mediastinum, axillary region, and retroperitoneal space.

Technical Aspects

CT uses x-rays (about 120 kVp with variable mAs) and computers to produce images that show anatomy in cross section. CT allows visualization of structures in sagittal, dorsal, transverse, and oblique planes without super-imposition artifact from fat, ribs, spine, pelvis, or any organs that may mask detail on a survey radiograph. Objects imaged by CT appear more clearly than those on conventional survey radiographs because the tomographic technology blurs the superimposed tissues. In general this is a static imaging modality, with images captured at a fixed moment in time. Images are saved and formatted to a smaller size so that they appear in sequence on a single piece of film.

The CT unit consists of a movable bed or cradle on which the patient lies and a gantry that contains the x-ray tube and detectors. The cradle moves through the opening (portal) in the doughnut-shaped gantry at specific distance increments (in millimeters) during scanning (Fig. 21-29). The cradle in standard CT units can support approximately 300 lb. CT for horses requires a specialized table to support and maneuver the larger patients into the gantry. Because of the small portal diameter of the gantry (20 to 25 inches), only the skull, neck, and distal parts of the extremities of horses can be scanned.

Within the gantry are the x-ray tubes, x-ray detectors, and x-ray collimators. The x-ray tube is positioned opposite the detectors. The x-ray tube and detectors can be moved 360 degrees around the patient. X-ray detectors absorb the photons emerging from the patient and convert these to electronic signals of varying intensity, depending on how much attenuation has occurred in the body. These electronic signals are assigned a number, which represents their intensity as they emerge from the patient. The computer reconstructs the information into a picture displayed on a television screen. A set of images or slices is acquired at each interval of movement through the gantry. The computer can further be used to reconstruct the internal structure of an organ from several projections of the organ.

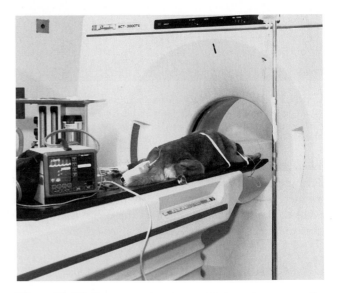

Figure 21-29   *Transverse-plane computed tomography scanner with a dog in the dorsoventral position in the cradle, which moves through the portal in the gantry.*

This examination requires general anesthesia to avoid excessive motion, which degrades the image more than in conventional radiography. The animal is placed on the cradle in dorsoventral, ventrodorsal, or lateral recumbency. To begin the procedure, a survey radiograph is taken with the animal positioned in the gantry to localize regional anatomic landmarks so that when the CT is programmed, patient movement will cover the appropriate region and slices can be obtained through the area of interest. The limits for cradle movement through the gantry are set to cover the area to be scanned.

The two-dimensional image that is produced is composed of many squares called **pixels,** or picture elements. The pixels are set in a framework of columns and rows called a matrix (256 × 512 pixels would equal about 0.7 to 1.5 mm in the patient). Each pixel represents an elongated block of tissue called a **voxel,** or volume element. When the computer assembles all the pixels of the image, the composite actually represents many three-dimensional voxels. The density of each voxel is compared with the density of water and then assigned a **CT number** that is proportional to the degree to which the volume of the block or tissue has attenuated the x-ray beam. CT numbers range from +3000 (metal) to +1000 (bone) to −1000 (air). Each CT number is assigned a gray-scale shade, which depicts the different types of tissues in the patient.

Because of CT numbers and computerized generation of the image, the tissues can be enhanced or subtracted to make relatively small differences more visible. To provide more contrast in tissue, radiographic contrast agents are often used. Many tumors show contrast enhancement because of increased blood supply, which results in a higher CT number after administration of contrast medium than without it.

Clinical Applications

Skull. The skull is a region where radiographs often fall short in identifying lesions. Intracranial lesions are easily demonstrated by CT. Normal brain tissue is relatively uniform and homogeneous, and the ventricular system, tentorium, falx cerebri, and pituitary fossa are easily seen on CT images. Indications for skull CT are seizure, blindness, vestibular signs, and change in disposition, which may be caused by brain masses, hydrocephalus, or trauma (Fig. 21-30). CT scanning is also effective in localizing nasal, sinus, and periorbital masses. Malignant nasal tumors are scanned to assess invasion into the frontal sinus and cranium (Fig. 21-31). CT images show the extent of the tumor in three planes, and this assists treatment planning when radiation therapy is being considered. The primary indications for CT in horses are to detect evidence of trauma; to assess the extent of nasal, sinus, and guttural pouch masses; and to identify congenital anomalies such as hydronephrosis.

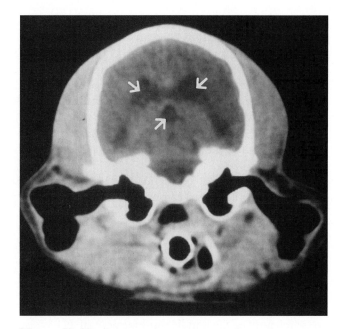

Figure 21-30 *Transverse-plane computed tomography scan of the brain of a dog with hydrocephalus. Both lateral ventricles and the third ventricle (arrows) are dilated.*

Spine. CT is helpful when myelography and standard radiographic procedures cannot completely outline a spinal lesion. Nerve root tumors are not well delineated by myelography, and CT provides good imaging of the paravertebral areas and nerve root foramina. Because of

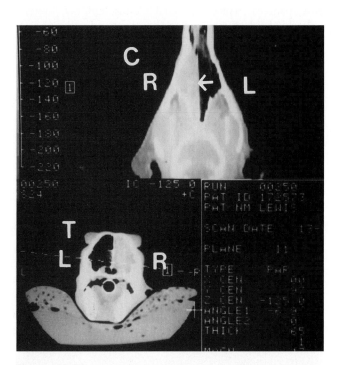

Figure 21-31 *Computed tomography scan of a dog with a nasal tumor. A radiopaque soft-tissue mass is seen in the right (**R**) nasal passage (arrow) in coronal-plane (**C**) and transverse-plane (**T**) scans. The left (**L**) nasal passage is normal, and no invasion of the brain is seen.*

the termination of the subarachnoid space in the caudal lumbar spine, myelography and epidurography are usually unpredictable for caudal spine lesions. CT is the modality of choice for imaging the spine caudal to L4-5, especially in the paravertebral areas and for lateralized spinal canal disease. In cases of lumbosacral degenerative disease, CT allows visualization of intervertebral disk protrusion at C6-7 and C7-S1, as well as nerve root compression by stenotic foramina and by intraspinal fibrous tissue.

Extremities. CT may be the method of the future for assessment of the ulnar coronoid process in cases of fragmented medial coronoid process in dogs. Both left and right elbow joints are scanned because the disease is often bilateral. CT provides good detail of this area that is not easily seen on radiographs. CT is also helpful for meniscal disease. Indications for CT in horses are fractures of the third carpal bone, supracondylar fractures of the distal third metacarpal, third phalanx fractures, and stress fractures of the middle third metacarpal. CT is also valuable for focal lesions such as infarct, osteochondrosis, and sequestra.

Thorax. Indications for CT in the thorax include pulmonary and mediastinal masses, mediastinal lymphadenopathy, thoracic mass invasion into spine or ribs, and detection of pulmonary metastases. Some advantages over ultrasonography may exist for detection of pericardial effusion and heart base masses.

Abdomen. The liver, gallbladder, stomach, small intestine, pancreas, spleen, adrenal glands, kidneys, ureters, urinary bladder, prostate, ovary, colon, and major vessels are easily identified on CT scans (Fig. 21-32). A suspected mass seen on radiographs or detected on palpation is a common indication for performing a scan. CT is

especially useful for canine adrenal masses. Vascular invasion from adrenal tumors may be determined by contrast-enhanced CT.

NUCLEAR SCINTIGRAPHY

Nuclear scintigraphy is a noninvasive imaging procedure that uses a small amount of radioactive material (radionuclide) administered intravenously, transcolonically, or by aerosol insufflation. Scintigraphy is more sensitive but less specific than standard radiographs or CT. Images do not provide the anatomic detail of radiographs or CT, but they do provide physiologic information about the function of specific organs. The studies are complementary to those of other imaging modalities.

Technical Aspects

Technetium 99m is a radioactive isotope that emits predominately gamma rays. Technetium radioactive pharmaceuticals are the most commonly used **labeled compounds** for imaging in veterinary medicine. The ideal **radiopharmaceutical** has a relatively short **half-life,** emits a low radiation dose to the patient and to personnel, is readily available from commercial producers, and is inexpensive. The radionuclide may be used alone or tagged to other compounds so that it is absorbed preferentially in a specific **target organ.**

A gamma scintillation camera (gamma camera) detects the gamma emissions (counts) from the radionuclide and forms a black-and-white image of the selected organ printed on x-ray film. Animals are sedated for the procedure. Horses may be placed in stocks. The animal is positioned so that the face of the detector is as close as possible to the area of suspected abnormality to detect the maximum number of counts (Fig. 21-33). It takes about

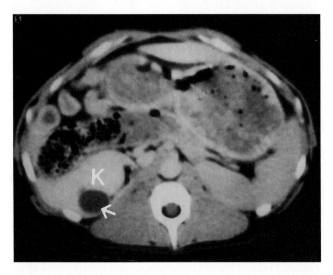

Figure 21-32 *Transverse computed tomography scan of the mid-abdomen of a dog showing a cyst (arrow) on the craniodorsal margin of the right kidney (K). This is the same patient as in Figure 21-24.*

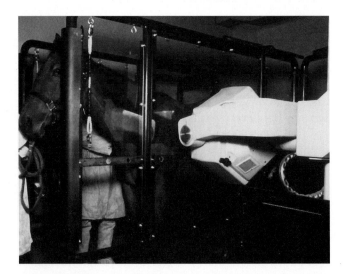

Figure 21-33 *Nuclear scan of a lame horse. The gamma camera seen to the right is raised to the level of the shoulder, which was the area of interest.*

1 to 2 minutes to detect enough emissions to produce an image.

Proper radiation protection such as restricted contact time with the patient, increased distance from the patient during scanning, and protective attire (laboratory coat, latex gloves) reduce the amount of personnel exposure. The radiopharmaceutical is excreted through urine and feces, so it is important to take precautions to avoid contamination during both scanning and the postscanning decay phase. Technetium 99m is a convenient isotope for veterinary practice because of the short half-life (6 hours). Animals can usually be released 24 to 72 hours after administration of the radiopharmaceutical, depending on the radiation safety and protection laws of the state in which the procedure is performed.

Clinical Applications

Thyroid. The most common indication for a thyroid scan is hyperthyroidism. Elevation of thyroid hormone (T_4) is often present when the gland is hyperactive. Thyroid scintigraphy is used mainly in hyperthyroid cats to confirm hyperactivity of the gland, determine relative activity and size of a hypersecreting nodule, and determine whether one or both lobes of the gland are involved. Imaging is also useful to identify ectopic thyroid tissue. This is especially important information if surgical removal of a thyroid lobe is being considered.

A dose of 1 to 5 millicurie (mCi) of technetium 99m is given intravenously, and imaging is performed 20 to 30 minutes after injection. Ventrodorsal and left and right lateral projections are performed. In the case of a thyroid gland that is hyperactive, uptake increases in active areas, called "hot spots" (Fig. 21-34). The image shows a blackened area in the involved lobe of the thyroid gland. Antithyroid drugs do not interfere with pertechnetate imaging.

Bone. The most common indication for a bone scan is lameness that cannot be localized by physical examination, survey radiographs, or ultrasound scan. In horses the primary indications are occult lameness, chronic lameness, stress fractures, osteochondrosis dissecans, early degenerative joint disease, navicular disease, bone or ligament injury, skull trauma, and osteomyelitis. There is greater accumulation of the radionuclide where there is increased blood flow or increased bone turnover. Bone scintigraphy is sensitive, and lesions can be seen at an earlier stage on a bone scan than on survey radiographs. "Hot spots" are areas of increased bone remodeling activity, produced by neoplasia, infection, or trauma. "Cold spots" are areas of decreased activity, for instance, from bone necrosis. Because of increased bone remodeling, young animals usually retain more isotope than older animals, especially in the growth plates. More activity is indicated by a darker image, which shows that more gamma emissions were detected (Fig. 21-35).

For bone scanning, technetium 99m is first linked to methylene diphosphonate (MDP) so that the radioisotope is preferentially absorbed by bone. Five to 20 mCi of the radionuclide is given intravenously for small animal imaging, and 100 to 300 mCi may be given to a horse. After the compound is injected intravenously, the radionuclide distributes first into the blood pool (soft tissue

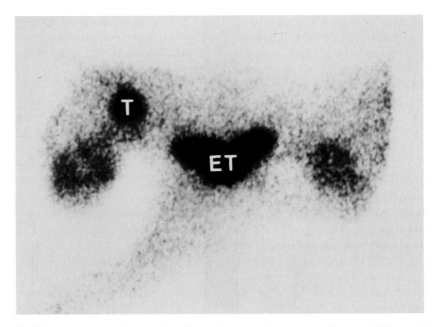

Figure 21-34 *Nuclear scan of a hyperthyroid cat. Notice that there are two "hot spots." The cranial one is a hyperactive thyroid gland (**T**); the other, located more caudally, is ectopic functional thyroid tissue (**ET**) in the thoracic inlet and cranial mediastinum.*

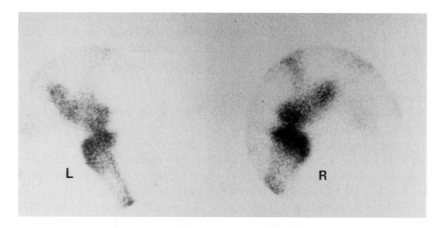

Figure 21-35 *Nuclear scan of both stifle joints in a lame horse. Notice the increased activity (blackness) of the right stifle joint (**R**) compared with the normal left stifle joint (**L**). The horse had degenerative joint disease (arthritis) in the right joint.*

phase). Later (after about 3 hours) the radionuclide clears from the bloodstream and redistributes into the hydroxyapatite crystals of bone (bone phase) in areas where there is active bone metabolism. Two-phased studies are performed to differentiate between soft tissue and bone lesions. After imaging, animals are isolated until the level of emitted radiation returns to a safe level (48 to 72 hours).

Liver. Liver scintigraphy is indicated in patients with a small liver or evidence of a liver mass, decreased liver function, biliary outflow obstruction, or abnormal hepatic blood flow. Technetium can be bound to any of several compounds that have selective uptake by the parenchyma, the biliary tree and outflow tract, or the vascular system. The most common indication for hepatic scintigraphy is congenital portosystemic shunt. The isotope is infused into the colon, absorbed through the colonic mucosa, and transported to the liver via the portal venous system. A vascular shunt diverts the portal flow away from the liver.

KEY POINTS

1. Portal veins have more echogenic walls than hepatic veins on an ultrasonograph of the liver.
2. The liver is less echogenic than the spleen but more echogenic than the renal cortex.
3. Nuclear scintigraphy can provide physiologic information about the function of specific organs and is a complementary imaging mode.
4. Lameness that cannot be localized by physical examination is the most common indication for a bone scan.

REVIEW QUESTIONS

1. Which of the following would cause acoustic shadowing?
   a. Urine
   b. Bone
   c. Air in the stomach
   d. Free blood in the abdomen

2. Which statement is false?
   a. The renal medullary papillae are more hyperechoic than urine.
   b. Urine causes more attenuation than renal medullary papillae.
   c. Echogenicity is an indication of liquid or solid composition of tissues.
   d. Anechoic tissue reflects more echoes than hyperechoic tissues.

3. What method of diagnostic imaging evaluates the cardiac wall and valvular movement in real time?
   a. Computed tomography
   b. Ultrasonography, B-mode
   c. Ultrasonography, M-mode
   d. Nuclear scintigraphy

4. Rate the echogenicity of the following, with the first being most echogenic and the last being the least echogenic.
   a. Spleen, renal cortex, liver
   b. Spleen, liver, renal cortex
   c. Liver, renal cortex, spleen
   d. Renal cortex, liver, spleen

5. Which of the following can be detected via ultrasonography?
   a. Normal, nonpregnant reproductive tract
   b. Hepatic masses
   c. Peristalsis
   d. Both b and c are correct.

6. What is the optimal earliest time to detect pregnancy in small animals?
   a. 17 days after the last breeding
   b. 11 days after the last breeding
   c. 48 days after the last breeding
   d. 30 days after the last breeding

7. A patient has lost vision in one eye. The veterinarian suspects a periorbital mass or a brain lesion. What imaging mode would identify the cause with the most detail?
   a. Computed tomography
   b. Radiographs
   c. Ultrasound
   d. Nuclear scintigraphy

8. What is the most reliable and common way to diagnose hyperthyroidism in cats?
   a. Computed tomography
   b. Radiographs
   c. Ultrasound
   d. Nuclear scintigraphy

9. Which of the following does not produce a hot spot in nuclear scintigraphy?
   a. Bone necrosis
   b. Infection
   c. Trauma
   d. Neoplasia

10. Which statement is true?
    a. M-mode ultrasound provides a static picture at a specific moment in time.
    b. Younger animals' bones usually have a darker image on nuclear scintigraphy.
    c. Nuclear scintigraphy provides a safe means of performing a biopsy of the liver.
    d. Abdominal ultrasound is fairly easy to interpret because all abdominal organs have equal acoustic impedance.

Suggested Readings

Burk RL, Ackerman N: *Small animal radiology and ultrasonography: a diagnostic atlas and text,* Philadelphia, 1996, WB Saunders.

Cartee RE et al: *Practical veterinary ultrasound,* Philadelphia, 1995, Williams & Wilkins.

Feeney DA, Fletcher TF, Hardy RM: *Atlas of correlative imaging anatomy of the normal dog: ultrasound and computed tomography,* Philadelphia, 1991, WB Saunders.

Herring DS: Diagnostic ultrasound, *Vet Clin North Am* 15:6, 1985.

Kaplan PM: Ultrasound, *Probl Vet Med* 3:4, 1991.

Mattoon JS, Nyland TG: *Veterinary diagnostic ultrasound,* Philadelphia, 1995, WB Saunders.

Rantanen N: Diagnostic ultrasound, *Vet Clin North Am* 2:1, 1996.

Saha GB: *Fundamentals of nuclear pharmacy,* New York, 1979, Springer-Verlag.

Shores A: Symposium on diagnostic imaging, *Vet Clin North Am* 23:2, 1993.

Steckel R: Advanced diagnostic methods, *Vet Clin North Am* 7:2, 1991.

chapter 22

Digital Radiography

John S. Mattoon

CHAPTER OUTLINE

History of Digital Radiography
Digital Radiography: An Overview
Limitations of Conventional Screen-Film Radiography
Advantages of Digital Radiography
Disadvantages of Digital Radiography
HIS, RIS, and PACS

Digital Imaging and Communications in Medicine
Image Management Software and Image Processing
Analog-to-Digital Radiographic Signal Conversion
Digital Computers
Pixels and Image Matrix

OBJECTIVES

Upon completion of this chapter the reader should be able to do the following:

- List the limitations of conventional screen-film radiography.
- Understand the advantages and disadvantages of digital radiography.
- Have a basic understanding of the interplay of the digital radiography system with hospital information systems (HIS), radiology information systems (RIS), and picture archiving and communication systems (PACS).
- Understand the meaning of digital imaging and communications in medicine (DICOM).
- Understand the concept analog-to-digital signal conversion.
- Have a basic understanding of digital language, the binary numerical system, and computers.

- Explain what a pixel is, how pixel size affects image quality, and how pixels are arranged in a matrix.
- Define indirect and direct digital radiography.
- Describe the technological principles of the three types of digital radiography image receptors that are currently available in veterinary medicine.
- Be aware of digital radiography artifacts.
- Understand that operator errors can create artifacts similar to those encountered with conventional screen-film systems.
- Be aware of x-ray dose considerations when converting to and using digital radiography.

GLOSSARY

ADC: Analog to digital converter. An electronic device that converts an analog voltage signal to a digital signal.

ALARA: As low as reasonably achievable. This acronym refers to a basic principle of radiation safety—to use the lowest amount of ionizing radiation as possible.

Analog: A voltage waveform that is continuous; at any point in time there is a voltage value.

Bit: A binary digit, either 0 or 1.

Bmp: Bit map. A representation of a graphic image stored in computer memory as rows and columns of dots; each dot is stored in one or more bits of information. Dot density, or resolution, is expressed as dots per inch (dpi). Images displayed on a monitor are converted from bit maps to pixels.

Byte: Composed of 8 bits.

CCD: Charged coupled device. A *small* flat panel device that is capable of creating images from visible light, used for digital radiography and digital photography.

CD-ROM: Compact disk, read-only memory. A CD-ROM (or CD) is a 5-inch diameter optical storage device with a capacity of approximately 700 megabytes (MB).

Compression: A mathematical reduction in size of digital data so that they are easier (faster) to transmit. *Loss-less* compression allows perfect decompression of compressed data without loss of information. With *lossy* compression, a portion of original digital data is lost and cannot be restored. The advantage of lossy compression is that higher compression levels can be attained.

Contrast resolution: The ability to distinguish between two structures of differing x-ray attenuation. The high-contrast resolution of digital radiography is vastly superior to conventional screen-film radiography.

CR: Computed radiography. A type of digital radiography that uses a photostimulable phosphor plate for image acquisition.

DICOM: Digital Imaging and Communications in Medicine. The global standard in the human medical industry for transmission of medical images and related information. A joint committee of the American College of Radiology and the National Electrical Manufacturers' Association (ACR-NEMA) is responsible for the continuous development of DICOM standards. DICOM is intended to realize the interoperability of multiple medical imaging devices manufactured by different vendors including the display and transmission of images and information.

Digital: To use digits (rather than numbers); data stored, displayed, or represented in numerical digits (binary). Images are converted into electronic bits.

DDR: Direct digital radiography. A digital radiography system in which there is direct conversion of x-ray energy into an electronic (digital) signal. Although DDR offers the best in digital radiography resolution, the technology is currently expensive and not yet commonly used.

DR: Digital radiography. Term used to denote any type of digital radiography including computed radiography, CCD technology, flat panel detectors, and direct radiography units.

DVD: Digital video (versatile) disk. A 5-inch diameter optical disk with approximately 5 gigabyte (GB) storage capacity.

Ethernet: A low-level networking standard used in local area networks. It defines wiring specifics and types of electrical signals transmitted.

Firewall: An electronic "security wall" that connects two or more computer networks yet secures one network from the other.

FTP: File transfer protocol. A high-level protocol designed for reliable transfer of digital files from computer to computer via the Internet. Transmission requires permission of both the sender and the recipient. A variant of FTP, *anonymous FTP*, allows information to be accessed by logging in a user name of anonymous. A Web database of anonymous FTP sites is termed "Archie."

HIS: Hospital information system. A computer-based information system necessary to manage a health care facility. Patient information, admission and discharge, billing, scheduling, medical procedures, and pharmacy are items that may be included in an HIS. Ideally, the HIS is integrated into the radiology information system.

HL-7: Health level 7. A nonprofit organization founded in 1987 that develops standards for transmission of electronic clinical, financial, and administrative data among health care computer systems.

HTTP: Hypertext transfer protocol. A high-level Internet protocol that defines the World Wide Web (www). This protocol allows Web browsers to speak to Web servers. Hypertext markup language (HTML) is the language used to transmit information.

Internet: Computers world wide connected by common high-level communication protocols using TCP/IP lower layer communication language.

Intranet: A private Internet.

IP: Internet protocol. A low-level protocol used to assign computer addresses. The addresses consist of 4 numbers between 0 and 255, each separated by a period (e.g., 199.193.45.7)

Jpeg (jpg): Joint Photographic Experts Group. A lossy compression technique and popular image format used to minimize file size and download time. It reduces file size to as low as 5% of the original size, with a loss of image resolution.

LAN: Local area network.

Matrix: A grid arrangement of pixels, expressed as numbers representing the amount of horizontal and vertical pixels used (e.g., 256×256).

PACS: Picture archiving and communication system. A broad term involving computers and components used to capture, transfer, store, and display medical digital information.

Pixel: Picture element.

PSP: Photostimulable phosphor.

RAID: Redundant array of inexpensive disks. Multiple inexpensive disk archives are configured such that storage, access, and redundancy of information can be increased more reliably than by use of a single, larger-capacity disk.

RIS: Radiology information system. A computer system that handles all of the information necessary to operate a radiology department. RIS manages patient information, scheduling of imaging procedures, radiology reporting, and a database allowing case search capabilities. HIS, RIS, and PACS systems must communicate effectively.

Scintillation devices: Materials that emit visible or ultraviolet light when exposed to x-rays.

SCP: Service class provider. The DICOM term for a server program.

SCU: Service class user. The DICOM term for a client program.

Server: A computer system that provides information upon request from a client (user).

SMTP: Simple mail transport protocol.

Spatial resolution: The ability to distinguish between two small, separate structures. Loss of spatial resolution renders two closely spaced small objects to appear as one structure. Usually measured as line pairs per millimeter. The best screen-film systems still have better spatial resolution than digital systems, but this is compensated for by the increased contrast resolution that digital radiography offers.

TCP: Transmission control protocol. A protocol for breaking information into smaller packets for data transmission.

TIFF: Tagged image file format. A popular public domain raster file format for image storage. Digital radiographic images stored in TIFF format are not compressed and therefore are large files (megabytes).

WWW: World Wide Web. Internet computers that exchange information via the HTTP protocol.

INTRODUCTION

Computers have become an integral part of our daily lives. More than half of the households in the United States have computers, and 60% of adults and an amazing 84% of young people (3 to 17 years) use a computer at work, school, or home. Not surprisingly, radiology has entered the computer age. What is surprising is that as the oldest imaging modality, radiography has been the last to make the conversion to the digital age. This speaks highly of how well conventional film-based radiography has served the medical profession since Conrad Roentgen's discovery of x-rays November 8, 1895.

HISTORY OF DIGITAL RADIOGRAPHY

Magnetic resonance imaging (MRI) and computed tomography (CT) began as digital imaging modalities with their inception in the 1970s, and ultrasound (US) and nuclear medicine (NM) have fully evolved into digital technologies. However, the evolution of digital radiography (DR) has been much slower, for two principle reasons. First and foremost, conventional screen film radiography has been used for decades and has served the medical profession well; there has not been a pressing need to convert to digital radiography. Secondly, the large field-of-view (e.g., 14×17 in radiographic image) and high spatial resolution of radiography require large amounts of digital data (4 to 32 MB) and demand high-quality monitors for viewing when compared with MRI, CT, and US.

Although conventional radiography has been a mainstay in diagnostic imaging, we are now wholly entrenched in an era of computers and digital data. Over the past 20 years digital radiographic image receptors have steadily replaced traditional screen-film cassettes as human medicine radiology departments transition to a filmless environment. In the early 1980s Fujifilm Medical Systems introduced the first digital radiography technology, known as *computed radiography* (CR). Traditionally, high cost has limited CR to human medical facilities and a few select veterinary colleges and private specialty veterinary practices. Maturation of digital technology, with lower costs and available veterinary-specific digital imaging equipment, has now enabled veterinary medicine to realize the benefits of digital radiography. Veterinary digital radiography is now growing at a frenzied pace.

DIGITAL RADIOGRAPHY: AN OVERVIEW

The concept of digital radiography is quite simple. The primary difference between conventional film-based radiology and digital radiology is that radiographic images are electronically captured, recorded, and viewed at a computer terminal, replacing radiographic film and the view box. The conventional screen-film cassette is replaced by a reusable image receptor (detector). The image receptor receives x-rays just as conventional intensifying screens do. Instead of exposing radiographic film, however, intensifying screens or other scintillation devices expose a "digital plate" that transforms emitted light to an electrical latent image. The different ways in which this is accomplished are discussed in detail in the following sections. The x-ray tube, generator, and peripheral x-ray machine hardware are essentially the same for conventional or digital radiography. Indeed, many of the available digital radiography systems use preexisting x-ray equipment (Fig. 22-1).

After the digital radiographic image is made, it is transferred to a dedicated digital radiography computer for "image processing" (Fig. 22-2). Here, the images can be adjusted as needed by the veterinary technologist. In small practices this may be the only computer available to view, but in most instances the processed image is finalized and then sent to another dedicated computer *workstation* for diagnostic interpretation by the veterinarian (Fig. 22-3). In large hospitals where multiple diagnostic workstations are necessary, the images will be sent to a main centralized computer (called a server) for storage and distribution to other workstation computers or sent off site via the World Wide Web for review.

The term *picture archiving and communication system* (PACS) is the broad term for computers and components used to capture, transfer, store, and display medical digital information. Digital images can also be printed on high-quality transparent film (laser printers) to be viewed at a conventional illuminated view box, though most practices that make the conversion to digital radiography opt to go "filmless," one of the major advantages of digital imaging.

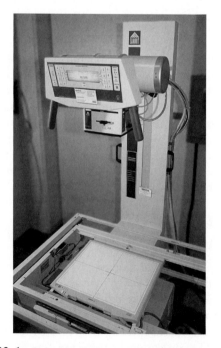

Figure 22-1 *Conventional x-ray machine with a flat panel detector digital radiography system. The tabletop of the x-ray machine has been removed to show the position of the detector panel.*

LIMITATIONS OF CONVENTIONAL SCREEN-FILM RADIOGRAPHY

Although conventional screen-film radiography has served the medical community well for many years, its limitations make digital radiography an attractive alternative. First, screen-film radiography requires fairly narrow exposure factors to produce a diagnostic quality radiograph. Because x-ray film has a limited linear response (recall the logarithmic toe, linear region, and shoulder of a radiographic film Hunter and Driffield curve), relatively small underexposure or overexposure may yield an unacceptable image. This is why a radiographic technique chart is required and radiographic technique adjustments are necessary for various anatomic areas (thorax, abdomen, skeletal); body part thicknesses (incremental changes in kilovoltage potential (kVp) per centimeter of body part thickness); and different screen-film speeds. In many instances the inherent latitude limitation of conventional screen film radiology means that some areas of the radiograph will be overexposed while other areas will be underexposed. Depending on technical factors chosen, the radiograph can be made with relatively high contrast (e.g., a low kVp bone technique) or wide latitude (more shades of gray, as desired for thoracic radiography), but not both. A compromise is always possible.

Another disadvantage with conventional screen-film radiography is that the radiographic image cannot be adjusted once made. The radiographic film is exposed and then processed and viewed. Any errors in the exposure cannot be remedied; the radiograph must be retaken. This leads to increase in radiation exposure to the technician and patient, increases the cost of the examination, and requires additional technician and veterinarian time. Because the digital image can be manipulated after it is made, overexposure and underexposure problems are essentially a thing of the past with digital radiography.

Traditional radiography requires handling of film for viewing, archiving (storage), and distribution to referring veterinary practices. Reviewing a radiographic examination from a remote location requires that the study either be copied and sent via courier or digitally scanned before electronic transmission. Film storage requires an area large enough to access and sort films, often a separate area from the patient's medical records.

ADVANTAGES OF DIGITAL RADIOGRAPHY

The Image

Unlike traditional screen-film radiography, kVp has little or no effect on the contrast or latitude of the digital image (this can be endlessly adjusted with software at the digital radiography computer terminal and diagnostic workstation). This flexibility is possible because of the

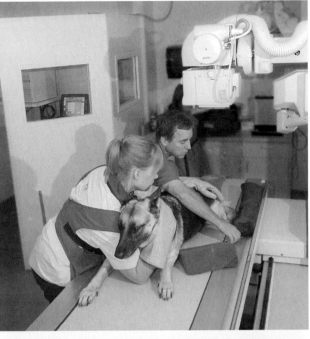

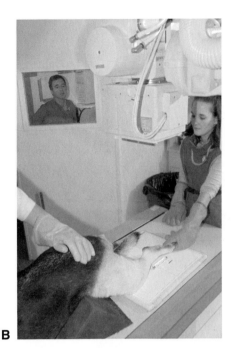

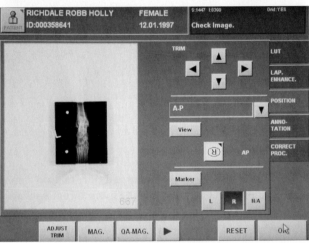

Figure 22-2 *Making the digital radiograph.* **A**, *This German shepherd is prepared for a caudocranial view of the tarsus. The local digital work station and radiology controls are in the background, behind a leaded glass and wall.* **B**, *The flat panel detector panel is positioned on the tabletop for caudocranial radiography of the left tarsus. A 10-cm bar marker has been placed lateral to the limb to allow for computer correction of magnification. In this application the detector panel is mobile and can be used for a multitude of positional studies including horizontal beam radiography. The panel can also be placed under the table for conventional radiography, with or without a grid. The radiology technologist is seen in the background in the control area.* **C**, *The local digital work station where the radiographic image of the tarsus appears following exposure. On this "Position" screen, the technologist can alter the orientation of the image, magnify the image, and make masking adjustments (black-out the white collimation). Note the tabs to the left of the screen that offer further choices on image manipulation.*

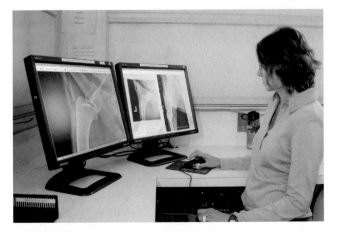

Figure 22-3 *Diagnostic workstation. This workstation uses a dual-monitor viewing system. The image of the humerus on the left monitor has been magnified for close scrutiny; two images on the right monitor are unmagnified. The workstation software applications allow the veterinarian to perform a multitude of image manipulations to optimize the image for diagnosis.*

linear relationship of the image receptors used for digital radiography. Simplistically, the number of electrons "trapped" by the digital image receptor during an x-ray exposure is linearly related to the intensity of the x-ray beam. Digital images have more latitude (more shades of gray) than film images and can display high-contrast body parts while simultaneously displaying soft tissues. This high gray-scale (high latitude) resolution is desirable because it allows observation of minor differences in radiation attenuation that may not be visible with film. When compared with conventional screen-film technique charts, digital technique charts do not vary greatly for the body part radiographed or patient thickness.

The higher-contrast resolution (or exposure latitude) of digital radiography has several tremendous advantages over conventional screen-film radiography. The need for retakes resulting from overexposure and underexposure is reduced, and for the most part eliminated. Images that

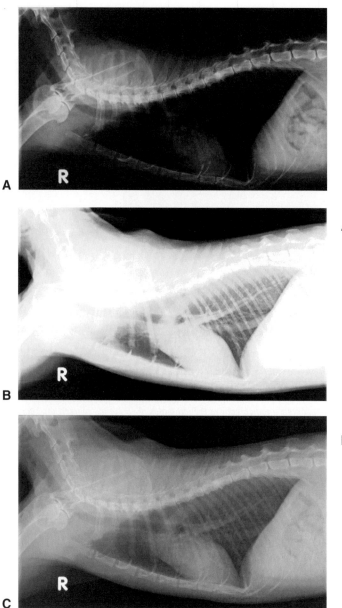

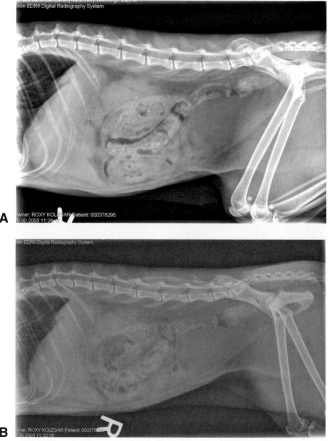

Figure 22-5 *Feline digital abdominal image.* **A,** *High contrast image. Note the high contrast between bone, soft tissue, and fat.* **B,** *High-latitude image.*

Figure 22-4 *Lateral thoracic radiographic image of a cat illustrates how overexposure (**A**) and underexposure (**B**) can be image processed to produce a perfectly exposed image (**C**). With conventional film-screen radiography, the improperly exposed studies would require retaking the radiographs.*

are too light or dark that would be discarded on radiographic film can be adjusted with the digital image management software (Fig. 22-4). Marginal radiographic images, which may have previously been deemed acceptable, are a thing of the past.

Computer manipulation of the digital image is a phenomenal advantage that digital radiography has over conventional screen-film radiography. Images can be altered for contrast or latitude (Fig. 22-5) and can be zoomed (magnified) (see Fig. 22-3) to scrutinize the image as if using a magnifying glass to view a radiographic film. Digital viewing software packages offer a variety of ways

to view digital images including subtraction tools that make it possible to view bone-only or soft-tissue-only images from a single exposure. Digital radiography makes it possible to see both soft tissue and bony detail in a single image. Because of the high exposure latitude, an unprocessed digital image usually does not look the same as a film/screen radiograph. Although digital images can be manipulated to mimic the appearance of conventional radiographs (Fig. 22-6), usually the image is adjusted to take advantage of simultaneous high contrast and high latitude. Curiously, the appearance of digital images is resisted by some veterinarians who are accustomed to viewing high-contrast radiographs. Getting accustomed to viewing digital images is one small initial disadvantage of digital radiography, but quickly overcome.

The spatial resolution of digital images is at best the same, but usually slightly lower than a high-quality radiographic film image. This is not a disadvantage in most instances because there is a limit to how much spatial resolution the human eye can discriminate. As digital technology advances, differences in spatial resolution between conventional and digital radiography have become almost negligible. Human medical studies have shown that digital images are equal to or better than traditional film for evaluating most body parts. This is

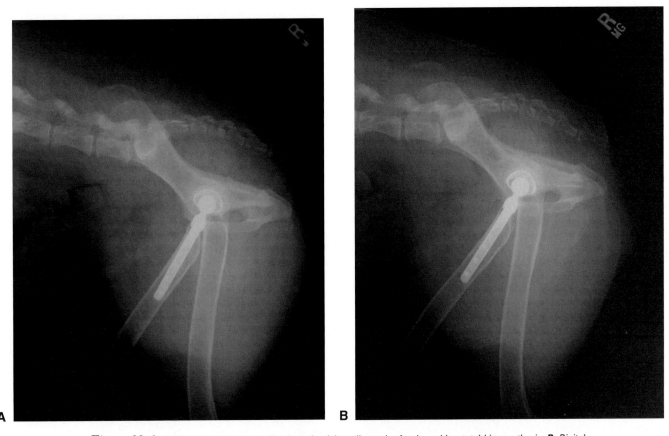

Figure 22-6 *A*, Conventional screen-film lateral pelvic radiograph of a dog with a total hip prosthesis. *B*, Digital radiographic image of the same patient. Note that high-quality conventional screen-film radiography can be similar to digital radiographic images.

because there is a point at which spatial resolution yields way to contrast resolution (the ability to separate two structures of different contrast, or x-ray attenuation), the hallmark of what makes digital radiography so diagnostic. Image quality and the ability to detect abnormalities are actually more dependent on postdigital image acquisition processing than on spatial resolution. Digital radiography has been clinically validated for 20 years in various human medical settings including mammography, indicating that its minimally lower spatial resolution is not a clinical limitation.

Digital radiography software not only allows an image to be manipulated for optimum viewing, but also measured, drawn on, and annotated. Heart dimensions (e.g., the vertebral heart score), pulmonary nodule size, or hip or tibial plateau angles can be measured and stored. These measurements and comments can be printed directly onto the image, with the original image retained as a separate, unaltered digital file. Highlighting suspect areas and noting comments on the image can make future readings easier. Additionally, templates used for total hip replacement and tibial plateau leveling osteotomy procedures (TPLO) have now become incorporated into some vendor software, allowing surgical planning directly from the diagnostic workstation.

Time Savings

Digital radiography will decrease the time it takes to make radiographic images. This is especially true of charged coupled devices (CCDs) and flat panel receptor digital imaging systems because images are literally available for viewing several seconds following the radiographic exposure. CR has an inherent disadvantage in that each CR cassette must be processed in a manner similar to a conventional radiographic film processor. Of course, CR is definitely faster when compared with manual film processing. Still, all of the digital modalities will save time due to better-quality images and a reduced number of retake radiographs caused by technical issues. Radiology-related case management should be more efficient, as the veterinarian can obtain the image more readily, render a diagnosis or list of differential diagnoses, and communicate with the client sooner. This is especially true for clinics with manual processing or mobile practices. Practices that have inefficient workflow patterns will not receive maximum benefit of the time savings afforded by digital radiography.

Repeating radiographs (the dreaded "retake") is common in veterinary medicine because of improper exposure techniques, patient motion, and positioning problems.

Repeat radiographs are significantly reduced with digital radiography. Specifically, exposure-related retakes should be essentially eliminated. Secondly, patient motion artifacts can be reduced by reducing radiographic exposure time (selecting a higher kVp and a corresponding lower mAs technique). Recall that kVp is no longer a factor in radiographic image contrast and latitude, so this can be done without altering image contrast. It should be obvious that repeat radiographs require additional veterinarian and technician time and are costly in terms of wasted film and film development chemicals. Patient resedation and additional radiation and film development chemicals exposure to personnel are yet further concerns of retaking radiographs. Repeat trips to the clinic for the client and additional farm visits or house calls for the veterinarian are added examples of the negative impact of retake radiographs.

Image Storage and Transport

Digital images are stored on the local computer dedicated to the digital system. Images are typically transferred to a second computer (or "server") for permanent storage and distribution (within large hospitals or distribution outside of the hospital). Image files can be stored or transferred in other formats (e.g., jpg, bmp, tiff) depending on the image management software. Like other computer files, these should be backed up to avoid loss or corruption of patient data. Backup strategies include copies to CD, DVD, additional hard drives, or outside archival sources.

One feature of digital image storage is that quick access and viewing is simply a computer search. No more hunting for lost radiographs! With today's demand for fast information, having access to a digital file offers veterinarians a distinct advantage over retrieving and viewing a conventional radiographic film.

Digital storage allows easy transferability of images via electronic mail (e-mail). Veterinarians commonly send cases via the World Wide Web to consulting or referring veterinarians. In emergency situations, nearly instantaneous consultation could be lifesaving for the patient. Large images must be sent off site via file transfer protocol (FTP) or custom teleradiology systems or converted to compressed formats (e.g., jpg) for effective transmission. Network PACS that allow access to the database are found in larger practices or universities and can solve some problems (e.g., veterinarians can access the larger system from a remote location and view the radiographs without downloading them onto their own computer).

A CD of the images can be made for the client or for a veterinary colleague. Laser printers are available to print digital images on transparent film, similar to a conventional radiograph that is viewed on a view box. Clients may request and be happy with a paper print copy for their records. Equine practices may wish to provide radiographic or paper copies for clients and their farriers when corrective shoeing is indicated.

Cost Savings and Increasing Profits

Much has been written and spoken regarding the cost benefits of digital radiography. By most accounts, digital radiography makes fiscal sense. Although the overall cost of purchasing a digital radiography system is higher than that of a film developer (processor), there are a number of cost savings associated with digital radiography. Fewer retakes result in reduced use of the x-ray machine, there are no film processor expenses (chemicals and maintenance), film purchasing is no longer required, and radiography is less labor intensive. For high-volume practices, the monthly cost of film, processor maintenance, and chemicals may be higher than the monthly lease of a new digital radiography system.

Another consideration is that in most practices, digital radiography improves the quality of the imaging studies. This in turn leads to better diagnostic information and potentially increased profitability. Increases in efficiency and diagnostic capability will probably lead to an increase in the number of radiographic studies performed. Some clients may actually demand it, especially equine clientele. Digital radiography vendors are well versed in showing how your practice can make digital radiography not only cost effective, but profitable.

Follow-up Radiography

Sequential or follow-up radiographs are a component of good case management, to assess response to therapy, monitor progression of disease, etc. Comparison of follow-up images is easier with digital radiography than with traditional radiography, as the images can be manipulated to have the same degree of contrast and latitude. Although differences associated with phase of respiration or poor positioning may still occur, subtle differences that may be masked or overinterpreted due to exposure differences should be minimized. Also, prior images can be quickly accessed from computer archives for comparison (remember, no more lost or misplaced radiographs to search for). Ambulatory veterinarians can access prior images on site rather than returning to the hospital to make comparisons.

DISADVANTAGES OF DIGITAL RADIOGRAPHY

Training and Learning Curve

Disadvantages of using digital radiography are minimal when compared with the advantages already outlined. These include changing and getting accustomed to a new imaging system, the need for personnel training, and cost. Manipulation of digital images takes time and practice and is somewhat dependent on the user's computer skills.

Digital manipulation cannot make all images useful. Gross errors in exposure factors or patient motion cannot be overcome with image enhancement. Veterinarians must also be careful not to overprocess an image and create artifacts (e.g., apparent lesions) through software manipulation. Comparing the unprocessed image with the manipulated one is a way of detecting processing artifacts.

Digital radiography will not compensate for poor radiographic techniques or poor staff training. Improper labeling or misidentification of patients will undermine image storage and retrieval functions. Investment in a new digital radiography system should establish a renewed commitment to diagnostic imaging.

Equipment Costs

Digital radiography systems are costly, although their prices are falling and they are affordable and economical for most practices. Direct costs include the computer hardware, software, and optional higher-quality paper for printing (images are to be viewed on the monitor for diagnosis and reading fine detail). The initial cost of the digital radiography system must be weighed against the benefits of becoming filmless, using less film and chemicals, and the important benefit of increased efficiency. The cost savings of a digital radiography system grows over time as the number of retakes is reduced.

The cost of consumables in conventional screen-film radiography includes film, film jackets, fixer, developer, and disposal of toxic chemicals. Digital technology eliminates those costs. Recall that digital images must be backed up just like other computer files. If veterinarians want printed copies of each image, hard-copy storage space will not be reduced.

HIS, RIS, and PACS

Nearly all veterinary practices now have some form of computerized hospital patient identification and medical record keeping or hospital information system (HIS). A HIS is a computer program that allows patient information to be entered into the hospital computer system upon admission. It can be used for electronic medical record keeping. Ideally, the HIS communicates with the digital imaging system directly or via a radiology information system (RIS). Patient information is thus entered into the hospital computer system only once, interfaced with the RIS for immediate access to patient identification and imaging procedure.

The type of imaging studies required, the scheduling and status of the radiography examination, and even the radiology report are functions of an RIS interfaced with HIS, with information stored, accessed, and distributed via the PACS. Digital images can also be placed into electronic patient records, one step closer to an integrated and totally digital (paperless) medical record system. The PACS server can accommodate all forms of digital imaging technology such as ultrasound, computed tomography, nuclear medicine, and magnetic resonance

imaging. Other digital imaging examinations such as endoscopy can also be stored and viewed via PACS.

As mentioned previously, the term PACS encompasses computers and related components used to capture, transfer, store, and display medical digital information. In addition to the multitude of PACS created for human medical use, veterinary-specific PACS have been developed by a number of vendors. PACS allow communication between computers. Some users of digital radiography do not use PACS but instead simply use the image software provided by the manufacturer to manipulate and view the data. However, this severely limits the ability to distribute digital images for consultation. For large practices, some form of PACS is necessary to realize all of the advantages of digital radiography.

Digital Imaging and Communications in Medicine

The American College of Radiology and the National Electrical Manufacturer's Association formed a joint committee to develop a global standard for Digital Imaging and Communications in Medicine (DICOM). DICOM was intended to realize the interoperability between multiple devices manufactured by different vendors (e.g., transmission of images or information, displaying of an image). DICOM's scope is diagnostic imaging. DICOM images are embedded, extensive, detailed, and specific information. DICOM embedded information cannot be altered. Each piece of DICOM equipment is uniquely identified such that a DICOM image can be precisely identified as to its origin; each DICOM image is unique.

The DICOM standard is now embraced by the veterinary imaging community, ensuring the highest possible standard of quality. DICOM compliance assures that digital images can be transferred and read safely by any DICOM workstation software.

IMAGE MANAGEMENT SOFTWARE AND IMAGE PROCESSING

Before digital image acquisition, patient information is entered into the digital radiography computer. If an HIS is interfaced to the digital radiography computer (this may be direct or more commonly via a RIS), this information is automatically entered into the digital radiography computer, a significant savings. In the best systems, there are preset selections available for species, body part of interest, and radiographic view to further identify the study type. Following acquisition, the digital image is viewed on the digital radiography computer for processing (see Fig. 22-2). Here, the image can be adjusted if necessary in a variety of ways using manufacturer-specific software. Image processing tools include brightness, contrast, magnification, inverting black and white, edge enhancement, a number of image processing curves (algorithms), and image cropping and masking. The digital radiography image processing software is manufacturer specific and is an area of rapid development in veterinary medicine. Use of equipment designed for human use requires adoption of software for veterinary use for optimum realization of digital imaging. Understanding and learning how to use this software is one of the biggest challenges for the veterinary technologist when converting to digital radiography.

In small practices the digital imaging computer may be the only computer available, especially if digital images are printed on transparent film for viewing. In most instances, however, the processed, finalized images are sent to a dedicated computer *workstation* for diagnostic interpretation by the veterinarian (see Fig. 22-3).

ANALOG-TO-DIGITAL RADIOGRAPHIC SIGNAL CONVERSION

A conventional radiograph is produced by a series of *analog* signals, from x-ray formation and interaction with the patient, to capture of x-rays by the intensifying screen, which in turn emit light that exposes the radiographic film. The final radiographic image results by development of silver halide contained within the emulsion of the x-ray film. As previously mentioned, the *origin* of a digital radiographic image is identical to a conventional radiographic image. The difference is conversion of the analog signal (light emitted from scintillation screens) to an electronic digital signal by use of a digital radiographic device, explained in detail shortly.

An analog signal is a waveform—a continuous electrical signal. Its electrical value is represented as a voltage value. A digital signal is produced from an analog signal by way of an analog-to-digital converter (ADC). The ADC samples the analog waveform and transforms it into a "stepped" representative signal. The more times the analog signal is digitally sampled, the closer the digital waveform is to the original analog waveform. The frequency of digital sampling is termed *sampling rate*. Sampling rates in the 10s to 100s of thousands per second are necessary to accurately digitally replicate an analog waveform. An analog waveform and its digital conversion are depicted in Figure 22-7.

DIGITAL COMPUTERS

For many people familiar with personal computers, terminology used for digital imaging computers is already part of their daily vocabulary. For others, a comprehensive review of digital computers is beyond the scope of this chapter. Nonetheless, is important for the veterinary radiology technologist to be at least familiar with the

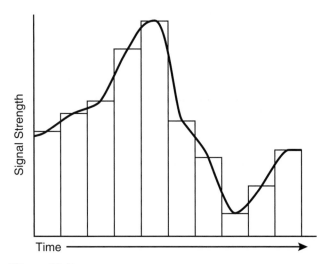

Figure 22-7 *Analog-to-digital (ADC) waveform conversion. The analog waveform is the curved continuous black line. Conversion of this analog waveform to a digital waveform is accomplished by a series of "steps." Note that the digital waveform only approximates the original analog signal. The number of digital "steps" per unit time (seconds) is termed sampling rate. The more digital samples per unit time, the higher the sampling rate and the closer the digital sample to the original. In this example the sampling rate is low. An ADC is used to make the conversion from analog to digital waveforms.*

concepts and terminology of computers as used in digital imaging.

The digital waveform is represented numerically for computer analysis by *binary numbers*. Unlike the base 10 (decimal) numerical language that we are all familiar with (ten digits, 0 through 9), the binary system uses only two digits (0 and 1) to represent numbers. The smallest binary number is termed a *bit* and has four numerical possibilities (0; 0.1; 1,0; 1,1, which correspond to the numbers 0, 1, 2, and 3, respectively). Electronically, this can be thought of in terms of an ON/OFF switch, where 0 is off and 1 is on. Large numbers are represented by a series of 0s and 1s. This is convenient because any given numerical value can be represented electronically by a series of ON/OFF switches.

Each digital sample is assigned a binary value on the basis of the voltage signal strength of the original analog waveform. Between 8 and 12 bits are used in digital imaging to represent digital voltage values. Depending on equipment specifications, each pixel (defined shortly) will be assigned a binary number between 0 and 255 (8 bits of information, or relatively poor resolution) to as high as 0 to 4095 (12 bits of information, high resolution). Digital radiography requires 10 or preferably 12 bits of numerical value per pixel for diagnostic resolution. The more bits available, the larger the range of possible numbers stored per pixel. This translates into increased contrast resolution, the various shades of gray between black and white. These numerical values are then displayed as a particular corresponding shade of gray on the video monitor. The more shades of gray, the better, and this is known as "image depth." As discussed later, many display options are available to maximize the diagnostic quality of the digital image. As an aside, lack of bit or image depth is one reason that a digital photograph of a conventional radiograph made from an illuminated view box is not satisfactory for all but the most obvious lesion. A digital photographic image of a radiograph is NOT of the same diagnostic quality as a true digital radiograph.

Computer memory and storage consist of *bits* (for **bi**nary dig**its**), each bit representing one binary digit. Eight (8) bits are grouped into a larger unit, termed *byte*. One byte (or 8 bits) has 256 number configurations of 0 and 1s (numerical values of 0 to 255), whereas 2 bytes (16 bits) has 65,536 possible configurations (numbers of 0 to 65,535). Computer capacity is described in kilobytes (2^{10} bytes, or 1000 bytes), megabytes (2^{20} bytes, a million bytes), gigabytes (2^{30} bytes, a billion bytes), and terabytes (2^{40} bytes, a trillion bytes). Terabyte storage capability is required for large hospitals using digital imaging modalities. Bits are also grouped into larger units, called *words*. This terminology is important when assessing computer usable memory, storage capacity, and digital radiography specifications.

As you can see, the computer is at the heart of digital image processing. Advances in imaging have gone hand-in-hand with increases in computer speed and storage capabilities. Computers allow digital information to be processed and viewed in the most diagnostic manner. It is emphasized that computer processing of digital images does not add any *new* information to the digital image; it only changes the way in which we view the image. Still, manipulation of the image allows a phenomenal variety and number of viewing options that may allow a diagnosis to be made that would otherwise go undetected.

PIXELS AND IMAGE MATRIX

In digital radiography the x-ray beam is converted into an electronic form that is digitized and numerically encoded into millions of tiny, discrete squares of digital information known as *pixels* (picture elements). Pixels are arranged in a *matrix* of rows and columns; each row and column is made up of pixels. Matrix sizes depend on the digital modality. For example, CT, US, and MRI are usually in a 512 pixel × 512 pixel matrix, while digital radiography requires smaller and more numerous pixels for higher spatial resolution demands (e.g., 2000 × 2500 matrix or more). Each pixel represents an electronic signal, corresponding to the intensity of the x-ray signal at any given location within the patient. Each pixel can only display a single value (shade of gray). The concept of pixels and matrix is shown in Figure 22-8.

It should be intuitive that the smaller the pixel, the better image resolution (think of a photograph made using 1000 ASA film versus one made with 100 ASA; the 1000 ASA photograph is grainy when compared with the 100 ASA photo). Pixel size is determined by the size of the image divided by matrix size. As an example,

if a thoracic image is 35 cm (roughly 14 inches) × 43 cm (17 inches) and the matrix size is 2000 × 2500, pixel size would be approximately 0.17 mm × 0.17 mm. Pixel size determines spatial resolution, the ability to separate two closely spaced objects. Actual spatial resolution of the digital image is further determined by the efficiency of the imaging plate and other design criteria.

VIEWING DIGITAL IMAGES

Display Monitors

All diagnostic review of digital images should be made through a high-quality display monitor. The ability of the viewer to appreciate the image quality obtained with digital radiography depends largely on the quality of the computer monitor.

Important considerations when assessing viewing station monitors include screen size, resolution, brightness, and gray-scale versus color capabilities. Although waning in popularity, the oldest and most familiar type of monitor is the cathode ray tube (CRT), which is similar to the picture tube in a conventional television set and uses an "electron gun" to illuminate each pixel. CRT monitors can be gray scale ("black and white") or color. Gray-scale monitors have a greater dynamic range (are brighter) than color CRT monitors and can yield higher resolution. This is because there is only one electron gun per monitor pixel. Conversely, a color monitor has a red, green, and blue electron gun for each pixel; therefore the pixels are larger. Although a color monitor is not necessary for digital radiography, it is necessary for viewing color Doppler ultrasound images and useful for nuclear medicine image viewing as well. Flat panel monitors use liquid crystal display technology (LCD) and have become popular over the past several years, superseding the CRT because of lower cost and smaller size (depth).

As an example, a high-resolution, diagnostic, gray-scale, 20-inch monitor may have 2048 × 1536 pixels (known as 3-megapixel), while a high-quality, color, 19-inch diagnostic monitor may have a matrix size of 1600 × 1200. Note that these monitors offer a matrix size that is smaller than that of many digital image receptors. Medical-grade, gray-scale monitors are expensive ($10,000 or more), while high-quality color monitors are one-tenth this price. Vendors of digital radiography equipment often prefer a particular brand of monitor.

Film and Paper

Alternatively, diagnostic hard-copy images can be made by printing to a high-quality laser film (transparent film that resembles standard radiographic film), viewed using an illuminated view box. Use of film-based digital imaging in place of a computer diagnostic workstation viewing counteracts one of the primary advantages of digital imaging (i.e., going filmless). Nondiagnostic-quality paper

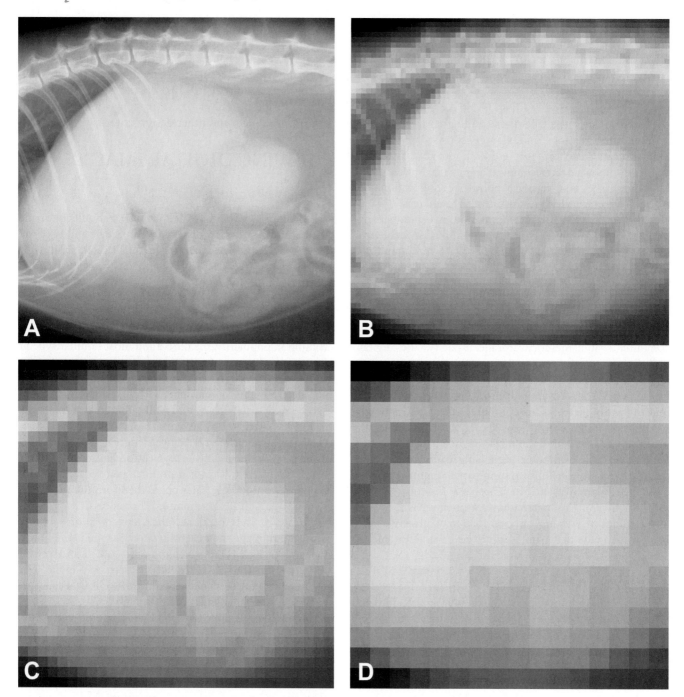

Figure 22-8 *The effects of matrix and pixel size on image resolution are illustrated in this series of otherwise identical lateral cat abdominal radiographic images. **A,** A high-quality digital image with a high matrix size (e.g., 2048 pixels on the vertical axis × 2048 pixels across the horizontal axis). **B,** The matrix size is reduced to 64 × 64 pixels. Note that individual pixels can be seen as small squares, and the image has a pixilated appearance. **C,** The pixilation becomes noticeably worse when the matrix size is reduced to 32 × 32. **D,** The matrix size is only 16 × 16 pixels, and the image of the cat abdomen is no longer recognizable. Note that each pixel only represents a single shade of gray, dependent on bit number.*

images can be made to print out digital images for record keeping purposes.

TYPES OF DIGITAL RADIOGRAPHY (DR)

Digital receptors are generally classified as *indirect* or *direct* digital conversion systems. Indirect systems use a two-part process, converting x-ray energy first to light and then to an electronic (digital) signal. The indirect digital systems include photostimulable phosphor (PSP) imaging plates (used in CR), CCDs, and silicon flat panel receptors. Direct systems convert x-ray energy directly into an electrical (digital) signal. Using selenium detectors, these are correctly referred to as direct digital radiography systems (DDRs). DDRs are not commonly used even in

human medicine due to great manufacturing costs. However, they yield the highest spacial resolution currently available.

Three principle types of digital image receptors are available to veterinarians: CR, flat panel detectors, and the CCD.

COMPUTED RADIOGRAPHY

CR was introduced to the medical community in the 1980s by Fujifilm Medical Systems. Although it has become common in human medicine over the past 20 years, CR has only recently been introduced to the veterinary community. Idexx markets a CR system designed for veterinary use. Agfa, Fuji, and Kodak are major human medical CR manufacturers that have shown an interest in the veterinary market.

CR is the term for digital imaging systems using a phosphostimulable phosphor (PSP) detector screen. The PSP screen *absorbs and stores* most of the incident x-ray energy (latent image), which is to be "read out" later. Because PSP screens store energy, they are also known as storage *phosphors* or *CR imaging plates*. By contrast, conventional screen-film intensifying screens do not *store* energy. Instead, they emit light instantaneously upon x-ray interaction, in turn exposing the radiographic film (latent image production), which is later developed into a radiograph.

PSP screens are composed of several layers—an outer protective layer, a phosphor layer (active component of system), a polyester support layer, a conductive layer (grounds plate to eliminate electrostatic interference and absorbs light, increasing image sharpness), and a light shield layer (prevents visible light from erasing data). The phosphor layer of a PSP screen is a barium fluorohalide phosphor composition (BaFlBr and BaFI).

The CR system can be thought of as using a filmless cassette. The PSP screens are thin, rigid yet flexible layered sheets (10×12, 14×17) and fit into a cassette, nearly identical to conventional screen-film cassettes. CR cassettes are used identically to conventional screen-film cassettes, placed on a tabletop or in a cassette ("Bucky") tray for under-table use, with or without a grid. One PSP imaging plate is used per exposure. Following exposure, the CR cassette is taken to a laser CR reader unit (also known as an *Image Reader Device* [IRD], *"CR processor,"* or *plate reader*, among others) for processing the latent image.

The following occurs after exposure of the CR cassette:

1. The CR cassette is placed into the CR reader, where it is automatically opened and the CR plate removed.
2. As the CR plate moves through the processor, it is scanned by a helium-neon laser beam. The laser light stimulates release of trapped x-ray energy stored in the CR plate as visible light.
3. The released visible light is collected by fiberoptics to a photomultiplier tube, producing an electrical signal.
4. The electrical signal is digitized and stored on a computer.
5. The CR plate is then exposed to a bright white light, *erasing* any residual latent image.
6. The CR plate is returned to the cassette, ejected from the CR reader, and ready to reuse.

CR readers vary in speed of processing. The simplest CR readers require the user to actually remove the CR plate and place it into the CR reader (a process similar to a fax or photocopy machine). The most robust units allow multiple CR cassettes to be "stacked," automatically feeding, processing, and ejecting each CR cassette following reading and erasing. The CR reading process is analogous to an automatic x-ray film processor used with conventional screen-film systems. Thus there is little or no time savings of CR over screen-film systems from an image development point of view. CR is well-suited for equine radiography as the cassettes are portable.

The digital image is stored temporarily on a local or dedicated hard disk. As local storage is limited (several thousand images), digital images must ultimately be transferred to permanent storage in a larger-capacity computer or PACS if they are to be stored and archived digitally. Alternatively, "hard copy" can be made. Most common is film (similar in look and feel to a conventional radiograph), but images may be printed on paper (for archival purposes only, not for diagnosis).

Other Computed Radiography Considerations

PSP screens maximally absorb x-rays in the 35 to 50 keV range, due to the barium k-edge. This is lower than conventional rare earth screen film systems. Below and above this range, however, absorption is inferior to rare earth systems and therefore more exposure may be necessary when using CR systems compared with 400-speed, screen-film systems.

The latent image is formed by attenuation of x-ray energy within the PSP plate, stored as light. Although PSP plates do *release* some light during x-ray exposure (i.e., they are not 100% efficient in capturing energy), enough energy remains to form a latent image. The latent image is converted to a digital image for computer storage and display. It should be noted that the latent image is temporary, losing 25% or more of its energy within 8 hours. Therefore CR cassettes must be processed in a timely manner, preferably within several hours of exposure. Also, because of their sensitivity to secondary radiation, they must be stored carefully and should routinely be "erased" before use. This is essential if CR plates have not been used for 24 hours or more. Failure to do so will result in artifacts and reduced signal-to-noise from spurious exposure.

CHARGED COUPLED DEVICE

A CCD is a *small* flat panel device that is capable of creating images from visible light. A CCD receives and stores incoming light energy in the form of trapped electrons. The CCD chip is an integrated circuit (IC) composed of crystalline silicon. It is photosensitive and divided into thousands of tiny electronically isolated pixels etched into its surface (e.g., a 1024 × 1024 or 2048 × 2048 matrix). Because of this, the CCD may be referred to as a *pixilated light detector.* CCD technology has been used for a number of years in digital camera and video recorder applications. When used in a digital radiology system, the CCD is coupled to a rather conventional rare earth or CsI intensifying (scintillation) screen. When the intensifying screen fluoresces following interaction with x-rays, the CCD captures this emitted light and stores the energy in the form of "trapped" electrons within each pixel. Once exposed, stored electrons are "read out" and converted from an analog electrical signal to a digital signal by an analog to digital converter (ADC).

One of the primary limitations of CCD technology is the size restriction of the chip, dictated by manufacturing obstacles and expense. CCD chips may be quite small (2.5 cm × 2.5 cm for digital dental applications), while the largest detectors are only 8 × 8 cm or so (and expensive). Small CCD chips can be directly coupled to the intensifying screen, with excellent transfer of light energy and radiographic image formation. However, larger areas such as the abdomen or thorax require a much larger field of view (FOV), considerably greater than the size of even the largest CCD currently available. To produce a real-size image, a high-quality focusing lens is used to couple a large intensifying screen (14 × 17 inches, or 35 × 43 cm) onto a considerably smaller CCD (this is termed *demagnification factor*).

Use of a coupling lens results in a substantial loss (>90%) of light energy reaching the CCD. The resultant radiographic image is degraded by a grainy appearance, a result of quantum mottle. Recall that quantum mottle occurs when there is insufficient number of photons to produce a quality image. These have been the limiting factors in the use of CCD technology for digital radiography, especially in cost-effective veterinary applications. Nonetheless, veterinary-specific systems are now marketed.

The CCD hardware is located under the tabletop of the x-ray machine, completely out of sight (Fig. 22-9). Most of the available systems are packaged as complete systems (with x-ray tube, generator, electronics, and table), though retrofitting a conventional x-ray system is possible. A CCD digital system is not suitable for ambulatory use, as the equipment is not portable.

Several manufacturers in the human imaging field producing high-quality, CCD-based digital radiography units (e.g., Swissray). Although offering state-of-the-art performance, this high-end equipment is usually not cost effective for most private veterinary practices. Currently available veterinary CCD digital radiography systems

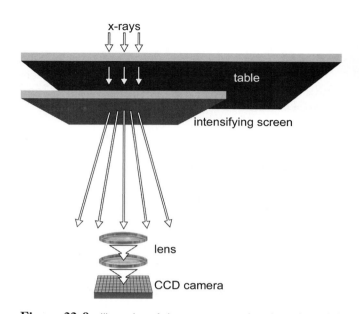

Figure 22-9 *Illustration of the components of a charged coupled device (CCD) digital x-ray system. An intensifying screen is placed underneath the x-ray table and coupled to the CCD via focusing mirrors. Notice the etched pixel matrix on the surface of the relatively small CCD device. NOTE: The "camera portion" of the CCD is not shown.*

include dental systems and systems designed for a small animal radiology suite. Veterinary specific manufacturers include Summit and HCMI.

FLAT PANEL DETECTORS

Large, full-size flat panel detectors have become popular over the past several years. They consist of a large (e.g., 10- × 12-inch or 14- × 17-inch) x-ray intensifying screen (cesium iodide or gadolinium and lanthanum oxysulfide scintillators) that is intimately coupled to an amorphous silicon flat panel serving as the light detector (photodiode).

Flat panel detectors are analogous to conventional screen film systems, but an electronic sensor layer, amorphous silicon, replaces x-ray film. The silicon detector consists of a matrix, composed of a large number of individual detector elements (Fig. 22-10). Each detector element is in turn composed of a light sensitive area and a smaller area of electronics, the ratio of which is termed "fill factor." Because each detector is an independent element, amorphous silicon detectors are more efficient and less susceptible to manufacturer imperfections than CCD technology.

Because the flat panel is a self-contained unit, it can be used for portable work (e.g., equine radiography) or permanently fixed beneath the x-ray tabletop for use in small animal radiology suites. The flat panel detector is hard-wired to the digital computer, which makes its use less flexible than CR for equine or field radiography. Current flat panel digital x-ray systems marketed for veterinary use include Eklin and Sound Technologies.

Because the flat panel is a self-contained unit, it can be used for portable work (e.g., equine radiography) or

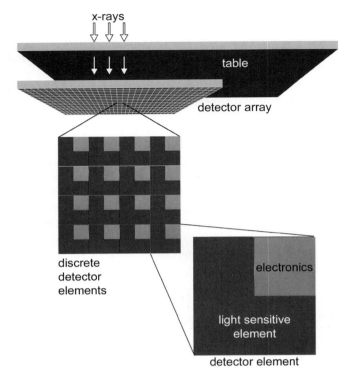

Figure 22-10 *Illustration of the components of a flat panel detector system. The complete detector panel is located underneath the tabletop. A close-up view of a section of detector elements and of an individual active pixel element is shown. The panel is composed of a matrix of these pixels (e.g., 2208 × 2688).*

permanently fixed beneath the x-ray tabletop for use in small animal radiology suites. The flat panel detector is hard-wired to the digital computer, which makes its use less flexible than CR for equine or field radiography. Current flat panel digital x-ray systems marketed for veterinary use include Eklin and Sound Technologies.

Digital Artifacts

The advent of digital radiography has brought forth a whole new set of unique imaging artifacts. Although not within the scope of this chapter to fully describe and illustrate them, the interested reader is referred to the bibliography for further information.

Image plate artifacts. CR image plates are susceptible to cracking as they bend inside the plate reader. Cracks occur first along the edges of the plate and progress centrally to interfere with the image. Cracks are areas without PSP and therefore show as white lines or "cracks" on the CR image. Debris within the CR cassette such as dirt or hair will block light and also appear as a sharp area of "white" image void. The latter is analogous to dirt within a conventional screen-film cassette. These white linear artifacts could be confused with a foreign body within the patient if not recognized.

Plate reader artifacts are caused when the CR plate has been improperly erased or not used for periods of 24 hours or longer. Ghost images from extraneous radiation from scatter radiation, "cosmic rays," etc. can cause a type of CR image fogging. This is why CR plates must be erased before use if they have been stored for prolonged periods (>24 hours). Flat panel detectors are less sensitive but not immune to ghost image artifacts.

Imaging processing artifacts. A number of operator-dependent imaging processing procedures can create artifacts if not applied properly. An example of this is a commonly encountered radiolucent "halo" around metallic orthopedic implants that can mimic implant infection and loosening. This is termed the *Uberschwinger* or *rebound effect* and occurs when the density of adjacent objects is significantly different (Figs. 22-11 and 22-12). Another

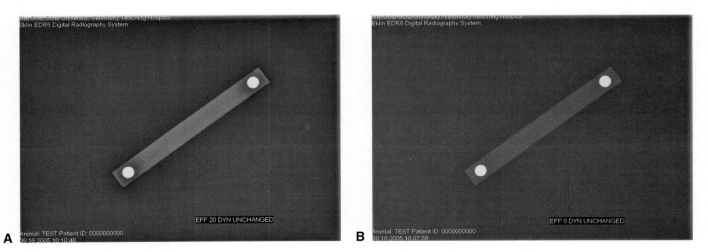

Figure 22-11 *Uberschwinger artifact. This acrylic bar with metal ball bearings placed precisely 10 cm center to center is used to illustrate the Uberschwinger artifact. **A,** The large dark "halo" around the ball bearings is an artifact due to digital image processing. Image processing included an "Effects" (EFF) setting of 20 and a "Dynamic Range" (DYN) of 15 (UNCHANGED) **B,** The dark "halo" is no longer present following digital image manipulation. In this example the EFF was reduced to 0 and the DYN value was UNCHANGED at 15, eliminating the artifact.*

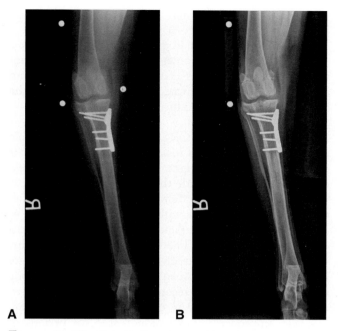

Figure 22-12 *Clinical utility of recognition of the Uberschwinger artifact.* ***A,*** *The caudocranial radiographic image of this healed tibial plateau leveling osteotomy procedure shows apparent bone lysis surrounding the tips of the bone screws and underneath the distal portion of the bone plate.* ***B,*** *Following proper image processing, the artifactual "lysis" is gone, indicating that the orthopedic implants are not loosening.*

example is a thoracic radiograph with extreme contrast that mimics lung pathology due to exaggerated edge enhancement (Fig. 22-13). Image processing parameters and application are CR manufacturer dependent. Image processing is a specific area of training that users of a new CR system should embrace.

OTHER OPERATOR ERRORS

Many operator errors mirror those made using conventional screen-film systems such as putting the CR plate upside down (the back of the CR plate is superimposed on the primary image) (Fig. 22-14) or misaligning the grid and causing grid cut-off or moiré lines (Fig. 22-15). Severe overexposure is possible even with digital radiography, to the point that processing cannot alleviate the artifacts (Fig. 22-16). Overexposure should be avoided at all costs.

X-RAY EXPOSURE FACTORS AND DOSE CONSIDERATIONS

Veterinarians must develop new technique charts for their digital systems on the basis of the manufacturer's guidelines because digital and screen-film have different characteristics and it cannot be assumed that the exposure techniques used for screen-film will be optimal for

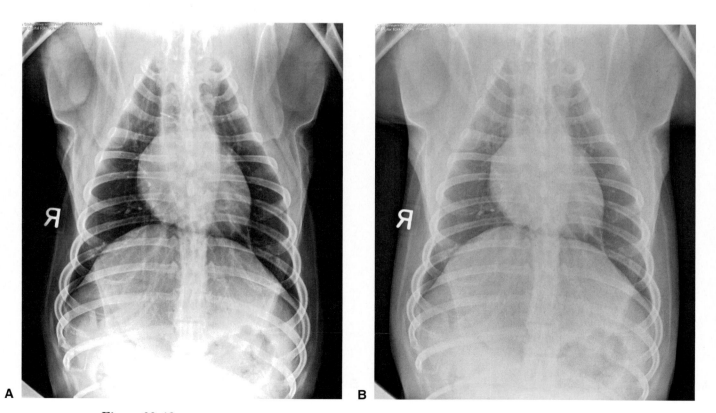

Figure 22-13 ***A,*** *The radiographic image of the thorax was processed to enhance image contrast. Note the dark lung parenchyma and the prominent white airways. This high-contrast processing mimics bronchial disease.* ***B,*** *Correctly processed digital image showing normal lung parenchyma.*

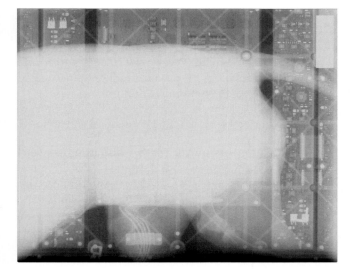

Figure 22-14 *Operator error artifact. This image was made when a conventional screen-film cassette was placed in the cassette tray underneath a flat panel detector and a radiographic exposure was made. The electronics of the flat panel detector can be seen in addition to an underexposed, faintly visible (underexposed) lateral dog abdominal image. Imagine the surprise of the radiology technologist when this radiograph was placed on the view box!*

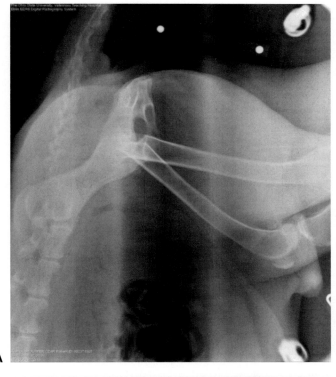

A

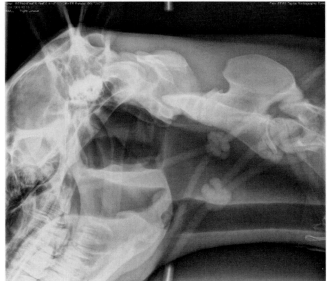

B

Figure 22-15 *Grid malalignment (cut-off) artifacts. **A,** Can you recognize the central dark black stripe artifact? This digital artifact was caused by an upside-down grid. The identical artifact can occur with screen-film radiography. **B,** Grid lines due to lateral decentering of the grid. This artifact can also occur when the digital radiography "Grid on" program is not activated. With "Grid on," a computer program recognizes the repeating grid lines and "eliminates" them from the image.*

digital imaging. Because of the greater latitude in exposure factors, digital technique charts are greatly simplified when compared with those used for conventional screen-film systems.

Most digital x-ray systems are not as efficient as a conventional 400-speed screen film system and therefore require an increase in radiation exposure to produce comparable images. Although direct comparison is difficult, most available digital systems can be compared with 200- to 300-speed screen film systems. This is countered with a reduced number of retake radiographic images from exposure errors, essentially eliminated with digital radiography. High radiation doses to both the patient and the radiology technician from overt overexposure are among the potential dangers when using digital radiography, perhaps not recognized because overexposed images can be corrected by computer manipulation, unlike a conventional radiograph. Purposeful overexposure "to be on the safe side" is irresponsible. The "as low as reasonably achievable" principle dictates that overt overexposures cannot be tolerated due to patient and technician exposure to radiation.

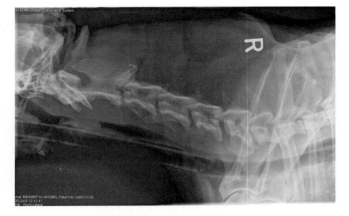

Figure 22-16 *Severe overexposure has caused the trachea, endotracheal tube, portions of the hyoid bone, and the cervical soft tissues to "fade away" and become black in this lateral cervical image taken during myelography. A black "halo" also exists around the periphery of the dog where the skin is "burned out." This degree of overexposure cannot be corrected at the digital workstation, and the exposure must be repeated. These errors should rarely, if ever, occur once a digital technique chart has been established.*

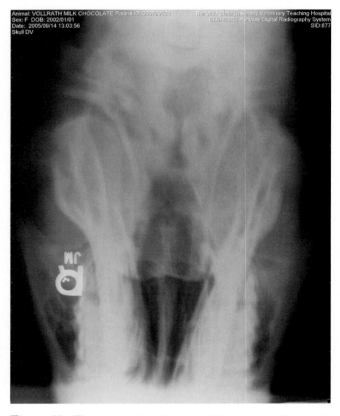

Figure 22-17 *Motion artifact. Blurring of this dorsoventral image of a horse skull was caused by head movement during the radiographic exposure. Note that the "R" marker is not blurred; this is because the leaded marker has been placed on the stationary image detector.*

KEY POINTS

1. Digital radiography uses advanced image capture and computer technology to produce radiographic images that are viewed on a computer monitor.
2. Digital radiography is advantageous because images can be adjusted on a computer to maximize diagnostic image quality.
3. Images can be archived on a computer and transmitted to other veterinarians via the Internet.
4. Digital image acquisition is often faster when compared with conventional screen-film radiography.
5. CR, CCDs, and flat panel detectors are digital radiography systems currently available.

REVIEW QUESTIONS

1. A disadvantage of conventional screen-film based radiography is that:
   a. it has a limited linear response to radiation.
   b. a radiograph may have underexposed and overexposed areas.
   c. it is difficult to have good contrast and good latitude on the same radiograph.
   d. all of the above

2. True or false (circle one):
   Spatial resolution of digital radiography systems is equal to or less than conventional screen film radiography, but contrast resolution is vastly superior.

3. PACS is an acronym for a:
   a. phosphor analog conversion system.
   b. pixel analog contrast software.
   c. picture archiving and communication system.
   d. photostimulable analog computer system.

4. Computed radiography is a(n) _____ imaging technology.
   a. indirect digital
   b. direct digital
   c. indirect analog
   d. direct analog

5. The latent image on a photostimulable phosphor plate is read by a computed radiography processor (image reader device, or plate reader) using:
   a. fluorescent light.
   b. a helium-neon laser.
   c. ultraviolet light.
   d. infrared light.

6. True or false (circle one):
   Digital radiography, with all of the available image manipulation tools, can make any radiographic image diagnostic, regardless of patient motion, malpositioning, or gross overexposure or underexposure.

7. A bit is:
   a. a small pixel.
   b. a binary number, composed of two digits, 0 and 1.
   c. a byte.
   d. a group of pixels arranged in a matrix.

8. True or false (circle one):
   Flat panel digital imaging systems allow you to use your existing x-ray machine in most instances.

9. Advantages of digital radiography over traditional screen-film radiography include:
   a. lower initial cost and burdensome image archival.
   b. easier image transport, archival, and ability to alter the contrast of the image.
   c. the ability to rotate the image on the screen to compensate for improper positioning.
   d. the ability to adjust any image, regardless of technical errors, to produce a diagnostic radiographic image.

10. Reducing the number of radiographs that must be retaken is advantageous because it:
    a. reduces radiation exposure of veterinary staff.
    b. reduces the potential amount of sedation necessary for the radiographic study.
    c. saves time.
    d. all of the above

Suggested Readings

Bushberg JT et al: *The essential physics of medical imaging*, Philadelphia, 2002, Lippincott Williams & Wilkins.

Carlton RR, Adler AM: *Principles of radiographic imaging*, ed 3, New York, 2001, Delmar.

Cesar LJ et al: Artefacts found in computed radiography, *Br J Radiol* 74;195-202, 2001.

Don S et al: Computed radiography versus screen-film radiography: detection of pulmonary edema in a rabbit model that stimulates neonatal pulmonary infiltrates, *Radiology* 213:455-460, 1999.

Greene RE, Oestmann J: *Computed digital radiography in clinical practice*, New York, 1992, Thieme Medical Publishers.

Hruby W, editor: *Digital (r)evolution*, New York, 2001, Springer-Verlag.

Launders J: Digital x-ray systems, part 1: health devices: an introduction to DX technologies and an evaluation of cassette DX systems, *Health Devices* 30(8):273-310, 2001.

Lund PJ et al: Comparison of conventional and computed radiography: assessment of image quality and reader performance in skeletal extremity trauma, *Acad Radiol* 4(8):570-576, 1997.

McLear RC et al: "Uberschwinger" or "rebound effect" artifact in computed radiographic imaging of metallic implants in veterinary medicine. In American College of Veterinary Radiology 2003 Annual Scientific Conference Proceedings, December 2-6, 2003, Chicago.

Murphey MD et al: Nondisplaced fractures: spatial resolution requirements for detection with digital skeletal imaging, *Radiology* 174 (3 Pt 1):865-870, 1990.

Ogoda M: DICOM 101. Understanding the basics of DICOM. Insights & images: the user's publication of computed radiography, Stamford, Conn, 2001, Fujifilm Medical Systems.

Reiner B et al: Evaluation of soft-tissue foreign bodies: comparing conventional plain film radiography, computed radiography printed on film, and computed radiography displayed on a computer workstation, *Am J Roentgenol* 167(1):141-144, 1996.

Roberts G, Graham J: Computed radiography. In Kraft S, Roberts G, editors: *Vet Clin North Am Equine Pract: Modern Diagnostic Imaging*. Philadelphia, 2001, WB Saunders.

Roberts G: Computed radiography: how it works and its advantages. The AAEP 2000 Resort Symposium Lecture Workbook, February 4-6, 2000.

Seigel EL, Kolodner RM, editors: *Filmless radiology*, New York, 1999, Springer-Verlag.

Swee RG et al: Screen-film versus computed radiography imaging of the hand: a direct comparison, *Am J Roentgenol* 168(2):539-542, 1997.

Wegryn SA et al: Comparison of digital and conventional musculoskeletal radiography: an observer performance study, *Radiology* 175(1):225-228, 1990.

World Wide Websites

All Pets Dental: *Why Radiology?* http://www.dentalvet.com/vets/basicdentistry/whywhenhow_radiology.htm.

Animal Insides: http://www.animalinsides.com

Eklin Medical Systems, Inc: http://www.eklin.com

Fujifilm Medical Systems: http://www.fujimed.com

HCMI: http://www.hcmixray.com, http://www.excelmedical.ca/digivet.htm

IDEXX Laboratories: http://www.idexx.com/animalhealth/digital

Kodak: http://www.kodak.com/global/en/health/productsByType/cr/crVet_Product.jhtml?pq-path=7630

Summit Innovet: http://www.innovet4vets.com, http://www.imagingdynamics.com

Swiss Ray: http://www.swissray.com

$\mathcal{A}$nswers to $\mathcal{R}$eview $\mathcal{Q}$uestions

Chapter 1
1. c
2. d
3. b
4. c
5. b
6. c
7. d
8. True: The new direction, however, is also in a straight line.
9. False: A radiograph is the radiographic record of an object on film produced by the passage of x-rays, a form of electromagnetic radiation, through that object.

Chapter 2
1. d
2. d
3. b
4. a
5. d
6. False: Air molecules interfere with the path of electrons, thus decreasing the number of electrons reaching the target.
7. a
8. d
10. b

Chapter 3
1. b
2. d
3. c
4. a
5. b
6. c
7. b
8. d
9. a
10. c

Chapter 4
1. c
2. a
3. c
4. b
5. b
6. b
7. d
8. c

9. a
10. c

Chapter 5
1. b
2. c
3. a
4. d
5. a
6. d
7. a
8. b
9. d
10. a

Chapter 6
1. c
2. a
3. b
4. d
5. d
6. False: The image seen on a view box is a negative image. X-rays are absorbed by structures with more density; therefore fewer x-rays pass through to the film. Bones appear white, and less-dense structures are darker. Remember that the degree of blackness on a radiograph depends on the amount of x-rays reaching the screen.
7. c
8. a
9. c

Chapter 7
1. d
2. b
3. a
4. c
5. d
6. b
7. a
8. c
9. False: Gold and silver refiners purchase fix solutions and films for reclamation of silver.
10. d

Chapter 8
1. d
2. a
3. c

4. c
5. b
6. d
7. a
8. a
9. d
10. c

Chapter 9
1. b
2. c
3. c
4. e
5. a
6. b
7. c
8. c
9. a
10. b

Chapter 10
1. a
2. d
3. b
4. b
5. c
6. a
7. d
8. d
9. d
10. c

Chapter 11
1. d
2. c
3. a
4. d
5. b
6. a
7. c
8. b
9. d
10. c

Chapter 12
1. b
2. a
3. d
4. False: Two views at 90 degrees are required because radiographs are two-dimensional views of three-dimensional structures.
5. a
6. c
7. d
8. b
9. a
10. d

Chapter 13
1. a
2. d
3. c
4. c
5. a
6. d
7. a
8. d
9. b
10. False: All radiographs require at least two views because radiographs are two-dimensional views of three-dimensional structures.

Chapter 14
1. b
2. d
3. d
4. a
5. d
6. c
7. a
8. b
9. d
10. c

Chapter 15
1. a
2. a
3. a
4. c
5. b
6. a
7. d
8. a
9. d
10. b

Chapter 16
1. b
2. a
3. d
4. c
5. c
6. a
7. d
8. b
9. c
10. c

Chapter 17
1. d
2. b
3. a
4. d
5. c
6. a

7. b
8. b
9. c
10. a

Chapter 18
1. a
2. c
3. d
4. c
5. d
6. a
7. b
8. b
9. c
10. d

Chapter 19
1. d
2. a
3. d
4. d
5. c
6. a
7. a
8. b
9. d
10. a
11. d
12. b
13. d
14. d
15. a

Chapter 20
1. d
2. a
3. c
4. d
5. b
6. c
7. b
8. a
9. d
10. b

Chapter 21
1. b
2. d
3. c
4. b
5. d
6. d
7. a
8. d
9. a
10. b

Chapter 22
1. d
2. True
3. c
4. a
5. b
6. False
7. b
8. True
9. b
10. d

Note: Page numbers followed by f indicate figures; those followed by t indicate tables.

3M. *See* Veterinary X-ray system

A
Abdomen, 231-232, 287. *See also* Large animals;
    Small animals
  abdominal ultrasound. *See* Dogs
  CT, usage, 324
  lateral view
    positioning, 231f
    radiograph, 231f. *See also* Dogs
  ventrodorsal view
    positioning, 230f
    radiograph, 230f
Abdominal palpation, 318
Abdominal radiograph (lateral view), exposure, 92f
Abdominal ultrasound, 316-321. *See also* Dogs
Absorbed dose, 25
  definition, 24
Acceleration. *See* Electrons
  definition, 10
Accelerators, 77
  definition, 74
Acetabulum, beam center/measurement, 175f
Acidifiers, 78
  definition, 74
Acoustic impedance, 313
  definition, 312
Acoustic shadow, definition, 312
Acoustic shadowing, 313
  presence, 313f
ACR-NEMA. *See* American College of Radiology and
    the National Electrical Manufacturers'
    Association
Actual focal spot, 14
  contrast. *See* Effective focal spot
  definition, 10
Acute gagging, 236
ADC. *See* Analog to digital converter
Adhesive, 69f
  tape, usage, 298
Adrenal glands, assessment, 319-320
Afterglow, 63-64
  definition, 60
Agfa film screen speed systems. *See* Film
ALARA. *See* As low as reasonably achievable
Alloy
  definition, 10

Alloy—cont'd
  usage, 13
Alternating current, waveforms. *See* Three-phase
    alternating current waveforms
Aluminum filter, placement. *See* X-ray tube
American College of Radiology and the National
    Electrical Manufacturers' Association
    (ACR-NEMA), 330
  joint committee, 337
Analog, definition, 330
Analog-to-digital converter (ADC), 338, 342
  definition, 330
Analog-to-digital radiographic signal conversion, 338
Analog-to-digital waveform conversion, 338f
Anatomic area measurement, caliper (usage), 148
Anatomic directional terms, 147f. *See also* Dogs; Horse;
    Humans; Oblique views
Anatomic orientation, markers (usage), 87
Anechoic, definition, 312
Anechoic cyst (C), 320f
Anechoic tissue, reflectance, 313
Anechoic urine, 321f
Anesthesia
  requirement, 248
  usage, 278
Angiocardiography
  definition, 234
  usage, 246
Angiography
  definition, 234
  usage, 246
Angulation
  indicator, test, 113
  verification, 113f
Anode, 5, 11f, 12-15. *See also* Rotating anode;
    Stationary anode
  bearing failure, 15
  damage, prevention, 16
  definition, 4, 10
  electrons, flow, 11f
  grid distance, decrease. *See* Grid cutoff
  side, 11
  target
    area, scatter radiation (result), 13f
    failure, 15-16
  types, 12-13
Anonymous FTP, 330

Antegrade cystourethrogram, lateral view, 247f
Antegrade urethrogram
    definition, 234
    performing, 244
Aorta (AO)
    echocardiogram, 314f
    presence, 321f
Aortic width (Ao), 317f
Arcing
    definition, 10
    phenomenon, 16
Arthritis. *See* Degenerative joint disease
Arthrogram, contraindication, 244, 246
Arthrography
    definition, 234
    usage, 244-246
Artifact. *See* Grid malalignment artfiacts; Motion
        artifact
    case studies, 128f-140f. *See also* Technical
        artifacts/errors
    causes, 126t-127t
    definition, 126
Artifact-free radiograph, 252-253
As low as reasonably achievable (ALARA), 25
    definition, 330
Atom
    definition, 4
    model, 5f
Atomic number, 5
    definition, 4
Attenuation, 313
    definition, 312
Ausonics Microimager. *See* Portable ultrasound machine
Automatic processing. *See* Film
Automatic processors, 83
    cross section, 83f
    maintenance, 84
        importance, 84f
    tanks/rollers, cross section, 83f
Autotransformer, 16
    definition, 10
Avian gastrointestinal contrast study,
        procedure/technique outline, 297
Avian radiography, 294-297
    considerations, 292-294
    equipment, 292
    exposure factors, 292, 293t
    introduction, 292
    patient restraint, 292-294
    readings, 309
    restraint, example, 292f
    review
        answers, 351
        questions, 308-309
    whole-body lateral view, 295
    whole-body ventrodorsal view, 294
    wing-caudocranial view, 296

B

Backscatter, 49
    definition, 44
Balloon tip, usage, 248
Barium
    administration, 238f
    enema
        lateral view, 241f
        ventrodorsal view, 241f
    preparations, 236
Barium fluorohalide phosphor (BaFlBr), 341
Barium sulfate, 237
    availability, 236
    definition, 234
    usage, 236
Base, 69f
    definition, 60
Base mAs factors, usage, 99. *See also* Technique
        chart
Bean scenario, illustration, 40f
Biliary tract, assessment, 317-318
Binary digit (bit), 339
    definition, 330
Biologic growth, 79
    inhibition, 79
Birds
    barium series. *See* Cockatiel
    beam center, 294f-296f
    gastrointestinal contrast study, 297
    ventrodorsal view, restraint/positioning, 294f
    whole-body lateral view
        positioning, 295f
        radiograph, 295f
    whole-body ventrodorsal view, radiograph,
        294f
    wing, caudocranial view, positioning, 296f
Bit. *See* Binary digit
Bit map (bmp), 336
    definition, 330
Bladder
    echoes, 321f
    overdistention, 244f
Blood clot, 321f
    arising, 320
Blue-light-sensitive film, 77
B-mode ultrasonography. *See* Brightness-mode
        ultrasonography
bmp. *See* Bit map
Bone
    nuclear scintigraphy, 325-326
    soft tissue/fat, contrast, 334f
Bone tissue
    penetration, 46
    whiteness, 47f
Bowed tendons, 321
Brain
    invasion, absence, 323f

Brightness-mode ultrasonography (B-mode ultrasonography). *See* Two-dimensional B-mode ultrasonography
 definition, 312
Bromide crystals, 60
Bucky tray distance, measurement, 108f
Buffers, 78
 definition, 74

C
C2, beam center, 286f
C3-C4, beam center, 210f, 211f
C4, beam center, 286f
C4-C5, beam center, 209f
C4-C6, measurement, 209f
C5, beam center, 286f
C7, measurement, 209f, 210f
Calcaneal tuberosity, 274f, 275f
Calcium tungstate, 5
Calculi, appearance, 320
Calibration, machine parameters, 118
Caliper
 definition, 36
 example, 38f
 usage, 38, 148f. *See also* Anatomic area measurement
Canines. *See* Dogs
 skull. *See* Lateral canine skull; Ventrodorsal canine skull
Carpal bones
 beam center, 272f
 distal row, beam center, 167f, 168f
Carpus. *See* Small animals
 beam center site, measurement, 168f
 DMPaLO, 146
 dorsopalmar view
  positioning, 168f
  radiograph, 168f
 lateral view
  positioning, 167f
  radiograph, 167f
 middle, measurement, 167f
 radiograph, collimation. *See* Cats
Carpus joint, 268-272. *See also* Large animals
 dorsopalmar view
  positioning, 268f
  radiograph, 268f
 flexed lateral view
  positioning, 270f
  radiograph, 270f
 lateral medial view
  positioning, 271f
  radiograph, 271f
 lateral oblique view
  positioning, 271f
  radiograph, 271f
 lateral view
  positioning, 269f
  radiograph, 269f

Carpus joint—cont'd
 limb, lateral aspect (beam center), 269f-270f
 middle, beam center, 268f-271f
 skyline view
  positioning, 272f
  radiograph, 272f
 true dorsopalmar plane, 268f
Cassette, 60-62. *See also* Closed cassette; Open cassette
 care, 62
 definition, 60
 dirt, impact, 63f
 film removal, 80f
  improper method, 131f
 fish, placement, 307f
 groove, 255
 hair, trapping, 68f
 holder. *See* Equine radiography
 lead letters, placement, 86f
 placement, 268
 positioning, 267
 quadrants, division, 61f
 screens
  mounting, 67
  setup match, 117f
 screen-to-film contact, 116f
 splitting, 149f
 tape adherence, 86f
 top/tabletop distance measurement, 108f
 tray, diagram, 53f
 tunnel, 253f
  patient position, 257f
  system, usage. *See* Nonselective cardioangiogram
 unloading, 79-80
 x-ray beam, perpendicularity, 269, 271, 273
Cathode, 5, 11-12, 11f
 definition, 4, 10
 electrons, flow, 11f
 failure, 15
 filament construction, 11f
 side, 11
Cathode ray tube (CRT), 339
Cats
 carpus (radiograph), collimation, 149f
 digital abdominal image, 334f
 echocardiogram, 315f, 316f
 hypertrophic cardiomyopathy, 315f, 316f
 lateral thoracic radiographic image, 334f
 nuclear scan. *See* Hyperthyroid cat
Caudal, definition, 146
Caudal border, beam center. *See* Scapula
Caudal spine. *See* Small animals
 beam center, 219f, 220f
 ventrodorsal view
  positioning, 219f
  radiograph, 219f
Caudocranial shoulder, position, 158
CCD. *See* Charged coupled device

CD-ROM. *See* Compact disk, read-only memory
Ceiling-mounted x-ray unit, 20f
Centering points, marking, 281f
Centimeter increments, 38f
Cervical spine, 208-211, 286. *See also* Large animals;
    Small animals
  flexed lateral view
    positioning, 210f
    radiograph, 210f
  hyperextended lateral view
    positioning, 211f
    radiograph, 211f
  lateral view
    positioning, 209f, 286f
    radiograph, 209f. *See also* Cranial cervical spine
  ventrodorsal view
    positioning, 209f
    radiograph, 209f
Channel film hanger, 76f
Charged coupled device (CCD), 335, 342
  components, 342f
  definition, 330
  technology, 342
Charged selenium plates, x-rays (interaction), 60
Charts. *See* Technique chart
  suggestion, 98
Cheek teeth, lateral oblique view
  positioning, 285f
  radiograph, 285f
Chemicals
  carryover, 81
  precipitation, 84, 85
  restraint, 28, 293-294
  stirring. *See* Hand processing
  temperature, 84
  usage. *See* Processing chemicals
Cholecystography
  definition, 234
  usage, 246-247
Chronic lameness, 325
C_i. *See* Curie
Clearing agents, 78
  definition, 74
Clip film hanger, 76f
  film, loading, 80f
Closed cassette, 61f
Cockatiel
  barium series, lateral view, 297f
  barium series, ventrodorsal view, 297f
Coffin, dorsopalmar/dorsoplantar oblique view, 253
Coiled wire filament, 11
Cold spots, 325
Collimation (coning down). *See* Cat carpus
  example. *See* Cones
Collimator, 19-20
  definition, 10
  lead shutters, inclusion, 19, 20f

Collimator—cont'd
  light field, penny placement, 115f
  setting, 8x10-inch field size, 111f
  test, 112
Compact disk, read-only memory (CD-ROM), 336
  definition, 330
Compression, definition, 330
Computed radiography (CR), 60, 331, 341
  considerations, 341
  definition, 330
  operator errors, 344
Computed tomography (CT), 321-324, 331
  clinical applications, 323-324
  number, 323
    definition, 312
  scan. *See* Dogs
  scanner. *See* Transverse-lane computed tomography
    scanner
  technical aspects, 322-323
  usage. *See* Abdomen; Extremities; Skull; Spine;
    Thorax
Cones
  collimation, example, 19f
  test, 112
Coning down. *See* Collimation
Contrast, 45-46. *See also* Double contrast; Radiographic
    contrast; Subject contrast
  alteration, 49f
  cystogram. *See* Double-contrast cystogram;
    Positive-contrast cystogram
  definition, 36, 44, 90
  enhancement. *See* Image
  guidelines, 46t
  long scale, 47f
  radiograph, 45f
  resolution, definition, 330
  review, 90-91
  short scale, 47f
  studies. *See* Birds; Gastrointestinal tract; Urinary
    system
    procedure/technique outline. *See* Avian
      gastrointestinal contrast study
Contrast media (medium), 235-236
  definition, 234
  leakage, 242
  ureteral reflux, 244f
  usage, 234-235
Control panel (console), 20-21. *See also* X-rays
Copper, 12f
Coronal-plane scan, 323f
Coronary band, beam center, 254f-257f
CR. *See* Computed radiography
Crane locks, test. *See* X-ray tube
Cranial, definition, 146
Cranial cervical spine, lateral view (radiograph), 286f
Cranial mediastinum, ectopic functional thyroid tissue,
  325f

Cranial midline, beam center, 276f
Cranial thorax, scapula (superimposition), 155
Cranioventral thorax, measurement, 155f
Cranium, 192f. *See also* Small animals
   high point, measurement, 193f
   rostrocaudal view
     positioning, 196f
     radiograph, 196f
Crisscross grid, helpfulness, 281
Crossed grid (crisscross grid), 52
   definition, 44
CRT. *See* Cathode ray tube
Crystal size, 64-65. *See also* Phosphor
CT. *See* Computed tomography
Curie (C$_i$), definition, 312
Cut-off artifacts. *See* Grid malalignment artifacts
Cystogram, lateral view, 244f. *See also* Double-contrast
     cystogram; Negative-contrast cystogram;
     Positive-contrast cystogram
Cystography
   definition, 234
   precautions, 242
   procedure, 245-246
   technique outline, 245-246
   usage, 242
Cystourethrogram, lateral view. *See* Antegrade
     cystourethrogram; Retrograde
     cystourethrogram

D

Darkroom
   dry side, 75, 75f
   fog test, 119
   layout, sample, 75f
   lightproofing, 76-77
   organization, 74-76
   QC, 118
   revolving door, 76f
   safelight, 76-77
   usage, 74-77
   wet side, 75-76, 75f
DDR. *See* Direct digital radiography
Degenerative joint disease (arthritis), 326f
Densitometry, test, 120-121
Density. *See* Radiographic density
   definition, 36, 90
   radiograph, 45f
   review, 90-91
Detail characteristics, radiograph, 45f
Detector array, 343f
Developer, 77-78
   definition, 74
   labeling, 79f
Developing agents, 77
   definition, 74
Developing tank, film immersion, 81f
Diaphragms, test, 112

DICOM. *See* Digital Imaging and Communications in
     Medicine
Digital, definition, 330
Digital abdominal image. *See* Cats
Digital artifacts, 343-344
Digital computers, usage, 338-339
Digital images
   computer manipulation, 334
   processing, 344f
   viewing, 339-340
Digital imaging. *See* Film-based digital imaging
Digital Imaging and Communications in Medicine
     (DICOM), 331, 337
   definition, 330
Digital radiograph, making, 333f
Digital radiographic image. *See* Dogs
Digital radiography (DR). *See* Direct digital radiography
   advantages, 332-336
   cost savings, 336
   definition, 330
   disadvantages, 336-337
   equipment, costs, 337
   glossary, 330-331
   Grid on program, nonactivation, 345f
   higher-contrast resolution, 333-334
   history, 331
   overexposure, 346f
   overview, 331-332
   profits, increase, 336
   readings, 347
   review
     answers, 351
     questions, 346-347
   software, 335
   time savings, 335-336
   training/learning curve, 336-337
   types, 340-341
   WWW sites, 347f
Digital video disk (digital versatile disk) (DVD),
     definition, 330
Digital waveform, representation, 338
Digital work station, 333f
Digits, beam center, 170f
Dilatory cardiomyopathy. *See* Dogs
Direct digital radiography (DDR), 340-341
   definition, 330
Direct safelight, 77f
Display monitors, usage, 339
Distal, definition, 146
Distal femurs
   enlargement, 56f
   gauze/tape, usage, 176f
Distal front leg, flexor tendons (ultrasound). *See* Horse
Distal humerus, measurement, 162f-164f, 166f
Distal phalanx (pedal bone), 254-256. *See also* Large
     animals
   beam center, 255f

Distal phalanx (pedal bone)—cont'd
    dorsopalmar/dorsoplantar oblique view
        positioning, 256f
        radiograph, 256f
    dorsopalmar/dorsoplantar view
        positioning, 255f
        radiograph, 255f
    inclusion, 256
    lateral view
        positioning, 254f
        radiograph, 254f
Distal tarsal joint, measurement, 188f, 189f
Distance. *See* Focal film distance; X-rays
Distant enhancement, 313
    definition, 312
    presence, 313f
Distortion. *See* Geometric distortion
Distraction device, placement, 179f
Diverticula, echoes, 320f
DNA, injury, 25
Dogs (canines)
    abdomen, abdominal ultrasound, 319f
    abdomen, lateral view (radiograph), 48f
        kV_p, underexposure, 49f
    abdominal ultrasound, 318f-321f
    anatomic directional terms, 147f
    anemia, history, 319f
    brain, transverse-plane computed tomography scan, 323f
    collapse, history, 319f
    digital radiographic image, 335f
    dilatory cardiomyopathy, 315f, 316f
    dorsoplantar view, radiograph, 149f
    dorsoventral position, 322f
    echocardiogram, 314f-316f
    echocardiography, performing, 314f
    forelimb, radiograph, 31f
    four-chamber view, 315f
    gestation, 321f
    hip dysplasia, positioning difficulty, 56f
    hydrocephalus, 323f
    kidney, cranial pole, 320f
    lower urinary tract infection, 313f
    mid-abdomen, transverse CT scan, 324f
    nasal tumor, CT scan, 323f
    screen-film lateral pelvic radiograph, 335f
    size, difference, 46f
    skull, kV_p (overexposure), 49f
    stifle joint, lateral view (radiograph), 47f, 48f
    tarsus, radiograph (lateral view), 149f
    testicles, shielding (example), 26f
    total hip prosthesis, 335f
    urinary bladder, ultrasound scan, 313f, 321f
    ventrodorsal extended view, 176f
    ventrodorsal frog-leg position, 176f
    ventrodorsal view, abdominal ultrasound, 317f
Doppler shift, 316
    definition, 312

Doppler studies, indications, 316
Doppler technique, application, 319
Dorsal, definition, 146
Dorsal recumbency, 226
Dorsopalmar-lateromedial oblique views, 168
Dorsopalmar view, 148f
Dorsoplantar view, radiograph. *See* Dogs
Dorsoventral intraoral maxilla, positioning/
        radiograph, 201f
Dose. *See* Absorbed dose; Maximum permissible dose
    equivalent, 25
        definition, 24
Dosimeter, 26. *See also* Thermoluminescent
        dosimeter
    definition, 24
Dosimetry, 26
    definition, 24
    services, 27t
Double contrast
    definition, 234
    usage, 236
Double-contrast cystogram
    definition, 234
    lateral view, 245f
Double-contrast gastrogram
    lateral view, 240f
    nonrecommendation, 238
    ventrodorsal view, 240f
DR. *See* Digital radiography
Drainage phase. *See* Intravenous pyelogram
Drying rack, 82f, 83f
Dry side. *See* Darkroom
DVD. *See* Digital video disk
Dysphagia, 236

E
Echocardiogram. *See* Cats; Dogs; Foal
Echocardiography, 313-316. *See also* Two-dimensional
        echocardiography
    performing. *See* Dogs
Echogenicity. *See* Tissues
    definition, 312
Echogenic landmark, 318f
Ectopic functional thyroid tissue (ET). *See* Cranial
        mediastinum; Thoracic inlet
Effective focal spot, 14-15
    actual focal spot, contrast, 14f
    definition, 10
Effects (EFF) setting, 343f
Eklin and Sound Technologies, usage, 342, 343
Elbow. *See* Small animals
    craniocaudal view
        positioning, 162f, 276f
        radiograph, 162f, 276f
    flexed lateral view
        positioning, 164f
        radiograph, 164f

Elbow—cont'd
  lateral view
      positioning, 163f, 277f
      radiograph, 163f, 277f
  measurement, 165f
  middle, beam center, 164f
Elbow joint, 276-277. *See also* Large animals
  beam center, 162f-163f, 276f-277f
Electrolytic recovery, 84, 85
Electromagnetic radiation
  definition, 4
  physical properties. *See* X-rays
Electromagnetic spectrum, 5f
Electrons
  acceleration, 11f, 12
      method, 10
  collision. *See* Target
  definition, 4
  flow, 11f
  interaction, 11
  obstacle-free path, 10
  production, relationship, 36f
  source, 10
  stream, 90
      air molecules, collision, 16f
      spreading, 13
Elongation
  definition, 44
  distortion, 55
Emulsion, 69f
  definition, 60
  scratching, 135
Epithelial tissues, 24
Equine pedal radiography, 253f
Equine radiography, cassette holder, 253f
Esophagography
  definition, 234
  precautions, 237
  procedure, technique outline, 237
  usage, 236-237
Esophagram, lateral view (radiograph), 237f
Etched pixel matrix, 342f
Ethernet, definition, 330
Excitation, 5
  definition, 4
Excretory urography, 240-243
  definition, 234
  precautions, 241-242
  procedure, 243
  technique outline, 243
Exotic radiography
  considerations, 292-294
  equipment, 292
  exposure factors, 292, 293t
  introduction, 292
  patient restraint, 292-294
  readings, 309

Exotic radiography—cont'd
  review
      answers, 351
      questions, 208-209
Exposure
  button, 21
  indicator, malfunction, 130
  modification. *See* Grid
  time settings, 98
  trials, 101t
      examples, 100-101
Exposure factors, 46-48. *See also* Avian radiography;
      Exotic radiography; Psittacine; Raptors; Reptiles;
      Rodents; Technique chart
  readings, 41
  review
      answers, 349
      questions, 40-41
Exposure technique evaluation flow chart, 92f
Exposure time
  definition, 36
  measurement, 37
Extended projection. *See* Pelvis
Extremities
  CT, usage, 324
  ultrasound examination, 321
Eyes
  lateral canthus
      beam center, 192f-194f
      measurement, 194f, 200f
  midpoint, beam center, 196f
  ultrasound examination, 321

F
False-positive reaction, induction, 242
Falx cerebri, 323
Femoral condyles, 180
  measurement, 182f
  patellae, centering, 175
Femurs. *See* Small animals
  appearance, 56f
  craniocaudal view
      positioning, 180f
      radiograph, 180f
  distal end, measurement, 181f
  extension, 176f
  lateral view
      positioning, 179f
      radiograph, 179f
  middle, beam center/measurement, 179f, 180f
Fetlock joint, 261-264. *See also* Large animals
  beam center, 261f-264f
  dorsopalmar view
      positioning, 261f
      radiograph, 261f
  flexed lateral view
      positioning, 263f

Fetlock joint—cont'd
  flexed lateral view—cont'd
    radiograph, 263f
  lateral oblique view
    positioning, 264f
    radiograph, 264f
  lateral view
    positioning, 262f
    radiograph, 262f
  medial oblique view
    positioning, 264f
    radiograph, 264f
Fetus, ultrasound, 321f
FFD. *See* Focal fillm distance
Fibula. *See* Small animals
  caudocranial view
    positioning, 185f
    radiograph, 185f
  lateral view
    positioning, 184f
    radiograph, 184f
  middle, beam center, 184f, 185f
Field light. *See* X-rays
Field of view (FOV), 342
Field size verification, 111f
Filament. *See* Coiled wire filament; Light bulb
  circuit. *See* Low-voltage circuit
  construction. *See* Cathode
  definition, 10
  mA, effect, 36f
File transfer protocol (FTP), 336
  definition, 330
Film. *See* Nonscreen film; Screen film; X-ray film
  automatic processing, 83
  badge, 26
    definition, 24
    example, 27f
  developing, 80-81
  development, unevenness, 80f
  drying, 82
    example, 82f
  exposure, 83
    risk, 76f
  filing, 87
  final rinse, option, 82
  fixing, 81-82
  hanger, 75. *See also* Channel film hanger; Clip film hanger
  identification, 85-87. *See also* Radiographs
    lead letters, placement, 86f
  immersion. *See* Developing tank; Fixer tank
  latitude, 70
    definition, 60
  lightness/darkness, determination, 92f
  loading. *See* Clip film hanger; Hanger
  manual processing procedure, 79-82
  preparation, 79

Film—cont'd
  processing, 98
    solutions, 77-79
    techniques, 79-83
  removal. *See* Cassette
  rinse, 81f
  rinsing, 81
  screen speed systems
    (Agfa), 71t
    (Kodak), 70t
  storage bin, 75f
  tautness, 80
  usage, 339-340
  washing, 82
    example, 82f
Film-based digital imaging, 339
Film processing
  glossary, 74
  readings, 88
  review
    answers, 349
    questions, 88
Film-screen systems, 70-71
Filtration, calibration, 118
Fine-needle aspiration, performing, 317-318
Firewall, definition, 330
First lumbar vertebral body, measurement, 216f, 217f
First molar, measurement, 204f
Fish
  body, middle (beam center), 307f, 308f
  dorsoventral whole-body view, 307-308
  lateral whole-body view, 307-308
  placement. *See* Cassette
  radiography, 307-308
  whole-body dorsoventral view, positioning (water bag, usage), 307f
  whole-body lateral view
    positioning, horizontal x-ray beam (usage), 307f
    positioning, water bag (usage), 307f
    positioning, wet paper towel (usage), 308f
    radiograph, 308f
Fistula, definition, 234
Fistulography
  usage, 247-248
Fistulography, definition, 234
Fixation, 78
  definition, 74
Fixed tube stand construction, example. *See* X-ray tube
Fixed x-ray unit, 37f
Fixer, 78
  definition, 74
  tank
    film immersion, 81f
    labeling, 79f
Fixing agents, 78
Flat panel detectors, 342-344
  DR system, inclusion. *See* X-ray machine

Flat panel detectors—cont'd
  electronics, presence, 345f
  system, components, 343f
Flexor tendons, ultrasound. *See* Horse
Fluorescence, 5
  definition, 4
Fluorescent screens, 61f
  light, emittance, 62f
Fluoroscopy, 67
  definition, 24, 60
  equipment, installation, 67
  radiation safety rules, 31-33
  unit, 67f
    schematic drawing, 33f
  usage, 31-32
Foal
  echocardiogram, 317f
  heart murmur, 317f
Foam block, 220
Foam wedge pad, placement, 167
Focal fillm distance (FFD), 36, 38
Focal spot, 13-15. *See also* Actual focal spot;
        Effective focal spot
  area, 14f
  contrast. *See* Effective focal spot
  definition, 10
  size, impact. *See* Image
Focal spot-to-grid distance, 52
Focused grid, 51f, 52. *See also* Unfocused grid
  definition, 44
  impact. *See* Grid cutoff
  lead strips, divergence, 52f
  unfocused grid, contrast, 52
Focusing cup, 11f
  definition, 10
  usage, 12
Fog test. *See* Darkroom
Follow-up radiography, 336
Forelimbs. *See* Small animals
  radiograph. *See* Dogs
Foreshortening, 56
  definition, 44
  distortion, 55f, 56f
Formulation methods. *See* Technique chart
Four-chamber view. *See* Dogs
Fourth lumbar vertebral body, beam center, 216f,
        217f
FOV. *See* Field of view
Freehand technique, 318
Frequency, definition, 4
Frog-leg position. *See* Dogs
Frog-leg projection. *See* Pelvis
Frog-leg view. *See* Pelvis
Frontal bones, 192f
Frontal sinuses. *See* Small animals
  beam center, 195f
  measurement, 196f

Frontal sinuses—cont'd
  rostrocaudal view
    positioning, 195f
    radiograph, 195f
FTP. *See* File transfer protocol
Full-wave rectification, 18
  definition, 10
  illustration, 18

G
Gallbladder (G)
  opacification, variation, 247
  ultrasound, 318f
Gamma rays, definition, 4
Gamma scintillation camera, 324
Gases, usage, 236
Gassy x-ray tube, 16f
Gastrogram
  lateral view. *See* Double-contrast gastrogram
  ventrodorsal view. *See* Double-contrast gastrogram
Gastrography, 238
  definition, 234
  precautions, 238
  procedure, 240
  technique outline, 240
Gastrointestinal contrast study. *See* Birds
  procedure/technique outline. *See* Avian
        gastrointestinal contrast study
Gastrointestinal tract
  assessment, 319
  contrast studies, 236-239
  evacuation, 236
  study, 297
Generators. *See* High-frequency generators;
        Three-phase generator
Genes, damage, 25
Genetic damage, 25
  definition, 24
Geometric distortion, 54-56
  definition, 44
Geometric projection position, 55f
Geometric unsharpness, 54
  definition, 44
German shepherd tarsus (caudocranial view),
        preparation, 333f
Glass envelope, 11f
  damage, 16
  definition, 10
  usage, 11
Gonad shield, example, 26f
Grain, quality, 65-66
Gray (Gy), definition, 24
Gray-scale resolution, 333
Greater femoral trochanter, beam center, 174f
Green-light-sensitive film, 77
Grid, 50-54. *See also* Crossed grid; Focused grid; Linear
        grid; Pseudofocused grid; Unfocused grid

Grid—cont'd
  absorption, 51f
  care, 54
  construction, drawing, 50f
  contrast. *See* Focused grid
  definition, 44
  device, 50
    usage, 50f
  diagram, 53f
  efficiency, 50-51
    definition, 44
  factor, 51
    definition, 44
  focus, 50
    definition, 44
  lines, direction, 53f
  pattern, 51-52
  ratio, 51, 99
    definition, 44
    illustration, 51f
  usage, exposure modification, 99
Grid cutoff
  anode/grid distance, decrease, 53f
  definition, 44
  focused grid, impact, 52f
  inclusion, example. *See* Radiographs
  occurrence, 50
Grid malalignment artifacts (cut-off artifacts), 345f
Guttural pouch, 283-284. *See also* Large animals
  beam center, 283f
  lateral view
    positioning, 283
    radiograph, 283f

H

Hair
  artifact, presence. *See* Radiographs
  trapping. *See* Cassette
Half-life ($t_{1/2}$), 324. *See also* Radiopharmaceutical
  definition, 312
Half-wave rectification, 17-18
  definition, 10
  illustration, 18
Halo, absence, 343f
Hand processing
  chemicals, stirring, 80f
  tanks, 79f
Hands, positioning (avoidance). *See* Primary x-ray beam
Hanger. *See* Channel film hanger; Clip film hanger
  film, loading, 80
  lead apron, draping, 32f
Hardeners, 77-78
  definition, 74
Health level 7 (HL-7), definition, 330
Heart (H)
  base, short-axis view, 315f
  murmur. *See* Foal

Heart (H)—cont'd
  presence, 321f
  right parasternal approach, 314f
Heel effect, 13, 13f
  definition, 10
  demonstration, 14f
Hemangiosarcoma, 318, 319f
Hemopoietic, 24
  definition, 24
Hepatomegaly, 317
Higher-contrast resolution. *See* Digital radiography
High-frequency generators, 18-19
High-frequency output (100 kHz), 19f
High-frequency technology, 18
High-ratio grids, absorption, 51f
High-voltage circuit, 16-17
Hind legs, support, 208f
Hips
  dysplasia, positioning difficulty. *See* Dogs
  extended view, 178f
  PennHIP distraction view, 178f
HIS. *See* Hospital information system
HL-7. *See* Health level 7
Hoof dorsal wall, vertical position, 257f
Hoof wall, beam center, 254f, 268f, 273f
Horizontal x-ray beam
  direction, 229
  inclusion. *See* Small animals; Thorax
  radiography, 333f
  usage. *See* Fish; Turtles
Horse
  anatomic directional terms, 147f
  distal front leg, flexor tendons (ultrasound), 322f
  nuclear scan, 324f
  skull, dorsoventral image (blurring), 346f
  stifle joints, nuclear scan, 326f
Hospital information system (HIS), 337
  definition, 330
Hot spots, 325
HTML. *See* Hypertext markup language
HTTP. *See* Hypertext transfer protocol
Humans
  anatomic directional terms, 147f
  hand, visibility. *See* Radiographs
Humerus. *See* Small animals
  caudocranial view
    positioning, 160f
    radiograph, 160f
  center, beam center, 159f
  centering, 160
  craniocaudal view
    positioning, 161f
    radiograph, 161f
  lateral view
    positioning, 159f
    radiograph, 159f
  measurement. *See* Distal humerus

Humerus—cont'd
    middle, beam center, 160f, 161f
    superimposition, elimination, 227
Hunter and Driffield curve. *See* Radiographic film
        Hunter and Driffield curve
Hyperactive thyroid gland (T), 325f
Hyperechogenic lumen (L), 319f
Hyperechogenic mass (M), irregularity, 321f
Hyperechogenic needle. *See* Liver
Hyperechogenic stone, 313f
Hyperechoic, definition, 312
Hyperechoic tissues, 313
Hypertext markup language (HTML), 330
Hypertext transfer protocol (HTTP), definition, 330
Hyperthyroid cat, nuclear scan, 325f
Hypertrophic cardiomyopathy. *See* Cats
Hypoechogenic mass (M). *See* Spleen
    irregularity, 321f
Hypoechoic, definition, 312
Hypoechoic tissues, 313

I

ICN Dosimetry Service, 27t
Identification. *See* Film
    card, placement, 87f
    methods, 87
Image
    accuracy, 55f
    contrast, enhancement, 344f
    distortion, 56f
    DR, advantages, 332-335
    intensifier, 33f
    magnification, 55f
    management software, 337-338
    matrix, 339
    plate artifacts, 343
    processing, 337-338
    resolution, matrix/pixel impact, 340f
    sharpness, focal spot size (impact), 14f
    storage/transport, 336
    viewing. *See* Digital images
Image-intensifying unit, 67
Image receptors
    distance. *See* X-rays
    glossary, 60
    readings, 72
    review
        answers, 349
        questions, 71-72
    rules, 64-68
    subject, parallelism, 55f
Image receptor screen
    care, 67-68
    construction, 63-64
    speed, 64-65
        ratings, 65-66
        summary, 66

Imaging processing artifacts, 343-344
Imaging technologies
    glossary, 312
    readings, 327
    review
        answers, 351
        questions, 326-327
Imprinter, closure, 87f
Incisor teeth, intraoral projection (positioning), 285f
Indirect safelight, 77f
Inferior, definition, 146
Information system. *See* Hospital information system;
        Radiology information system
Infrared rays, definition, 4
Inhalant anesthetics, 293
Injectable sedatives, 293
Intensifying screens, 62-64
    base, support, 63
    construction, 63-64
    crack, 63f
    cross section, 63f
    definition, 60
    usage, 342f
Internet, definition, 330
Internet protocol (IP), definition, 330
Interspacers, structure. *See* Radiolucent interspacers
Interventricular septum (S)
    defect, 317f
    echocardiogram, 314f-316f
Intervertebral space
    beam center, 209f-211f
    measurement, 209f
Intraoral radiography, sedation (requirement), 285
Intravenous pyelogram (IVP)
    definition, 234
    drainage phase
        lateral view, 243f
        ventrodorsal view, 243f
    nephrogram phase, ventrodorsal view, 243f
    pyelogram phase
        lateral view, 243f
        ventrodorsal phase, 243f
    usage, 240
Intravenous urogram (IVU)
    definition, 234
    usage, 240
Inverse square law
    definition, 36
    illustration, 39f
    usage, 38-39
Iodinated contrast media, 237
    amount, 241
Iodinated oral contrast agent, usage, 237
Iodine compounds, 239
Iohexol, 235
Ionization, 5
    definition, 4

Ionizing radiation, hazards, 24-25
Iopamidol, 235
IP. *See* Internet protocol
Ischium, caudal portion (beam center), 177f
IVP. *See* Intravenous pyelogram
IVU. *See* Intravenous urogram

J
Joint Photographic Experts Group (JPEG/jpg),
336
    definition, 330

K
Kidneys
    assessment, 319-320
    cranial pole. *See* Dogs
    enlargement, 320f
    presence, 319f
Kilovoltage, 37-38
    application, 12
    calculation, 100, 101
    definition, 10, 36
    impact, 48
    measurement, 38
    selector, 20
Kilovoltage peak (kV$_p$), 16, 38
    calibration, 118
    control, 90
    definition, 10, 90
    impact. *See* Penetration
    importance, 292
    increase, 45
    maximum, 252
    necessity, 281
    overexposure. *See* Dogs
    technique chart. *See* Variable kV$_p$ technique chart
    underexposure. *See* Dogs
Kinetic energy, definition, 36
Kodak. *See* Film; Photo-Flo 200 solution

L
Labeled compound
    definition, 312
    usage, 324
Label system. *See* Photoimprinting
Labrador retriever abdomen, ventrodorsal view
        (radiograph), 46f
Large animal radiography
    considerations, 252-253, 287
    equipment, 252
    introduction, 252
    patients
        preparation, 252-253
        restraint, 252
    positioning devices, 253
    radiation safety, 253
    readings, 289

Large animal radiography—cont'd
    review
        answers, 351
        questions, 288-289
Large animals
    abdomen, 287
    carpus joint, 268-272
        dorsopalmar view, 268
        flexed lateral view, 270
        lateral view, 269
        oblique views (lateral/medial), 271
        skyline view, 272
    cervical spine, lateral, 286
    distal phalanx, 254-256
        dorsopalmar/dorsoplantar oblique view, 256
        dorsopalmar/dorsoplantar view, 255
        lateral view, 254
    elbow joint, 276-277
        craniocaudal view, 276
        lateral view, 277
    fetlock joint, 261-264
        dorsopalmar/dorsoplantar view, 261
        flexed lateral view, 263
        lateral view, 262
        oblique views (lateral/medial), 264
    larynx
        dorsoventral view, 284
        lateral view, f283
    metacarpus/metatarsus
        dorsopalmar/dorsoplantar view, 265
        lateral view, 266
        oblique views (lateral/medial), 267
    navicular bone, 257-258
        dorsopalmar/dorsoplantar oblique view, 257
        flexor bone, 258
    pelvis, ventrodorsal view, 281
    pharynx
        dorsoventral view, 284
        lateral view, 283
    proximal phalanges, 259-260
        dorsopalmar/dorsoplantar view, 260
        lateral view (short/long pastern), 259
    shoulder joint, lateral view, 278
    skull, lateral view, 282
    stifle joint
        caudocranial view, 279
        lateral view, 280
    tarsus joint, 273-275
        dorsoplantar view, 273
        lateral view, 274
        oblique views (lateral/medial), 275
    teeth (mandibular/maxillary), oblique views, 285
    thoracic spine, 287
    thorax, 287
Larynx, 283-284. *See also* Large animals
    lateral view
        positioning, 283f

Larynx—cont'd
  lateral view—cont'd
    radiograph, 283f
Latent image, 77
  definition, 60, 74
Lateral. *See* Mediolateral
  definition, 146
  view, 148f
Lateral canine skull, 192f
Lateral canthus, beam center. *See* Eyes
Lateral cervical image, 346f
Lateral spine study, positioning alterations, 208f
Lateral thoracic radiographic image. *See* Cats
Lead
  blocker, usage. *See* Photographic identification
  lead-impregnated tape, 85-86
    usage, 86f
  letters, placement. *See* Cassette; Film
  markers, 85
  placement, 149
  sheet, usage, 149f
  shutters, inclusion. *See* Collimator
  wall. *See* Portable lead wall
Lead aprons
  draping. *See* Hanger
  vertical storage, 32f
Lead gloves
  circulation, cans (usage), 32f
  horizontal storage, 32f
  lead lining (crack, appearance), radiograph (usage), 33f
  usage, 296
  vertical storage, 32f
Lead-impregnated tape, 86
Lead strips
  divergence. *See* Focused grid
  placement, 50f
  structure, 50f
Left atrium (LA)
  dilation, 317f
  echocardiogram, 314f, 315f
Left ventricle (LV)
  dilation, 315f, 316f
  echocardiogram, 314f, 315f, 317f
Left ventricle wall (LW), echocardiogram, 316f
Left ventricular lumen, 315f
Leukopoietic, 24
  definition, 24
LGI. *See* Lower gastrointestinal
Light bulb, filament, 11f
Light emissions, irregularity, 63f
Light field
  alignment, 115
    verification, 115f
  size, 111
Light-sensitive emulsion, 68
Limbs, positioning, 175

Linear array probe, definition, 312
Linear grid, 51-52
  definition, 44
Line-focus principle, 14
  definition, 10
Lines per centimeter, 51
  definition, 44
Line-voltage compensator, 17
  definition, 10
Lips, commissure
  beam center, 198f
  measurement, 198f, 203f
Liquid barium, administration, 237f-239f
Liver (L)
  assessment, 317-318
  echogenicity, 319f
  enzymes, elevations, 317
  nuclear scintigraphy, 326
  ultrasound, 318f
  ultrasound-guided biopsy, hyperechogenic needle, 318f
Lizards, 303-304
  body, beam center, 303f, 304f
  skeletal system, inclusion, 303f
  thorax/abdomen, inclusion, 303f, 304f
  vertebral column, inclusion, 304f
  whole-body dorsoventral view, 303
    positioning, 303f
  whole-body lateral view, 304
    positioning, 304f
Local area network (LAN), 331
Long-axis view. *See* Two-dimensional long-axis view
  definition, 312
Long pastern. *See* Large animals; Proximal phalanges
Lower gastrointestinal (LGI) study, 239
  definition, 234
  precautions, 239
  procedure, 241
  technique outline, 241
Lower urinary tract infection. *See* Dogs
Low-osmolar contrast media, 235
Low-voltage circuit (filament circuit), 17
Lumbar spine. *See* Small animals
  lateral view
    positioning, 217f
    radiograph, 217f
  ventrodorsal view
    positioning, 216f
    radiograph, 216f
Lymphatic system, impairment, 248
Lymphography
  definition, 234
  usage, 248

M

mA. *See* Milliamperage
Magnetic resonance imaging (MRI), 331

Magnification, 54-56
  definition, 44
Mandible, 192f. *See also* Small animals
  beam center, 203f, 204f, 283f
  dorsoventral oblique open-mouth view
    positioning, 204f
    radiograph, 204f
  joint. *See* Temporomandibular joint
  ventrodorsal intraoral view
    positioning, 203f
    radiograph, 203f
Manual processing, procedure. *See* Film
Manual restraint, 292, 306
Manual restraint, posture
  correctness, 30f
  incorrectness, 29f, 30f
Markers, 86. *See also* Lead
  usage. *See* Anatomic orientation
Matrix. *See* Image
  definition, 331
  impact. *See* Image
  size, reduction, 340f
Maxilla, 192f. *See also* Small animals
  beam center, 201f
  positioning/radiograph. *See* Dorsoventral intraoral
    maxilla
  ventrodorsal open-mouth oblique view
    positioning, 202f
    radiograph, 202f
Maximum permissible dose (MPD), 25-26
  definition, 24
  exceeding, 29
  per calendar year, 26t
MDP. *See* Methylene diphosphonate
Measurement, caliper (usage). *See* Anatomic area
    measurement
Medial view, 148f
Mediolateral, definition, 146
Medullary papillae (M), 320f
Metacarpal bones
  middle, beam center/measurement, 169f
Metacarpus
  dorsopalmar view
    positioning, 265f
    radiograph, 265f
  lateral view
    positioning, 266f
    radiograph, 266f
  oblique view
    positioning, 267f
    radiograph, 267f
Metacarpus/metatarsus, 265-267. *See also* Large
    animals
  middle, beam center, 267f
  midpoint, beam center, 265f-266f
  true dorsopalmar/dorsoplantar projection, 267f

Metacarpus-phalanges. *See* Small animals
  dorsopalmar view
    positioning, 169f
    radiograph, 169f
  lateral view
    positioning, 170f
    radiograph, 170f
Metal clips/buckles, 282
Metal housing, 11f
Metallic replacement, 84-85
Metatarsus-phalanages. *See* Small animals
  dorsoplantar view
    positioning, 189f
    radiograph, 189f
  lateral view
    positioning, 188f
    radiograph, 188f
Methylcellulose, usage, 253
Methylene diphosphonate (MDP), 325
Metrizamide, 235
Mid-abdomen, transverse CT scan. *See* Dogs
Midcervical region, support, 208f
Middle phalanx, measurement, 170f
Midfemur region, measurement, 177f
Midlumbar region, support, 208f
Midmetatarsal region, beam center, 188f, 189f
Milliamperage (mA)
  application, 12
  definition, 10
  effect. *See* Filament
  necessity, 281
  selector, 20
  time, relationship, 36-37
Milliamperage-seconds (mAs)
  calculation, 37, 100, 101
  change. *See* Technique chart
  chart, 99t
  control, 909
  definition, 36, 90
  factors, usage. *See* Base mAs factors
  impact, 47
  overexposure, 49f
  technique chart. *See* Variable mAs technique chart
  underexposure, 48f
Milliampere
  definition, 36
  measurement, 36
Mineralizations, location (determination), 319
Mitral valve, 314f
M-mode ultrasonography. *See* Motion-mode
    ultrasonography
Mobile x-ray unit, 37f
Molybdenum, 12
  definition, 10
Motion artifact, 346f
Motion-mode image (M-mode image), 316f, 317

Motion-mode ultrasonography (M-mode ultrasonography), 313
   definition, 312
Motion-mode ultrasound (M-mode ultrasound), 315
MPD. *See* Maximum permissible dose
MRI. *See* Magnetic resonance imaging
Myelography
   definition, 234
   usage, 248
Myocardial disease, 316

N
Nares, demonstration, 192f
Nasal bones, 192f
Nasal cavity. *See* Small animals
   ventrodorsal open-mouth view
      positioning, 197f
      radiograph, 197f
Nasal notch, measurement, 192f
Nasal passage, normal appearance, 323f
Nasal sinuses, measurement, 195f
Nasal tumor, CT scan. *See* Dogs
National Committee on Radiation Protection and Measurements (NCRP), 25
Navicular bone, 257-258. *See also* Large animals
   dorsopalmar oblique view
      positioning, 257f
      radiograph, 257f
   flexor view
      positioning, 258f
      radiograph, 258f
Navicular disease, 325
NCRP. *See* National Committee on Radiation Protection and Measurements
Negative-contrast agents, 236
   definition, 234
   usage, 235
Negative-contrast cystogram, lateral view, 245f
Negative-contrast media, 236, 237
Nephrogram
   definition, 234
   usage, 240
Nephrogram phase, ventrodorsal view. *See* Intravenous pyelogram
Network PACS, 336
Neutron, definition, 4
Nine-penny test, radiograph, 115f
NM. *See* Nuclear medicine
Nonimage-forming x-rays, absorption, 50
Nonscreen dental film, usage. *See* Teeth
Nonscreen film, 69-70
   definition, 60
Nonselective cardioangiogram, cassette tunnel system (usage), 247f
Nose stop, measurement, 195f
Nuclear medicine (NM), 331

Nuclear scan. *See* Horse
Nuclear scintigraphy, 60, 324-326
   clinical applications, 325-326
   technical aspects, 324-325

O
Object-film distance, 161
Oblique views, anatomic directional terms, 148f
Occult lameness, 325
OFA. *See* Orthopedic Foundation for Animals
Oily agents, usage, 235-236
Oily contrast media, 235
Oily iodinated contrast agents, 248
On/off switch, 20
Open cassette, 61f
Operator errors. *See* Computed radiography artifact, 345f
Orthopedic Foundation for Animals (OFA) ratings, 178f
Osteochondrosis dissecans, 325

P
PACS. *See* Picture archiving and communication system
Palmar, definition, 146
Palmarodorsal view, 148f
Pancreas, assessment, 319
Pancreatitis, 319
Paper
   image processing, 344f
   usage, 339-340
Papillary muscles (P), echocardiogram, 314f
Parallel grid. *See* Unfocused grid
Parasympathetic agents
   definition, 234
   usage, 236
Patella, 279f, 280f
   skyline projection, sunrise view, 183
   skyline view
      positioning, 183f
      radiograph, 183f
Pathologic conditions, 102
Patients
   care, 147-148
   exposure. *See* Radiation
   motion, radiograph (illustration), 54f
   position. *See* Cassette
      PennHIP distraction procedure, 179f
   positioning, criteria, 146-150
   preparation, 150, 236. *See also* Large animal radiography
   restraint, 150. *See also* Avian radiography; Exotic radiography; Large animal radiography
PDA. *See* Persistent ductus arteriosus
Pedal bone. *See* Distal phalanx
Pelvic radiograph. *See* Dogs

Pelvis, 174-179, 281. *See also* Large animals; Small
    animals
  beam center, 281f
  extended projection, 175
  frog-leg projection, 175
  lateral view
    positioning, 174f
    radiograph, 174f
  rotation, absence, 175
  ventrodorsal extended view, 176f
    positioning, 177f
    radiograph, 177f
  ventrodorsal frog-leg view
    positioning, 175f
    radiograph, 175f
  ventrodorsal view
    positioning, 281f
    radiograph, 281f
Penetration, kV$_p$ (impact), 38f
Penetration evaluation. *See* Radiographs
PennHIP
  distraction procedure. *See* Patients
  method, 178
  phenotype, 178
  procedure, 179f
  view. *See* Hips
Penumbra
  definition, 10
  effect, 14f
  formation, 14
Pericardial effusion, 316
Perpendicularity, 109f
  test, 109
Persistent ductus arteriosus (PDA), 316
Personnel monitoring devices, 26-27
Phalanges. *See* Metatarsus-phalanages
Phalanx. *See* Distal phalanx
Pharynx, 224, 283-284. *See also* Large animals; Small
    animals
  beam center, 224f
  lateral view
    positioning, 224f, 283f
    radiograph, 224f, 283f
Phosphor
  absorption rate, 64
  crystal layer, 63
    dyes, 65
    thickness, 65
  crystal size, impact, 64
  intensifying screen, 64
  types. *See* Screens
Phosphostimulable phosphor (PSP) detector screen, 341
Photo-Flo 200 solution (Kodak), 82
Photographic identification, lead blocker (usage), 62
Photoimprinting, 87f
  label system, 86

Photons, 5
  definition, 4
Photostimulable phosphor (PSP), 340-341
  definition, 331
  detector screen, 341
Physical restraint, 292-294, 306
Picture archiving and communication system (PACS),
    332, 337, 341
  definition, 331
Picture elements (pixels), 323, 339
  definition, 312, 331
  impact. *See* Image
  matrix. *See* Etched pixel matrix
Pituitary fossa, 323
Pixilation, decrease, 340f
Plantar, definition, 146
Play-Doh, usage, 253
Pneumocystogram, definition, 234
Pneumoperitoneography
  definition, 234
  usage, 248
Pocket ionization chamber, 27
  definition, 24
Portable lead wall, 30f
Portable ultrasound machine (Ausonics Microimager),
    313f
Portable X-ray unit, 12f
Portal veins, defining, 317
Positional studies, 333f
Positional terminology, 146
Positioning
  aids, 150
    assistance, 29f
    examples, 29f
  criteria. *See* Patients
  devices. *See* Large animal radiography
  guidelines, 149-150
Positioning principles
  glossary, 146
  readings, 151
  review
    answers, 350
    questions, 151
Positive-contrast agents
  definition, 234
  usage, 235
Positive-contrast cystogram
  definition, 234
  lateral view, 246f
Positive-contrast media, 237
Potter-Bucky diaphragm, 52-53
  definition, 44
  diagram, 53f
Power, availability, 18
Preservatives, 77, 78
  definition, 74

Primary x-ray beam
  definition, 24
  exposure, 27
  hands, positioning (avoidance), 30f
  intensity, 39f
  table top, interaction, 28f
Procedures. *See* Special procedures
  flowchart. *See* Technique chart
Processing chemicals, usage, 83-84
Processor maintenance. *See* Automatic processors
Propyliodone, suspension, 235
Prostate, assessment, 320
Prostatomegaly, 320
Protective apparel, maintenance, 30-31
Protective aprons, usage, 30
Protective coating, 69f
Proton, definition, 4
Protractor, usage, 113f
Proximal, definition, 146
Proximal hard palate, measurement, 202f
Proximal phalanges, 259-260. *See also* Large animals
  beam center, 259f, 260f
  dorsopalmar view
    positioning, 260f
    radiograph, 260f
  lateral view
    positioning, 259f
    radiograph, 259f
Proximal tail, measurement, 219f, 220f
Proxtronics, Inc., 27t
Pseudofocused grid, 51f, 52
  definition, 44
Psittacine, exposure factors, 293t
PSP. *See* Phosphostimulable phosphor; Photostimulable phosphor
Pubis, beam center, 175f
Pulmonic valve, 315f
Pyelogram
  definition, 234
  phase, 240-241. *See also* Intravenous pyelogram
  usage, 240

Q
Quality assurance/quality control (QA/QC)
  definition, 106
  glossary, 106
  introduction, 106
  processing chart, 122f-123f
  quality control, definition, 106
  readings, 124
  review
    answers, 350
    questions, 124-125
  tests. *See* X-rays
  umbrella, 106f
  usage. *See* Veterinary radiography

Quanta, 5
  definition, 4
Quantum mottle, 66
  definition, 60

R
Rack, usage. *See* Turtles
Radiant energy, definition, 4
Radiation. *See* Secondary radiation
  detection device, example, 27f
  exposure units, 25-26
  hazards. *See* Ionizing radiation
  mortality, 25
  patient exposure, 26
Radiation Detection Company, 27t
Radiation safety. *See* Large animal radiography
  application, 27-33
  glossary, 24
  practice, 30f
  readings, 34
  review
    answers, 349
    questions, 33-34
  rules. *See* Fluoroscopy
    checklist, 31
Radiation-sensitive film, 26, 27f
Radiographic artifact, 136-137
  dirt, impact, 63f
Radiographic contrast, 45-46, 90
  definition, 44
Radiographic density, 44-45, 90
  absence, 51f
  definition, 44
  difference, 46f
  factors, 45
  tissue density, impact, 47f
Radiographic detail, 54-56
  definition, 44
Radiographic exposure, 345f
Radiographic film, blackening, 44
Radiographic film Hunter and Driffield curve, 332
Radiographic output, 83
Radiographic quality
  definition, 44
  glossary, 44
  readings, 57
  reference, 44
  review
    answers, 349
    questions, 56-57
Radiographic studies, performing, 300
Radiographic technique evaluation, 91-92
  error considerations, 95
  glossary, 90
  practical applications, 92-95
  questions, 91

Radiographic technique evaluation—cont'd
  readings, 96
  review
    answers, 349-350
    questions, 95-96
  scenarios, 93f-95f
Radiographs
  definition, 4
  evaluation
    case studies, 93f-95f
    practical applications, 92-95
  examination, case studies, 93f-95f, 128-140
  examples, 46f
  exposures, 66f
  film identification, 150
  gray appearance, 47f
  grid cutoff, inclusion (example), 51f
  hair artifact, presence, 68f
  high contrast, 48f
  human hand, visibility, 31f
  lateral view. *See* Dogs
    exposure. *See* Abdominal radiograph
  penetration evaluation, 91-92
  repetition, 335-336
  screen types, impact, 66f
  usage. *See* Lead gloves
  viewing, 6, 91
  views, requirement, 148-149
Radiography. *See* Avian radiography; Computed
      radiography; Digital radiography; Exotic
      radiography; Large animal radiography
  cassette holder. *See* Equine radiography
  physics, review, 90
  process, 39-40
Radiology information system (RIS), 337
  definition, 331
Radiolucent interspacers, structure, 50f
Radiolucent mouth gag, 202
Radiolucent sheet, usage, 292f
Radiolucent tube, usage. *See* Rodents
Radionuclide, clearance, 326
Radiopharmaceutical
  definition, 312
  half-life, 324
  injection, 60
Radius. *See* Small animals
  craniocaudal view
    positioning, 166f
    radiograph, 166f
  lateral view
    positioning, 165f
    radiograph, 165f
  middle, beam center, 165f, 166f
RAID. *See* Redundant array of inexpensive disks
Raptors, exposure factors, 293t
Rare-earth elements, 64

Rare-earth phosphors, fluorescence, 5
Rats
  whole-body dorsoventral view, 298
  whole-body lateral view, 299
Real-time images, capture, 313
Rebound effect. *See* Uberschwinger effect
Rectification, 17-18. *See also* Full-wave rectification;
      Half-wave rectification
  definition, 10
Recumbent, definition, 146
Redundant array of inexpensive disks (RAID),
      definition, 331
Reflective layer
  definition, 60
  efficiency, 65
Regurgitation, 236
Renal parenchyma, diffuse opacification, 240
Reproductive tract, assessment, 320-321
Reptiles
  exposure factors, 293t
  radiography, 300-306
Restrainer, 77
  avoidance, 29f
  definition, 74
Reticulation, 77
  definition, 74
Retrograde cystourethrogram, lateral view, 247f
Retrograde urethrogram
  definition, 234
  performing, 244
Right atrium (RA), echocardiogram, 315f
Right ventricle (RV), echocardiogram, 314f, 315f,
      317f
Rinse bath, 78
  definition, 74
Rinse tank, labeling, 79f
RIS. *See* Radiology information system
Rodents
  exposure factors, 293t
  radiography, 298-299
    radiolucent tube, usage, 299f
  whole-body dorsoventral view
    positioning, 298f
    radiograph, 298f
  whole-body lateral view
    positioning, 299f
    radiograph, 299f
Roentgen, Wilhelm Conrad, 6, 6f
Rope halter, usage, 282
Rostral, definition, 146
Rostrocaudal open-mouth view. *See* Tympanic bullae
Rotating anode, 13
  definition, 10
  example, 13f
Rotor, 13f
R.S. Landaurer Jr. & Company, 27t

S

Sacrum. *See* Small animals
  beam center, 218f
  measurement, 218f
  ventrodorsal view
    positioning, 218f
    radiograph, 218f
Safelight, 118. *See also* Darkroom; Direct safelight;
    Indirect safelight
Sagittal crest, 192f
Saint Bernard abdomen, ventrodorsal view (radiograph),
    46f
Sandbags, usage, 194, 230
Santes' rule
  definition, 36, 98
  usage, 99
Scapula
  beam center, 154f-156f
  caudal border
    beam center, 212f, 225f-229f
    measurement, 225f-229f
  caudocranial view
    positioning, 156f
    radiograph, 156f
  dorsal to vertebral column, 154-155
  lateral view, dorsal to vertebral column
    positioning, 154f
    radiograph, 154f
  measurement, 154f
  superimposition. *See* Cranial thorax
Scapulohumeral joint, measurement, 156f
Scatter radiation, 49-50
  absorption, 50f, 51f
  definition, 44
  example, 28f
  impact, 48
  production, 49f
  result. *See* Anode
Scintigraphy, 324. *See also* Nuclear scintigraphy
Scintillation devices, definition, 331
SCP. *See* Service class provider
Screen-film cassette, placement, 345f
Screen-film contact, 62
Screen-film lateral pelvic radiograph. *See* Dogs
Screen-film radiography, limitations, 332
Screens. *See* Image receptor screen
  cleaner, usage, 68f
  contact test, radiograph, 116f
  cross section, 65f
  film, 69. *See also* Nonscreen film
    definition, 60
  film contact, 116
  glow, process, 62f
  mounting. *See* Cassette
  phosphor types, 63-64
  setup match. *See* Cassette

Screens—cont'd
  specialization, 67
  speed
    systems (Kodak). *See* Film
    uniformity, 117-118
  types, 99
    impact. *See* Radiographs
Screen-to-film contact. *See* Cassette
SCU. *See* Service class user
Seashell, radiograph, 45f
Secondary radiation, 28
  definition, 24
Sector probe, definition, 312
Sedation
  recommendation, 279
  requirement. *See* Intraoral radiography
Selenium detectors, usage, 340
Sensitometer, usage. *See* Test strip exposure
Sensitometry, test, 120-121
Server, definition, 331
Service class provider (SCP), definition, 331
Service class user (SCU), definition, 331
Seventh rib, measurement, 213f
Seventh thoracic vertebral body, beam center, 213f
Sheep, radiography, 132
Shell, 5
  definition, 4
Short-axis scans, 314
Short-axis view. *See* Two-dimensional short-axis
    view
  definition, 312
Short pastern. *See* Large animals; Proximal phalanges
Shoulder. *See* Small animals
  caudocranial view
    positioning, 158f
    radiograph, 158f
  lateral view
    positioning, 157f, 278f
    radiograph, 157f, 278f
  point, beam center, 157f
  region, measurement, 160f, 161f
Shoulder joint, 278. *See also* Large animals
  beam center, 158f, 278f
  measurement, 157f-159f
Sialography
  definition, 234
  usage, 248-249
SID. *See* Source-image distance
Sievert (Sv), 25
  definition, 24
Silver halide, 69
  crystals, 60, 68
  definition, 60
Silver recovery, 84-85
  system. *See* Vault Junior trickle silver recovery
    system

Simple mail transfer protocol (SMTP), definition, 331
Skull, 192-194, 282. *See also* Large animals; Small
    animals
  base, measurement, 224f
  beam center, 282f
  CT, usage, 323
  dorsoventral view
    positioning, 193f, 284f
    radiograph, 193f, 284f
  lateral view
    positioning, 192f, 282f
    radiograph, 192f, 282f
  midline, beam center, 284f
  region, support, 208f
  rotation, 194
  ventrodorsal view
    positioning, 194f
    radiograph, 194f
  views, 283
Skyline projection, sunrise view. *See* Patella
Small animals
  abdomen, 231-232
    lateral view, 231
    ventrodorsal view, 230
  carpus, 167-168
    dorsopalmar view, 168
    lateral view, 167
  caudal spine, 219-220
    lateral view, 220
    ventrodorsal spine, 219
  cervical spine, 208-211
    extended lateral view, 208-209
    flexed lateral view, 210
    hyperextended lateral view, 211
    ventrodorsal view, 208
  cranium, rostrocaudal view, 196
  elbows, 162-164
    craniocaudal view, 162
    flexed lateral views, 164
    lateral view, 163
  femur, 179-180
    craniocaudal view, 180
    lateral view, 179
  fibula, 184-185
    caudocranial view, 185
    lateral view, 184
  forelimbs
    readings, 171
    review answers, 350
    review questions, 171
  frontal sinuses, rostrocaudal view, 195
  humerus, 159-161
    caudocranial view, 160-161
    lateral view, 159
  lumbar spine, 216-217
    lateral view, 217
    ventrodorsal view, 216

Small animals—cont'd
  mandible, 203-204
    lower dental arcade, 204
    ventrodorsal intraoral view, 203
  maxilla, 201-202
    dorsoventral intraoral view, 201
    upperdental arcade, 202
  metacarpus-phalanges, 169-170, 188-189
    dorsopalmar view, 169
    dorsoplantar/plantarodorsal views, 189
    lateral view, 170, 188
  nasal cavity, ventrodorsal open-mouth view, 197
  pelvis, 174-179
    lateral view, 174
    ventrodorsal view, 175-179
  pelvis/hind limb
    readings, 190
    review answers, 350
    review questions, 190
  pharynx, lateral view, 224
  radius, 165-166
    craniocaudal view, 166
    lateral view, 165
  sacrum, ventrodorsal view, 218
  scapula, 154-156
    caudocranial view, 155-156
    lateral view, 154-155
  shoulder, 157-158
    caudocranial view, 158
    lateral view, 157
  skull, 192-194
    dorsoventral view, 193
    introduction, 192
    lateral view, 192-193
    readings, 206
    review answers, 350
    review questions, 206
    ventrodorsal view, 194
  soft tissue
    readings, 232
    review answers, 350-351
    review questions, 232
  spine
    readings, 221
    review answers, 350
    review questions, 221
  stifle joint, 181-183
    caudocranial view, 181
    lateral view, 182
  tarsus, 186-187
    lateral view, 186
    plantarodorsal/dorsoplantar views, 187
  teeth, lateral intraoral view, 205
  temporomandibular joint, ventrodorsal oblique view,
    200
  thoracic spine, 212-213
    lateral view, 213

Small animals—cont'd
    thoracic spine—cont'd
        ventrodorsal view, 212
    thoracolumbar spine, 214-215
        lateral view, 215
        ventrodorsal view, 214
    thorax, 225-229
        dorsoventral view, 225
        lateral decubitus view, 229
        lateral view, 227
        lateral view, horizontal x-ray beam (inclusion), 228
        ventrodorsal view, 226
        ventrodorsal view, horizontal x-ray beam (inclusion), 229
    tibia, 184-185
        caudocranial view, 185
        lateral view, 184
    tympanic bullae
        lateral oblique view, 199
        rostrocaudal open-mouth view, 198
    ulna, 165-166
        craniocaudal view, 166
        lateral view, 165
Small intestines, loops, 319f
Smith, Gail, 178
SMTP. *See* Simple mail transfer protocol
Snakes, 305-306
    beam center, 305f, 306f
    lateral view
        positioning, 306f
        radiograph, 306f
    whole-body dorsoventral view, 305
        positioning, box (usage), 305f
        positioning, plastic tube (usage), 305f
        radiograph, 305f
    whole-body lateral view, 306
Sodium iodide crystal gamma camera, 60
Softened soap, usage, 253
Soft tissue. *See* Small animals
    description, 224
    fat, contrast. *See* Bone
Soft x-rays, absorption, 28f
Solution
    replacement, 79
    replenisher, 78-79
Solvent, 78
    definition, 74
Somatic damage, 24-25
    definition, 24
Soot and whitewash (gray-and-white) appearance, 48
Source-image distance (SID), 38, 52
    change, 39
    decrease, 53f, 292
    definition, 36
    increase, 54, 287
    marks, 108f

Source-image distance (SID)—cont'd
    measurement, 99
    reduction, 201, 203, 258
Spatial resolution, definition, 331
Special procedures
    glossary, 234
    indications, 234-235
    readings, 250
    review
        answers, 351
        questions, 249-250
    techniques, overview, 244-249
Spindle, 13f
Spine. *See* Caudal spine; Cervical spine; Lumbar spine;
        Small animals; Thoracic spine; Thoracolumbar
        spine
    CT, usage, 323-324
    study, positioning alterations. *See* Lateral spine study
Spleen (S)
    assessment, 318
    echogenicity, 319f
    hypoechogenic mass (M), 319f
    ultrasound, 318f
Splints, visualization, 267f
Sponge pad, placement, 188
Sponges, usage, 208f
Sponge wedge
    elevation, 213
    pad, placement, 215, 217
    placement, 184, 200, 210
Static electrical charge, release, 129
Stationary anode, 12-13
    construction, 12f
    definition, 10
    limitation, 13
Step-down transformer, 17
    definition, 10
Step-up transformer, 16
    definition, 10
Sternum
    caudal tip, beam center, 294f, 295f
    measurement, 212
    support, 208f
Stifle joints, 181-183, 279-280. *See also* Large animals;
        Small animals
    activity, increase, 326f
    beam center, 181f, 182f, 279f
    caudocranial view
        positioning, 181f, 279f
        radiograph, 181f, 279f
    lateral view
        positioning, 182f, 280f
        radiograph, 182f, 280f
    measurement, 184f, 185f
    nuclear scan. *See* Horse
    rotation, 176f
    space, beam center, 280f

Stop bath, 78
    definition, 74
Stress fractures, 325
Stripe artifact, recognition, 345f
Subject contrast, 46
    definition, 44
    factors, 46t
Sunrise view. *See* Patella
Supercoat, 69
    definition, 60
Superior, definition, 146
Suspensory ligament tear, 321
Sv. *See* Sievert
Synbiotics Corporation, 178

T
T-1, measurement, 211f
$t_{1/2}$. *See* Half-life
T-6, measurement, 212f
Table, test. *See* X-rays
Tagged image file format (TIFF), 336
    definition, 331
Tail, securing, 175
Target, 11f
    area. *See* Tungsten
        scattered radiation, result. *See* Anode
    definition, 10
    electrons, collision, 14f
    failure. *See* Anode
    organ, 324
        definition, 312
    surface, unevenness (impact), 13f
Tarsal joint
    measurement, 186f, 187f. *See also* Distal tarsal joint
    middle, beam center, 187f, 274f
Tarsus. *See* Small animals
    craniocaudal view, preparation. *See* German
        shepherd tarsus
    dorsoplantar view, positioning, 187f
    lateral oblique view
        positioning, 275f
        radiograph, 275f
    lateral view
        positioning, 186f, 274f
        radiograph, 186f, 274f
    medial oblique view
        positioning, 275f
        radiograph, 275f
    middle, beam center, 186f
    plantarodorsal view
        positioning, 187f
        radiograph, 187f
Tarsus joint, 273-275. *See also* Large animals
    dorsoplantar view
        positioning, 273f
        radiograph, 273f
    middle, beam center, 273f

Tarsus joint—cont'd
    true dorsoplantar plane, 273f
TCP. *See* Transmission control protocol
TCP/IP, 330
Technetium, 325
Technical artifacts/errors, case studies
    glossary, 126
    introduction, 126-127
    readings, 141
    review
        answers, 350
        questions, 141
Technique chart. *See* Variable mAs technique chart
    definition, 98
    development
        glossary, 98
        readings, 104
        review answers, 350
        review questions, 103-104
    exposure factors, 99
    formulation, 98-99
        methods, 101-102
    mAs change, 102t
    modification, recommendations, 102-103
    plotting, 100, 101
    procedure flowchart, 99-101
    trial exposure, 101t
        examples, 100-101
Technique evaluation. *See* Radiographic technique
        evaluation
Teeth, 205, 285. *See also* Large animals; Small animals
    beam center, 205f, 285f
    intraoral projection, positioning. *See* Incisor teeth
    lateral-intraoral view
        positioning, nonscreen dental film (usage), 205f
        radiograph, nonscreen dental film (usage), 205f
    lateral oblique view. *See* Cheek teeth
Teledyne Isotopes, 27t
Television monitor, usage, 67f
Temporomandibular joint, 192f. *See also* Small animals
    beam center, 200f
    oblique projection, 199
    ventrodorsal oblique view
        positioning, 200f
        radiograph, 200f
Tenosynovitis, 321
Tentorium, 323
Test strip exposure, sensitometer (usage), 120f
Thermionic emission, 36
    definition, 36
Thermo Analytical, Inc., 27t
Thermoluminescent dosimeter (TLD), 27
    badges, 31
    definition, 24
Third premolar, beam center, 202f
Third upper premolar, beam center/measurement,
    197f

Thirteenth rib, caudal aspect
  beam center, 230f, 231f
  measurement, 230f, 231f
Thoracic cavity, ribs (superimposition), 155
Thoracic inlet
  ectopic functional thyroid tissue, 325f
  measurement, 209f-211f
Thoracic spine, 212-213, 287. *See also* Large animals;
      Small animals
  lateral view
    positioning, 213f
    radiograph, 213f
  ventrodorsal view
    positioning, 212f
    radiograph, 212f
Thoracic vertebrae, dorsal spinous processes,
      154-155
Thoracic vertebral body, beam center. *See* Seventh
      thoracic vertebral body
Thoracolumbar junction
  beam center, 214f, 215f
  measurement, 214f, 215f
Thoracolumbar spine. *See* Small animals
  lateral view
    positioning, 215f
    radiograph, 215f
  ventrodorsal view
    positioning, 214f
    radiograph, 214f
Thorax, 225-229, 287. *See also* Large animals; Small
      animals
  CT, usage, 324
  dorsoventral view
    positioning, 225f
    radiograph, 225f
  lateral view
    positioning, 227f
    radiograph, 227f
  radiographic image, 344f
  recumbent lateral view (positioning), horizontal x-ray
      beam (usage), 228f
  standing lateral view (positioning), horizontal x-ray
      beam (usage), 228f
  ventrodorsal decubitus view, horizontal x-ray beam
      (usage)
    positioning, 229f
    radiograph, 229f
  ventrodorsal view
    positioning, 226f
    radiograph, 226f
Three-phase alternating current waveforms, 19f
Three-phase generator, 18
Three-phase output, 19f
Thyroid
  gland. *See* Hyperactive thyroid gland
  nuclear scintigraphy, 325
Tibia. *See* Small animals

Tibia—cont'd
  caudocranial view
    positioning, 185f
    radiograph, 185f
  lateral view
    positioning, 184f
    radiograph, 184f
  middle, beam center, 184f, 185f
Tibial plateau, caudocranial radiographic image, 344f
Tibial plateau leveling osteotomy (TPLO) procedures,
      335
Tibiotarsal joint, visualization, 274
TIFF. *See* Tagged image file format
Timer, 21
  calibration, 118
Timer switch, 17
  definition, 10
Tissues
  biologic changes, x-rays (impact), 5
  density, impact. *See* Radiographic density
  echogenicity, 313
TLD. *See* Thermoluminescent dosimeter
Tongue depressor, superimposition, 197
Toxicity, concern, 235
TPLO. *See* Tibial plateau leveling osteotomy
Trachea, barium aspiration, 297f
Transducers, usage, 313, 321
Transformer. *See* Step-down transformer; Step-up
      transformer
Transmission control protocol (TCP), definition, 331
Transverse CT scan. *See* Dogs
Transverse-plane computed tomography scan. *See* Dogs
Transverse-plane computed tomography scanner, 322f
Transverse-plane scan, 323f
Triceps, superimposition (elimination), 227
Tricuspid valve, 315f
Tricuspid valvular insufficiencies, 316
Triiodinated compounds
  definition, 234
  usage, 235
Trochanter
  beam center. *See* Greater femoral trochanter
  measurement, 174f
True dorsopalmar/dorsoplantar projection. *See*
      Metacarpus/metatarsus
True dorsopalmar plane. *See* Carpus joint
True dorsoplantar plane. *See* Tarsus joint
True ventrodorsal position, 212, 214
Tube. *See* X-ray tube
Tungsten
  definition, 10
  target area, 12f
  usage, 11
Turtles, 300-302
  body, beam center, 301f
  head, middle (beam center), 302f
  preparation, 300

Turtles—cont'd
  shell, beam center, 300f
  whole-body craniocaudal view, 302
    positioning, horizontal x-ray beam (usage), 302f
    positioning, rack (usage), 302f
    radiograph, 302f
  whole-body dorsoventral view, 300
    positioning, 300f
    radiograph, 300f
  whole-body lateral view, 301
    positioning, horizontal x-ray beam (usage), 301f
    positioning, rack (usage), 301f
    radiograph, 301f
Two-dimensional B-mode ultrasonography, 313
Two-dimensional echocardiography, 314
Two-dimensional image, 323
Two-dimensional long-axis view, 314f
Two-dimensional scans, 314-315
Two-dimensional short-axis view, 314f, 315f
Tympanic bullae, 192f. *See also* Small animals
  beam center/measurement, 199f
  impact, 199
  lateral oblique view
    positioning, 199f
    radiograph, 199f
  rostrocaudal open-mouth view
    positioning, 198f
    radiograph, 198f

U

Uberschwinger artifact, 343f
  recognition, clinical utility, 344f
Uberschwinger effect (rebound effect), 343
UGI. *See* Upper gastrointestinal
Ulna. *See* Small animals
  craniocaudal view
    positioning, 166f
    radiograph, 166f
  lateral view
    positioning, 165f
    radiograph, 165f
Ultrasonography, 312-321. *See also* Brightness-mode
      ultrasonography; Motion-mode ultrasonography
  clinical applications, 313-316
  technical aspects, 313
Ultrasound
  examination. *See* Extremities; Eyes
  machine. *See* Portable ultrasound machine
  principles/artifacts, 313f
  scan. *See* Dogs
Ultrasound-guided biopsy
  hyperechogenic needle. *See* Liver
  performing, 317-318, 318f
Ultraviolet rays, definition, 4
Unfocused grid (parallel grid), 51f
  contrast. *See* Focused grid
  definition, 44

United States Testing Company, 27t
Upper gastrointestinal (UGI) study
  definition, 234
  lateral view, 238f, 239f
  precautions, 237-238
  procedure, 238-239
  technique outline, 238-239
  usage, 237
  ventrodorsal view, 238f, 239f
Ureteral reflux. *See* Contrast media
Urethrogram. *See* Antegrade urethrogram; Retrograde
      urethrogram
Urethrography
  definition, 234
  precautions, 244
  procedure, 247
  technique outline, 247
  usage, 244
Urinary bladder (B)
  assessment, 320
  presence, 321f
  ultrasound scan. *See* Dogs
Urinary system, contrast studies, 239-244
Urine, leakage, 242
U.S. food and Drug Administration approval, 235

V

Vacuum, 6, 11f
  definition, 4
  environment, 11
Vaginography
  definition, 234
  usage, 249
Valve tubes
  definition, 10
  usage, 18
Variable kV_p technique chart, 99-101
Variable mAs technique chart, 102t
Vault Junior trickle silver recovery system, 85
Ventral, definition, 146
Ventricular septal defect (VSD), 316
Ventricular system, 323
Ventricular wall (W), echocardiogram, 315f
Ventrodorsal canine skull, 192f
Ventrodorsal open-mouth view. *See* Nasal cavity
Ventrodorsal projection, exposure, 243
Veterinary radiography
  Murphy's law, 37
  QA/QC, usage, 106-123
    equipment, 106-107
    procedures, 107
    tracking charts, 107
Veterinary X-ray system (3M), 71t
View-box uniformity, test, 114
Views, exposure, 61f
Viscous agents, usage, 235-236
Voltage compensator, 20

Voltage pulses, production, 60
Volume element (voxel), 323
  definition, 312
VSD. *See* Ventricular septal defect
V trough
  placement, 219, 230
  usage, 194

W
Warning light, 21
Wash bath, 78
Wash tank, labeling, 79f
Water-soluble agents, usage, 235
Water-soluble contrast agents, 235
Water-soluble iodinated contrast medium, 240
Water-soluble iodine compound, 244
Waveforms. *See* Three-phase alternating current
    waveforms
Wavelength
  definition, 4
  motion, 4f
Waves, points, 4f
Wet side. *See* Darkroom
Wetting agent, 78
  example, 82f
White image, void, 343
Window, 11f
Wood block, usage, 257f
World Wide Web (WWW), definition, 331

X
Xeroradiography, 60
X-ray beam, 5
  aiming, 261
  angle, 272
  centering, 286
  collimation, 263
  definition, 4
  direction, 33f, 146, 265, 274, 298
  divergence, 52
  film, perpendicularity, 205
  filtration, 98
  horizontal direction, 277, 278
  inclusion. *See* Small animals; Thorax
  intensity. *See* Primary x-ray beam
  line, 182
  object interaction, 50f
  parallel direction, 301
  penetration, 38f
  quantity/intensity, 36
  table top, interaction. *See* Primary x-ray beam
  usage. *See* Thorax
  vertical direction, 303, 304
X-ray film, 68-70
  composition, 69
  cross section, 69
  latent image, 60

X-ray film—cont'd
  speed, 70
  supply, 134
  types, 69-70
X-ray machine, 21f
  anatomy
    glossary, 10
    readings, 22
    review answers, 349
    review questions, 21-22
  calibration, 129
  electrical components, 16-18
  flat panel detector DR system, inclusion, 332f
  technical components, 16-21
X-ray production, 10-12
  glossary, 4
  readings, 7
  review
    answers, 349
    questions, 6-7
X-rays
  absorption. *See* Soft x-rays
  apparatus, QA/QC tests, 108f-123f
  console, 21f
  definition, 4-5
  discovery, 6
  dose considerations, 344-346
  electromagnetic radiation, physical properties, 5
  emission, 67f
  exposure
    blockage, 62
    factors, 344-346
  field
    alignment, 115
    alignment verification, 115f
    light test, 110
  generation, 5-6
  interaction. *See* Charged selenium plates
  source, image receptor (distance), 38-39
X-ray system (3M). *See* Veterinary X-ray system
X-ray table
  diagram, 53f
  exposure, 29f
X-ray tube, 10-15. *See also* Gassy x-ray tube
  angle, 285
  bird's-eye view, 193
  collimator, aluminum filter (placement), 28f
  construction, 11f
  definition, 10
  direction, 218
  failure, areas, 15-16
  fixed tube stand construction, example, 20f
  focal spot/table distance, measurement, 108f
  housing anomalies, 16
  illustration, 20f
  level/parallelism, level (usage), 109f
  life, prolongation, 15

X-ray tube—cont'd
  location, 33f
  positioning, 279, 280, 284
  rating, 18
  rotation, verification, 113f
  stand, 20
  table/crane locks, test, 110

X-ray unit. *See* Ceiling-mounted x-ray unit; Fixed x-ray unit; Mobile x-ray unit; Portable X-ray unit

Z
Zygomatic arch, 192f
  measurement, 192f